MEDICAL RADIOLOGY

Diagnostic Imaging

Softcover Edition

Editors:
A. L. Baert, Leuven
K. Sartor, Heidelberg
J. E. Youker, Milwaukee

Springer
Berlin
Heidelberg
New York
Barcelona
Hong Kong
London
Milan
Paris
Singapore
Tokyo

A. Heuck · M. Reiser (Eds.)

Abdominal and Pelvic MRI

With Contributions by

A. L. Baert · J. O. Barentsz · H.-J. Brambs · M. A. Cuesta · T. Doesburg · T. H.M. Falke
R. Forstner · S. Gryspeerdt · T. Helmberger · A. Heuck · N. Holzknecht · H. Hricak
G. P. Kerstin · W. Luboldt · G. Marchal · H. B. Marcos · P. J. Mergo · U. G. Müller-Lisse
R. H. Oyen · P. R. Ros · E. J. Rummeny · M. P. Sandler · P. Sattlegger · J. Scheidler
R. C. Semelka · M. Steinborn · R. F. Thoeni · A. P. van Gils · L. Van Hoe

Foreword by
A. L. Baert

With 255 Figures in 579 Separate Illustrations

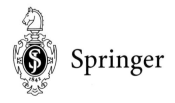

Springer

ANDREAS HEUCK, MD
Professor, Radiologisches Zentrum
München-Pasing
Pippinger Strasse 25
81245 München
Germany

MAXIMILIAN REISER, MD
Professor, Institut für Klinische Radiologie
Ludwig-Maximilians-Universität
Klinikum Großhadern
Marchioninistrasse 15
81377 München
Germany

MEDICAL RADIOLOGY · Diagnostic Imaging and Radiation Oncology

Continuation of
Handbuch der medizinischen Radiologie
Encyclopedia of Medical Radiology

ISSN 0942-5373
ISBN 3-540-67216-8 Springer-Verlag Berlin Heidelberg New York

CIP data applied for

Die Deutsche Bibliothek - CIP-Einheitsaufnahme
Abdominal and pelvic MRI / A. Heuck; M. Reiser (ed). With contributions by A. L. Baert ... Foreword by A. L. Baert. – Berlin;
Heidelberg; New York; Barcelona; Hong Kong; London; Milan; Paris; Singapore; Tokyo: Springer, 2000 (Medical radiology)
ISBN 3-540-67216-8

Springer-Verlag is a company in the BertelsmannSpringer publishing group.
© Springer-Verlag Berlin Heidelberg 1998, 2000

Printed in Germany

Typesetting: Best-set Typesetter Ltd., Hong Kong

SPIN: 107 632 44   21/3135 – 5 4 3 2 1 0 – Printed on acid-free paper

Foreword

While MRI has proved itself to be an excellent diagnostic noninvasive modality for imaging of the brain, medulla, and musculoskeletal system due to its high intrinsic contrast resolution and tissue characterisation potential based on the judicious application of specific sequences, this has not been the case in the abdomen and pelvis. The reasons are the long exposure time and the lower spatial resolution, inherent to MRI. However, during recent years considerable process has been achieved in MRI of the abdominal and pelvic organs due to the development of new and more rapid imaging sequences and the routine clinical application of specific magnetic resonance contrast media. Consequently for some anatomical areas such as the female genital organs and the biliary system MRI is already the best performing morphological diagnostic modality. However, the question arises as to wether MRI, given its performance capabilities, should not also be considered a primary diagnostic modality for the study of parenchymal organs like the liver, spleen, and pancreas, and not merely as a complentary modality to solve residual problems after ultrasonography and computed tomography have been performed. Although the future role of MRI in respect of the gastrointestinal tube itself is still somewhat unclear, some possibilities for routine clinical use are becoming visible even in this abdominal field.

All these problems and questions are fully addressed in this excellent book, edited by A. Heuck and M. Reiser with the help of an international group of well-known abdominal MRI specialists. The editors have been able to provide us with a much-needed update on the progress achieved in the rapidly evolving and fascinating field of abdominal MRI. The volume will be of benefit to all radiologists eager to maintain their experience in MRI as well as to gastroenterologists, abdominal surgeons, and gynecologists who want to remain informed about new diagnostic noninvasive possibilities in their organ area.

As current editor-in-chief of this volume series I express my gratitude to the editors for the very expert and rapid preparation of this high-quality volume.

Leuven   ALBERT L. BAERT

Preface

In many fields of science and technology, periods of fast growth alternate with times of gradual consolidation. Problems which long seemed to be insurmountable may suddenly become irrelevant when new solutions are found. MRI of the abdomen and pelvis may be cited as an example for this. Following the introduction of NMR into medical imaging, numerous attempts were made to overcome the major obstacle that the long acquisition time of MRI rendered it almost impossible to avoid motion artifacts in abdominal and pelvic imaging due to pulsation, respiration, bowel motion, etc. Methods to compensate for these artifacts, such as cardiac gating, respiratory gating, and bowel compression, made the examinations laborious and highly dependent on the specific setting. Recently, however, major advances have been made in MR technology: Stronger gradients with rapid rise times allow for fast acquisition of imaging data within one breath hold. Coil technology, e.g., with phased array coil systems, has contributed to better signal-to-noise ratios. Moreover, contrast media targeted to specific organs have been introduced into medical practice.

With these and other advances, high image quality in MRI of the abdomen and pelvis has become possible and robust imaging protocols have been established. Now, the unique potential advantages of MRI, e.g., superior soft-tissue contrast, multiplanar capabilities, and tissue characterization, can also be utilized for abdominal and pelvic imag-ing. Moreover, in addition to cross-sectional imaging, specific techniques, such as MR-cholangiopancreatography, MR-urography and MR-angiography, make MRI a versatile modality which can be adapted to the specific clinical question.

In many fields of abdominal and pelvic imaging, MRI has provided its superiority over other modalities. Even if there are still relatively few studies on large patient groups that permit extensive comparison with other modalities, it can be expected that MRI will play a dominant role in the future.

This book was prepared by a group of distinguished experts in the field of abdominal and pelvic MRI from Europe and North America. It attempts to convey the latest knowledge on this rapidly evolving and fascinating field of radiology. We are deeply grateful to the authors who have contributed to this book with their expertise and well-structured and highly informative chapters. They have made it possible to achieve a comprehensive overview on all aspects of advanced MRI of the abdomen and pelvis.

We would like to thank Prof. A. L. Baert for encouraging, inspiring and supporting us in this project. The high quality and acknowledged professionalism of Springer-Verlag has permitted the publication of this book after a relatively short period of preparation, thereby ensuring that all the information provided is up-to-date and of current relevance.

Munich, February 1998

ANDREAS HEUCK
MAXIMILIAN REISER

Contents

Retroperitoneum

Gastrointestinal Tract

Pelvis

1 Imaging Strategies for the Detection of Liver Lesions

G. Marchal

1.1 Introduction

Of all the organs in the abdomen, the hepatobiliary system is the most frequent site of pathology. This is not surprising since the liver is the metabolic factory of the body with important anabolic and catabolic activity. All components of the liver, the afferent and efferent vessels, the parenchyma, and the biliary system, can be affected by disease. Though pathology can be limited to the liver as such, quite often it is either the result or the cause of extrahepatic pathology. The detection of such extrahepatic disease is often as important as the detection of the hepatic pathology itself. For instance in cirrhotic patients the presence of large gastroesophageal varices can be the life-threatening condition. Therefore, and independently of the modality used, an imaging strategy for the liver should provide diagnostic information not only on the liver as such but also on all the other organs which can be at the origin of or affected by the liver disease included in the volume studied. In MRI this means that the sequences used should ideally offer diagnostic information on all the abdominal organs.

G. Marchal, MD, Professor, Department of Radiology, University Hospitals K.U. Leuven, Herestraat 49, B-3000 Leuven, Belgium

1.2 Hepatic MRI: Imaging Strategies and Technical Evolution

1.2.1 Fast and Ultrafast MRI

Although since their inception MRI systems have been built as total body scanners, for a long time they did not perform like this because artifacts related to the long acquisition times prevented the routine acquisition of images of diagnostic quality of organs subject to motion. Respiratory motion induces volume averaging with a reduction in lesion contrast to noise (C/N) ratio and therefore a lower conspicuity, often rendering difficult the characterization of small lesions. On the other hand, classical multislice spin-echo (SE) sequences offer an excellent signal to noise (S/N) ratio. Non-breath-hold imaging performs better at lower field strengths.

With the introduction of scanners with fast high-power gradient systems, appropriate antennas, and fast and ultrafast T1- and T2-weighted imaging sequences, organ motion is no longer problematic. Unfortunately, not all equipment in clinical use today relies on this state-of-the-art technology. The exact value of T1- and T2-weighted techniques depends on the field strength: at higher field strength, T2-weighted images become more important. It has been shown, for instance, that at 1.5 T only a minority of hypovascular metastases are identified only on T1-weighted images (Semelka et al. 1994). Nevertheless, most investigators use both T1- and T2-weighted sequences for liver imaging, not only because the addition of T1-weighted images may occasionally make possible the detection of additional lesions, but also because they may be helpful for lesion characterization (hepatocellular carcinomas and adenomas, for instance, are often predominantly or partially hyperintense on T1-weighted images, a feature which virtually excludes other types of lesions such as hemangiomas and metastases from gastrointestinal tumors or breast

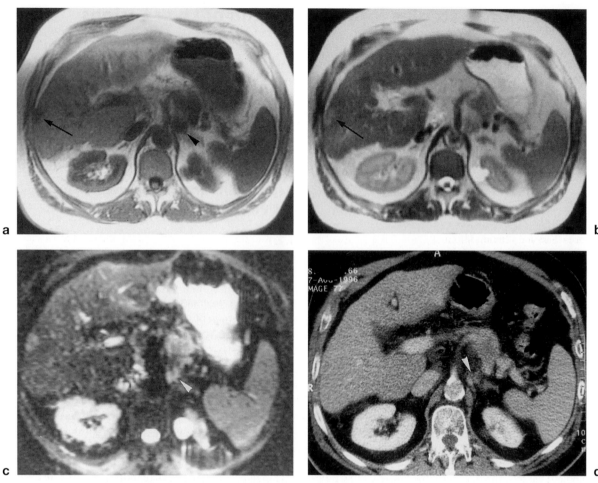

Fig. 1.1 a–d. Liver metastasis of pancreatic adenocarcinoma: comparison of SE and GE ultrafast sequences for T2-weighted images (HASTE and EPI) and usefulness of T1-weighted imaging. **a** T1-weighted image obtained with an ultrafast sequence (turbo FLASH acquisition time/slice 300 ms) shows a hypointense lesion (*arrow*) in the right liver lobe. Also well depicted are a hypointense pancreatic mass and an enlarged para-aortic lymph node (*arrowhead*). **b** T2-weighted image obtained with an ultrafast sequence (HASTE acquisition time/slice 400 ms) depicts the liver lesion as a slightly hyperintense focus (*arrow*). The pancreatic tumor was nearly isointense relative to normal pancreatic tissue. **c** T2-weighted image obtained with an ultrafast sequence (EPI acquisition time/slice 30 ms) shows the primary pancreatic tumor as well as the hepatic metastasis and the lymphadenopathy (*arrowhead*) as hyperintense masses. Fat saturation was applied to avoid chemical shift artifact. Note the suboptimal image quality and the limited spatial resolution. The thickness of the gastric wall cannot be assessed, due to the use of the saturation (compare with b). **d** Helical CT image obtained late in the portal venous phase: the hepatic metastasis is not well seen. On the other hand, the pancreatic adenocarcinoma is well visualized as a hypodense mass. The lymphadenopathy (*arrowhead*) is also well delineated due to the high contrast relative to the retroperitoneal fat

carcinoma). Furthermore, T1-weighted images may be required for the optimal detection of extrahepatic disease (Fig. 1.1).

Slower systems using classical T1- and T2-weighted SE sequences with motion compensation can solve a number of diagnostic problems. Techniques used to suppress motion artifacts are averaging of multiple excitations, phase reordering, gradient moment nulling, fat saturation (to suppress ghost artifacts originating from fat), and gating (SPRITZER et al. 1996). It has, for instance, been demonstrated that, compared with nontriggered images, respiratory-triggered fast spin-echo (FSE) images provide sharper anatomic detail, equal or less phase ghosting, and measurable improvement in lesion-to-liver contrast (Low et al. 1997).

In this regard fast breath-hold imaging could be considered a major breakthrough (REINIG 1995). Its main advantage is obviously the decrease in respiratory-induced volume averaging and therefore theoretically a higher spatial and contrast resolution. It should be stressed, however, that breath-hold imaging is not necessarily superior to non-breath-hold imaging. In the study by SOYER et al. (1996), breath-hold FSE offered lower lesion-to-liver C/N and S/N ratios than non-breath-hold FSE, a finding most likely relate to the fact that changes in technical parameters such as the number of averages, effective TE, matrix size, and echo train length, necessary to reduce imaging times, may negatively influence the quality of the resulting images.

With gradient-echo (GE) acquisitions characterized by short TR/TE, e.g., 100 ms/5 ms, a few T1-weighted images can be acquired within a single breath-hold period of about 16 s. This acquisition has to be repeated several times to cover the whole liver or upper abdomen. If parallel saturating slabs are applied to overcome flow artifacts, or if fat suppression pulses are used, the number of slices per breath-hold is further reduced. A common problem is that small lesions can be missed in this way. A first approach to overcome this disadvantage is to acquire both transverse and coronal or sagittal images (DE LANGE et al. 1996). Another technique would be to let the patient breathe quietly and incorporate navigator echoes that force the data acquisition during a specific fraction of the respiratory cycle only (WANG et al. 1996). The S/N and C/N ratios in GE acquisitions depend on the choice of TR, TE, and flip angle. Due to a short TR and the use of a high bandwidth to shorten TE, S/N and C/N ratios can be lower than with conventional SE techniques. Currently, the best available antennas (e.g., phased array body coils) should always be used to minimize the S/N problems. SE acquisitions can also be performed within a breath-hold, using TR/TE 240 ms/15 ms. Such acquisitions yield T1-weighted images with S/N and SD/N ratios (SD: signal difference) that are slightly inferior to breath-hold GE measurements (SEMELKA et al. 1991; SIEWERT et al. 1994).

Using regular GE techniques, it is difficult to obtain T2-weighted images. Hence, with longer TE, the T2* effects rapidly dominate the T2 effects.

T2-weighted SE acquisitions can only be obtained during a single breath-hold by using FSE methods [also called turbo spin echo (TSE)]. In these acquisitions, multiple echoes or "echo trains" are collected per RF excitation pulse and, therefore, the whole imaging process is accelerated by a factor equal to the echo train length. As an example, using an echo train length of 15, a T2-weighted acquisition with TR/TE 2000 ms/90 ms can be obtained in 2.1 min (matrix 160 × 256). With good patient cooperation,

image contrast can be excellent (SIEWERT et al. 1994; GIOVAGNONI et al. 1996; PEARLMAN and EDELMAN 1994). While FSE techniques offer a significant time saving, one concern has been the decreased C/N and signal intensity ratios of solid lesions, which may be partially related to magnetization transfer effects (CATASCA and MIROWITZ 1994). While such effects may theoretically decrease the conspicuity of solid lesions, they may be beneficial too, because they facilitate the differentiation of solid lesions and hemangiomas, at least if a sufficiently large TE is used. Another particular feature in T2-weighted FSE is the paradoxical brightening of fat; this effect increases as the number of refocusing pulses increases and the time between refocusing pulses decreases.

Ultrafast sequences are just a further evolution of the above-mentioned sequences (PEARLMAN and EDELMAN 1994). T2-weighted images are acquired using only one excitation pulse. The echo train can consist of gradient echoes, in which case the acquisition belongs to the class of echo planar imaging (EPI) techniques (BUTTS et al. 1993) (Fig. 1.1). In another implementation, it can consist of spin echoes, using half-Fourier reconstruction techniques to decrease the echo train length. This acquisition is called HASTE (half-Fourier single-shot turbo spin-echo) (KIEFER et al. 1994) or half-Fourier RARE (Fig. 1.1).

Both HASTE and EPI measurements are so short that respiratory and even cardiac motion is frozen in the images. Freezing cardiac motion is possible even if the acquisition window is relatively long (e.g., 300 ms), because motion significantly degrades images quality only if it occurs during acquisition of the central lines of k-space. Although breath-hold imaging may produce similar image quality in cooperative patients, single-shot imaging is clearly superior in critically ill patients or anyone unable to cope with the breath-hold requirements (VAN HOE et al. 1996). Single-shot T2-weighted EPI has the shortest acquisition times (down to 30 ms), but it suffers from even small field inhomogeneity. The use of EPI in the abdomen is therefore rather limited to larger organs. The images of other organs are often heavily degraded by susceptibility artifacts due to in nearby bowel loops. Distortion can be so severe that the organs may no longer even be recognized. In practice, the magnet has to be shimmed first, making the whole procedure rather time consuming. Furthermore, the use of fat saturation techniques is a must to reduce N/2 ghosting and chemical shift artifacts. Moreover, EPI images suffer from high noise levels (high bandwidth) and poor spatial resolution (pixel size 2–3 mm). HASTE acquisitions, on the other

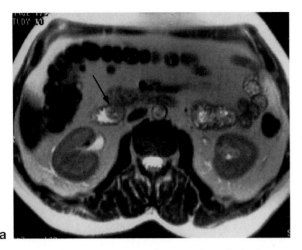
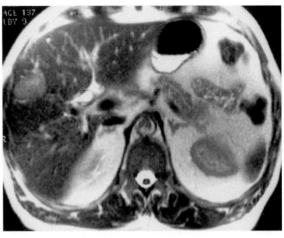

a   b

Fig. 1.2 a,b. Malignant ampulloma: Value of ultrafast SE (HASTE) for the detection of extrahepatic disease. **a** Small tumor (*arrow*) protruding in the fluid-filled duodenum. The stenotic distal common bile duct inside the mass suggests the diagnosis of ampulloma. **b** Solitary liver metastasis seen as a moderately hyperintense mass in the right liver lobe. Note also the dilated hepatic duct. Since ultrafast SE images do not suffer from susceptibility artifacts, the wall of the air-filled stomach is well appreciated

hand, are very robust. They are sensitive neither to susceptibility artifacts nor to motion (Fig. 1.2). GAA et al. (1996) compared single-shot and multishot T2-weighted SE EPI sequences with conventional T2-weighted FSE and inversion recovery SE EPI sequences with conventional T2-weighted SE imaging for the detection of focal liver lesions. These authors found that lesion-to-liver C/N ratios were highest on fat-suppressed HASTE images. HASTE may also be used to diagnose extrahepatic diseases. The stationary fluids in the biliary system and in the renal pelvis, and the fluid-filled bowel loops, are shown with high intensity. The presence of air in the bowel does not degrade the images because of the low sensitivity of these sequences to susceptibility artifacts. Therefore, the pancreaticobiliary, the genitourinary, and even the gastrointestinal system are properly imaged (AERTS et al. 1996).

Recently, a double-echo version of HASTE has been developed (BOSMANS et al. 1997). In this technique, two images are calculated at the same anatomic level after a single excitation pulse. The first image has a relatively short echo time (e.g., 60 ms), while the second image has a longer echo time (e.g., 378 ms). Combined evaluation of these two corresponding images with variable T2 weighting leads to improved differentiation of focal liver lesions (particularly cysts and hemangiomas) and improved detection of other abnormalities such as acute pancreatitis or rupture of the common bile duct (BOSMANS et al. 1997).

T1-weighted EPI or HASTE can only be obtained with special preparation pulses. In practice, ultrafast T1-weighted acquisitions are realized using a 180° inversion recovery pulse, followed by a fast (conventional) GE acquisition ("turbo FLASH") (Fig. 1.1). C/N and S/N ratios can be excellent, and further increased using "segmented turbo FLASH," in which case a specific segment of the k-space is acquired per inversion recovery pulse (EDELMAN et al. 1990; WALLNER et al. 1992).

Although ultrafast sequences do not necessitate breath-holding to freeze the motion, a multislice acquisition during breath-holding represents a true volume acquisition, avoiding the slice misregistration which can occur during a non-breath-hold slice by slice acquisition. In the future, a non-breath-hold respiratory gated ultrafast acquisition could be worked out. Besides ultrafast two-dimensional imaging, the new state-of-the-art technology also allows ultrafast projective and three-dimensional (3-D) imaging.

In many centers projective imaging is routinely used for MR cholangiopancreatography, MR urography, and myelography (REUTHER et al. 1996). The principle is simple: a single thick slab is acquired with an extremely heavily T2-weighted sequence that produces an image in which only the signal intensity of the stationary water is displayed. This can be a single-shot T2-weighted SE acquisition (RARE) or an FISP type acquisition. The combination of ultrafast techniques such as HASTE that provide multiple

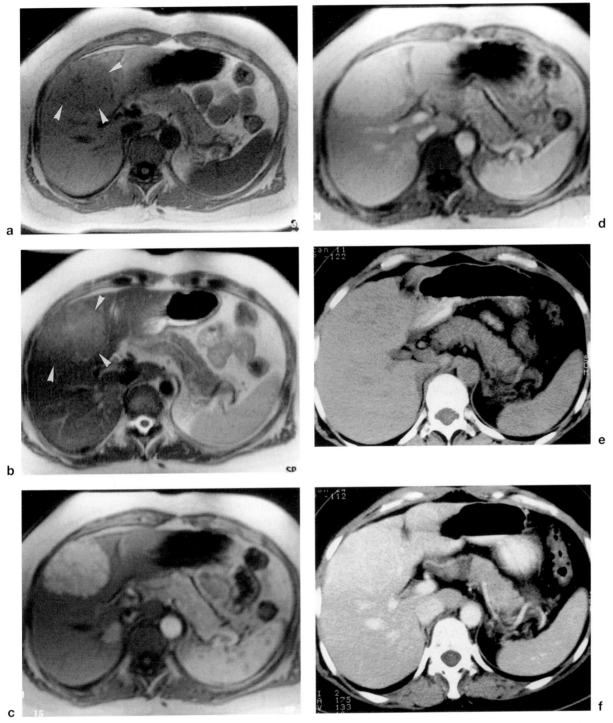

Fig. 1.3 a–f. Focal nodular hyperplasia (FNH): usefulness of contrast enhancement for the detection and characterization of primary hepatocyte-derived liver lesions. **a** Turbo FLASH T1-weighted image shows a relatively large lesion in the right liver lobe that is only slightly hypointense relative to normal liver tissue (*arrowheads*). This feature points to the diagnosis of a primary hepatocyte-derived mass (FNH, adenoma, or HCC). **b** HASTE image shows the lesion as a slightly hyperintense area (*arrowheads*). **c** Dynamic contrast-enhanced im-age obtained in the arterial phase shows homogeneous uptake of contrast material. The lesion is now markedly hyperintense. Based on these morphologic features, the diagnosis of FNH can be proposed. Because of the homogeneous appearance, adenoma and HCC are unlikely. **d** Contrast-enhanced MR image obtained in the portal venous phase shows the lesion as slightly hyperintense. **e** Non-contrast-enhanced CT image: the lesion is invisible. **f** Contrast-enhanced CT image obtained in the portal venous phase: the lesion is slightly hyperdense

cross-sectional slices within a short time and projective techniques such as RARE that offer an overall view of the anatomy of water-containing structures appears quite promising.

1.2.2
Contrast-Enhanced MRI

During the early years of MRI, it was believed that the intrinsic contrast in this new modality would be sufficient to achieve superior sensitivity and specificity and hence that contrast agents would not be required. The first contrast agent routinely tested in hepatic MRI was the nonspecific extracellular agent Gd-DTPA (Magnevist, Schering). This contrast agent has many similarities to those used in CT. Dynamic ultrafast 3-D imaging is the new trend in contrast-enhanced MR angiography and is also used in hepatic MRI. The approach consists in the acquisition of a 3-D volume with thin slices after the injection of a bolus of a T1 relaxation agent. These sequences use an ultrashort TR to allow breath-hold acquisition and an ultrashort TE to avoid flow dephasing (LEUNG et al. 1996). The acquisition times can be further reduced by acquiring multiple echoes per excitation pulse. This technique has been applied to MR angiography, and enables acquisition of 3-D abdominal angiograms in a breath-hold period of less than 10 s. It is obvious that all these technical improvements will dramatically change the role of body MRI in general and liver MRI in particular. It has been shown that dynamic contrast-enhanced MRI is much more accurate than non-contrast-enhanced MRI in the detection of hypervascular liver tumors, e.g., metastases of hepatocellular carcinoma (OI et al. 1996) (Fig. 1.3). Gadolinium-enhanced MRI also improves the characterization of focal liver lesions. While dynamic techniques are particularly useful in the diagnosis of hemangiomas, delayed images may offer additional information in some patients, by showing peripheral wash-out (pointing to the diagnosis of metastasis) or a homogeneous hyperdense aspect (hemangioma).

For liver imaging, the strategies are further influenced by the development and progressive commercial introduction of a number of liver-specific MR contrast agents. The substances closest to clinical introduction are directed either to the hepatocytes or to the reticuloendothelial system (RES). Hepatocyte-specific agents are all T1 relaxation agents with gadolinium or manganese as the active element, and all show biliary excretion. Gd-EOB-DTPA is a lipophilic

modification of the chelate Gd-DTPA with receptor-specific uptake in the hepatocytes and subsequent biliary excretion. It has been shown in phase I clinical studies that the product is safe and efficient for MRI of the liver (HAMM et al. 1995). A particular advantage of this contrast agent is that it can be administered as a bolus, which makes it suitable for use in dynamic MRI studies. The degree and time course of signal intensity enhancement might be used as a measure of liver function. Furthermore, biliary structures are strongly enhanced secondary to biliary excretion, which indicates the potential usefulness of this product in the evaluation of biliary disease. Gd-BOPTA is another lipophilic ligate which has been shown to be a safe contrast agent that helps in the detection of small metastases (CAUDANA et al. 1996). The paramagnetic ion manganese has a natural affinity for hepatocytes and is largely excreted in the bile. In order to reduce toxicity, manganese is bound to ligands, e.g., DPDP. In clinical studies, Mn-DPDP has yielded a significant improvement in the C/N ratio of normal liver tissue to tumorous tissue and improved lesion detection (HAMM et al. 1992). Interestingly, Mn has been reported to increase the signal of the normal pancreas and adrenal glands. The agent is currently under evaluation for the detection not only of liver lesions but also of pancreatic tumors and adrenal malignancies.

The RES-specific agents consist of suspensions of small iron oxide particles which, once injected, rapidly accumulate in the lysosomes of the macrophages of the liver, spleen, and bone marrow. There two major groups: superparamagnetic iron oxide particles (SPIOs), which have a high R2/R1 relaxivity ratio and a short blood half-life (minutes), and ultrasmall superparamagnetic iron oxide particles (USPIOs), which have a longer R2/R1 relaxivity ratio and a longer blood half-life (hours). SPIO agents efficiently accumulate in the liver (approximately 80% of injected dose) and spleen (WEISSLEDER 1994). The drug is relatively safe when infused slowly over 30 min. In comparison with the well-known nonspecific gadolinium chelates, this agent offers clear advantages for both lesion detection and characterization. Its administration improves the lesion C/N ratio and therefore detectability (HAGSPIEL et al. 1995). It tends to accumulate not only in liver parenchyma but also in primary hepatocyte-derived tumors (adenoma, focal nodular hyperplasia), allowing differentiation from metastases. While undifferentiated HCC does not take up contrast medium, well-differentiated HCC may show a distinct uptake. Quantitative evaluation of the percentage signal intensity loss (PSIL) after contrast administration may be the most useful approach to distinguish well-differentiated HCCs from benign lesions. VOGL et al. (1996) reported a threshold PSIL of at least 10% to be the best criterion in order to obtain a specific diagnosis of benignity.

USPIOs have some distinct advantages over SPIOs. Firstly, they also accumulate in normal lymph nodes, which makes them potentially valuable in evaluating lymph node enlargement. Secondly, they can be used as blood pool contrast agents in MR angiography, Finally, it has been shown that malignant tumors frequently show ring enhancement after administration of USPIOs. This feature is probably related to their prolonged blood-pool phase within collateral vessels surrounding malignant tumors. Irrespective of the exact mechanism involved, this feature may be another useful criterion for the characterization of liver lesions (MERGO et al. 1996).

1.2.3
Other Technical Aspects

The systematic use of fat saturation has been proposed to improve the S/N and C/N ratios. LU et al. (1994) compared fat-suppressed and non-fat-suppressed SE MR images and concluded that fat suppression should be routinely used in T2-weighted MRI of the upper part of the abdomen. Noise is lower on fat-suppressed SE images because fat signal does not contribute to motion-related phase-encoding artifacts. In patients with fatty livers, the lesion-to-liver contrast improves because of reduction of hepatic signal on fat-suppressed images. Furthermore, fat suppression makes lesions adjacent to fat (e.g., lesions next to the porta hepatis) more conspicuous. Frequency-based fat suppression has a minor drawback, however: fat located anterior in the liver is usually not completely suppressed. Inhomogeneous fat suppression can be avoided by using an inversion recovery techniques. In breath-hold and ultrafast sequences, the role of fat suppression is less clear. Since respiratory artifacts are no longer a problem, the advantages of obtaining fat-suppressed T2-weighted images are less important. While fat-suppressed images may enhance the detection of focal liver lesions in some patients, they make evaluation of other features such as bowel wall thickness more difficult (Fig. 1.1). Moreover, the contours of solid organs such as the liver and spleen are less well delineated. It is clear that determination of the exact

role of fat suppression in ultrafast MRI warrants further study.

In single-shoot acquisitions, the selection of an optimal echo spacing is critical. Because successive echoes are obtained during T2 decay (in SE techniques such as HASTE) or T2* decay (in EPI), use of a long echo train is only justified if a short echo spacing can be selected. The major problem is low-resolution imaging of tissues with short T2s. This feature may become problematic if superparamagnetic contrast media are used. HASTE images, for instance, offer poor resolution after administration of iron oxides. In such a situation, the use of a multishot sequence may be justified.

1.3
Comparison with Other Imaging Modalities

In an era of cost containment, comparison of the diagnostic accuracy of different imaging modalities is of critical importance. Currently, only a few studies comparing state-of-the-art hepatic MRI with helical CT are available. In one preliminary study, it was found that non-contrast-enhanced ultrafast- T2-weighted MRI is essentially as accurate as contrast-enhanced helical CT in the detection and characterization of focal liver lesions (VAN HOE et al. 1996). DE LANGE et al. (1996) showed that non-contrast-enhanced breath-hold T1-weighted magnetization-prepared GE MRI was superior to contrast-enhanced CT in the detection and localization of focal liver lesions. However, these authors used conventional dynamic CT scanning, not helical CT. There is little doubt that iron oxide-enhanced MRI is more sensitive than unenhanced MRI and helical CT. Moreover, it has been shown that iron oxide-enhanced MRI is at least as accurate as CT arterial potography (CTAP) for the detection of hepatic metastases (SENETERRE et al. 1996). This result is of critical importance because CTAP, which is an invasive techniques, has long been considered the imaging technique of choice in patients regarded as potential candidates for partial liver resection. When comparing MRI and CT, it should be kept in mind, however, that MRI currently has some limitations. Firstly, MR images usually offer a lower spatial resolution than CT images, with the image matrix of MR images typically 128 × 256 versus 512 × 512 for CT. Secondly, with the sue of body phased array coils, imaging of the entire abdomen in one session is currently impossible without patient repositioning.

Furthermore, the detection of lymphadenopathy may be more difficult on MRI than on CT. Finally, contrast-enhance MRI is certainly more expensive than contrast-enhanced CT. With the use of ultrafast sequences and simplified acquisition protocols (both enabling increased patient throughput), the real cost of unenhanced MRI could decrease significantly in the near future, thereby making this technique a potentially cost-effective noninvasive alternative to helical CT in a larger number of patients.

Iron oxide-enhanced MRI is still inferior to intraoperative ultrasonography in the detection of liver metastases. The detection of lesions <1 cm in diameter remains a particular problem, even after the administration of targetted contrast media. In one study, it was found that iron oxide-enhanced MRI depicted only 36% of lesions between 5 and 10 mm (HAGSPIEL et al. 1995).

1.4
Conclusion

Obviously the ongoing improvements in MR technology and in contrast agent research are dramatically changing the role of body MRI in general and liver MRI in particular. There is little doubt that in the near future MRI will outperform other imaging modalities for the detection of liver lesions.

References

Aerts P, Van Hoe L, Bosmans H, Oyen R, Marchal G, Baert AL (1996) Technical note. MR urography using the HASTE technique. AJR 166:543–545

Bosmans H, Gryspeerdt S, Van Hoe L, et al. (1997) Preliminary experience with a new double echo HASTE acquisition in the characterization of liver lesions. MAG*MA (in press)

Butts K, Riederer SJ, Ehman RL, Felmlee JP, Grimm RC (1993) Echo-planar imaging of the liver with a standard MR imaging system. Radiology 189:259–264

Catasca JV, Mirowitz SA (1994) T2-weighted MR imaging of the abdomen: fast spin-echo versus conventional spin-echo sequences. AJR 162:61–67

Caudana R, Morana G, Pirovano GP, et al. (1996) Focal malignant hepatic lesions: MR imaging enhanced with Gadolinium-BOPTA-preliminary results of phase II clinical application. Radiology 199:513–520

de Lange EE, Mugler JP, Gay SB, DeAngelis GA, Berr SS, Harris EK (1996) Focal liver disease: comparison of breath-hold T1-weighed MP-GRE imaging and contrast-enhanced CT-lesion detection, localization, and characterization. Radiology 200:465–473

Edelman RR, Wallner B, Singer A, Atkinson DJ, Saini S (1990) Segmented turboFLASH: method for breath-hold MR imaging of the liver with flexible contrast. Radiology 177:515–521

Gaa J, Habatu H, Jenkins RL, Finn JP, Edelman RR (1996) Liver masses: replacement of conventional spin-echo MR imaging with breath-hold MR imaging. Radiology 200:459–464

Giovagnoni A, Paci E, Valeri G, Ercolani P, Gesuita R, Carle F, Piga A (1996) MRI in characterization of focal liver lesions: comparison of T2 weighting by conventional spin-echo and turbo spin-echo sequences. Magn Reson Imaging 6:589–595

Hagspiel KD, Neidl KFW, Eichenberger AC, Weder W, Marincek B (1995) Detection of liver metastases: comparison of superparamagnetic iron oxide-enhanced and unenhanced MR imaging at 1.5 T with dynamic CT, intraoperative US, and percutaneous US. Radiology 196:471–478

Hamm B, Vogl TJ, Branding G, et al. (1992) MR imaging with Mn-DPDP-initial clinical results in 40 patients. Radiology 182:167

Hamm B, Staks T, Mühler T, et al. (1995) Phase I clinical evaluation of Gd-EOB-DTPA as a hepatospecific MR contrast agent: safety, pharmacokinetics, and MR imaging. Radiology 195:785–792

Kiefer B, Grässner J, Hausman R (1994) Image acquisition in a second with half-Fourier acquisition single-shot tubo spin echo (abstract). J Magn Reson Imaging 4(p):86–87

Leung DA, McKinnan GC, Davis CP, Pfammatter T, Krestin GP, Debastin JF (1996) Breathhold, contrast-enhanced, three-dimensional MR angiography. Radiology 200:569–571

Low RN, Alzate GD, Shimakawa A (1997) Motion suppression in MR imaging of the liver: comparison of respiratory-triggered and nontriggered fast spin-echo sequences. AJR 168:225–231

Lu DSK, Saini S, Hahn PF, et al. (1994) T2-weighted MR imaging of the upper part of the abdomen: should fat suppression be used routinely? AJR 162:1095–1100

Mergo PJ, Helmberger T, Nicolas AI, Ros PR (1996) Ring enhancement in ultrasmall superparamagnetic iron oxide MR imaging: a potential now sign for characterization of liver lesions. AJR 166:379–394

Oi H, Murakami T, Kim T, Matsushita M, Kishimoto H, Nakamura H (1996) Dynamic MR imaging and early-phase helical CT for detecting small intrahepatic metastases of hepatocellular carcinoma. AJR 166:369–374

Pearlman JD, Edelman RR (1994) Ultrafast magnetic resonance imaging. Segmented turboflash, echo-planar, and real-time nuclear magnetic resonance. Radiol Clin North Am 32:593–612

Reinig JW (1995) Breath-hold fast spin-echo MR imaging of the liver: a technique for high quality T2-weighted images. Radiology 194:303–304

Reuther G, Kiefer B, Tuchmann A (1996) Cholangiography before biliary surgery: single-shot MR cholangiography versus intravenous cholangiography. Radiology 198:561–566

Semelka RC, Simm FC, Recht M, Deimling M, Lenz G, Laub GA (1991) T1-weighted sequences for MR imaging of the liver: comparison of three techniques for single-breath, whole-volume acquisition at 1.0 and 1.5 T. Radiology 180:629–635

Semelka RC, Bagley AS, Brown ED, Kroeker MA (1994) Maligant lesions of the liver identified on T1- but not on T2-weighted MR images at 1.5 T. J Magn Reson Imaging 4:315–318

Semelka RC, Kelekis NL, Thomasson D, Brown MA, Laub GA (1996) HASTE MR imaging: description of technique and preliminary results in the abdomen. Magn Reson Imaging 6:698–699

Senéterre E, Taourel P, Bouvier Y, et al. (1996) Detection of hepatic metastases: ferumoxides-enhanced MR imaging versus unenhanced MR imaging and CT during arterial portography. Radiology 200:785–792

Siewert B, Muller MF, Foley M, Wielopolski PA, Finn JP (1994) Fast MR imaging of the liver: quantitative comparison of techniques. Radiology 193:37–42

Soyer PH, Le Normand S, Clement de Givry S, Gueye C, Somveille E, Scherrer A (1996) T2-weighted spin-echo MR imaging of the liver: breath-hold fast spin-echo versus non-breath-hold fast spin-echo images with and without fat suppression. AJR 166:593–597

Spritzer CE, Keogan MT, DeLong DM, Dahlke J, Macfall JR (1996) Optimizing fast spin-echo acquisitions for hepatic imaging in normal subjects. Magn Reson Imaging 1:128–135

Van Hoe L, Bosmans H, Aerts P, Baert AL, Fevery J, Kiefer B, Marchal G (1996) Focal liver lesions: fast T2-weighted MR imaging with half-Fourier RARE. Radiology 201:817–823

Vogl TJ, Hammerstingl R, Schwarz W, et al. (1996) Superparamagnetic iron oxide-enhanced versus gadolinium-enhanced MR imaging for differential diagnosis of focal liver lesions. Radiology 198:881–887

Wallner B, Friedrich JM, Goldman A, Edelman RR (1992) Magnetic resonance tomography of the liver with TurboFLASH and segmented acquisition. Fast imaging with flexible image contrast. Fortschr Geb Röntgenstr Neuen Bildgeb Verfahr 157:180–184

Wang VW, Rossman PJ, Grimm RC, Riederer SJ, Ehman RL (1996) Navigator-echo-based real-time respiratory gating and triggering for reduction of respiration effects in three-dimensional coronary MR-angiography. Radiology 198:55–60

Weissleder R (1994) Liver MR imaging with iron oxides: toward consensus and clinical practice (editorial comment). Radiology 193:593–595

2 Diffuse Disease of the Liver

P.J. Mergo and P.R. Ros

CONTENTS

2.1 Introduction

While magnetic resonance imaging (MRI) is utilized primarily in the liver for evaluation and characterization of focal lesions, it also has utility in the assessment of diffuse disease of the liver. It can offer a noninvasive means of establishing the presence of diffuse liver disease, characterizing the extent of disease, and, in certain instances, identifying the underlying cause of the disease.

The presence of cirrhosis is a common link among many diffuse diseases of the liver. Entities resulting in cirrhotic change include alcoholic liver disease, hepatitis, hemochromatosis, Wilson's disease, Budd-Chiari syndrome and hepatic venous congestion, schistosomiasis, sarcoidosis, amyloidosis, biliary cirrhosis, and hereditary disorders, such as α_1-antitrypsin deficiency, glycogen storage disease, and tyrosinemia.

P.J. MERGO, MD, Assistant Professor, Division of Body Imaging and MRI, Department of Radiology, University of Florida College of Medicine. P.O. Box 100374, 1600 SW Archer Road, Gainesville, FL 32610, USA
P.R. Ros, MD, Professor and Associate Chairman, Division of Body Imaging and MRI, Department of Radiology, University of Florida College of Medicine, P.O. Box 100374, 1600 SW Archer Road, Gainesville, FL 32610, USA

Some diffuse processes, such as fatty change and hepatocellular carcinoma (HCC), may occur concomitantly with cirrhosis, but are not direct causative agents of cirrhosis. In fact, they occur secondarily as a result of the same toxic insult that causes the cirrhosis. In addition, both may occur as isolated findings, without concomitant cirrhosis.

Other entities, such as malignancy from either metastases or lymphoma, form a third subset of diffuse disease which occurs predominantly in the noncirrhotic liver.

In this chapter, the imaging findings and pertinent features of these entities will be discussed. The focus is on the MR findings for those entities which can be primarily distinguished by imaging findings.

2.2 Cirrhosis

Since cirrhosis is a common thread among many of the diffuse liver diseases, it is important for the radiologist to understand the underlying pathologic changes that ensue in the liver, as well as to recognize the imaging findings of cirrhosis. Cirrhosis is a chronic response to repeated episodes of hepatocellular insult, characterized by phases of impaired circulation, injury, inflammation, and regeneration and fibrosis (BRENNER and ALCORN 1992).

Microscopically, cirrhosis may be characterized as either micronodular, macronodular, or mixed. Micronodular cirrhosis has diffuse nodules less than 3 mm in size, with thin fibrous septa, and is seen in alcoholic (Laënnec's) cirrhosis and hemochromatosis. In contrast, macronodular cirrhosis has nodules greater than 3 mm in size, with thick fibrous septa, and is most commonly associated with viral hepatitis. Both micronodular and macronodular cirrhosis result in progressive fibrosis of the liver, which may manifest as hepatic failure and portal hypertension, with associated complications of ascites, variceal hemorrhage, and hepatocellular carcinoma.

The corresponding changes in the size, configuration, and contour of the liver that ensue with progressive cirrhosis are manifest on cross-sectional imaging. These findings have been classically described on computed tomography (CT), but are also evident with MR imaging; they include a small fibrotic right lobe of the liver, with regenerative enlargement of the caudate and left lobes (Fig. 2.1). A caudate to right lobe ratio equal to or greater than 0.65 is a finding which is 90% specific for the presence of cirrhosis (HARBIN et al. 1980). Another specific imaging sign of cirrhosis is a portal vein diameter greater than 1.3 cm. While changes in the overall size and shape of the liver are relatively easy to see by cross-sectional imaging, the underlying nodularity of the liver is often difficult to appreciate, owing to the small size of the regenerative nodules. With current imaging techniques, when nodularity is present, the finding is most likely attributable to the presence of underlying macronodular change. The nodularity and fibrosis combined may result in a "hobnail" appearance of the liver contour (Figs. 2.1, 2.2).

While regenerative nodules can account for many of the contour changes in the liver, dysplastic nodules and HCC may also manifest as similar contour irregularities and also occur concomitantly in the cirrhotic liver. Their distinction from regenerative nodules is important since dysplastic nodules are thought to be a premalignant condition and since the presence of HCC has a poor prognosis and may preclude liver transplantation. MRI is potentially the most useful imaging modality for evaluation of the cirrhotic liver, since it allows better characterization of these underlying nodular changes than CT or ultrasonography and at the same time can provide pertinent information about portal venous flow direction and patency.

Dysplastic nodules have a low signal intensity on T2-weighted and gradient-echo sequences, with a slight increase in signal intensity on T1-weighted

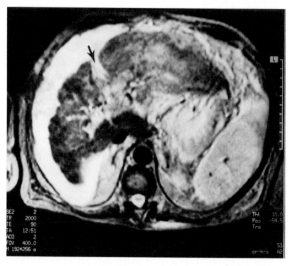

Fig. 2.1. MRI findings of cirrhosis. The liver has a nodular contour. The right lobe is small and fibrotic and the left lobe is enlarged. There is widening of the interlobar fissure (*arrow*) and ascites, in addition

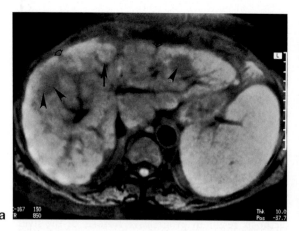

a

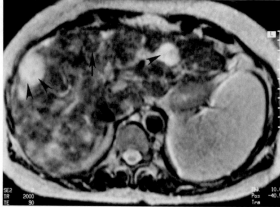

b

Fig. 2.2. a Fat suppression T1-weighted imaging shows the nodular contour of this cirrhotic liver. A rounded nodule of slightly increased signal intensity is representative of a dysplastic nodule (*arrow*). Two foci of decreased signal intensity are noted which are representative of HCC (*arrowheads*).

Note that the bands of confluent fibrosis are also hypointense (*open arrows*). **b** T2-weighted imaging shows the dysplastic nodule to be mildly hypointense relative to the liver (*arrow*), while the foci of HCC are hyperintense (*arrowheads*)

sequences (Fig. 2.2). The low signal intensity on T2-weighted imaging is attributable to the accumulation of iron and hemosiderin products within the nodules. HCC is distinguishable by its appearance as a mass of increased signal intensity on T2-weighted imaging (Fig. 2.2b). Thus, while the overall signal intensity of the cirrhotic liver is not significantly changed, discrete nodules can be further characterized as being secondary to HCC or regenerative nodules and/or adenomatous hyperplasia by the differences they exhibit in T2 relaxation time. Additionally, MR angiography (MRA) provides useful information regarding the presence of portal vein thrombosis and collateralization of flow in portosystemic shunts. These findings have been shown to correlate well with those seen with color Doppler ultrasound examination (KRAUS et al. 1993).

Ultrasonography remains the modality of choice, however, for the focused evaluation of portal venous flow, since it is the most cost-effective means of assessment. Distinction of mass lesions in the liver is less reliable with ultrasonography, however, often requiring further evaluation with MRI. Screening examinations, such as are needed in pre-liver transplant evaluations, are cost-effectively performed with ultrasonography to assess for portal venous flow, and further imaging with MRI and/or CT is obtained when either the α-fetoprotein level is elevated, suggesting HCC, and/or ultrasonography suggests an underlying mass lesion in the liver.

Additional associated signs of hepatocellular dysfunction, evident by MRI and other modalities, include splenomegaly, widening of the hepatic interlobar fissure, colonic interposition (Fig. 2.1), and ascites and small bowel edema, resulting from hypoproteinemia.

Overall, the diagnosis of cirrhosis by imaging requires recognition of changes in the size, configuration, and texture of the liver, combined with the secondary signs of portal hypertension and hepatocellular dysfunction mentioned above. Once the diagnosis of cirrhosis is suggested, the etiology of any focal lesions can be further assessed. MRI is most helpful in this regard, allowing the distinction of regenerative nodules and dysplastic nodules (hypointense on T2-weighted images) from HCC (hyperintense on T2-weighted images). In this setting, a solid hyperintense lesion on a T2-weighted image is most suggestive of HCC, since other focal hyperintense lesions, such as metastasis or hemangioma, are not usually seen in cirrhotic livers.

2.3
Iron Overload

Iron overload states may result in either hepatic parenchymal or reticuloendothelial deposition of iron. Hepatic parenchymal deposition of iron occurs with hereditary hemochromatosis, which is an autosomal recessive disorder of iron metabolism, with deposition also present in the pancreas, myocardium, endocrine glands, joints, and skin. Parenchymal deposition of iron can also be seen in patients with cirrhosis and intravascular hemolysis. Hepatic parenchymal deposition is usually distinguishable from chronic iron overload states, such as thalassemia, in which reticuloendothelial deposition of iron occurs. Although reticuloendothelial deposition of iron may also result in hepatic injury and cirrhosis, it is often less ominous than parenchymal deposition, which results in eventual cirrhosis, with an associated risk of the development of HCC.

The MRI findings of iron deposition are characteristic. The paramagnetic effects of iron cause the liver to have markedly decreased signal intensity on T2-weighted imaging (Fig. 2.3) (STARK et al. 1985). In the absence of administration of contrast, such as superparamagnetic iron oxide (SPIO) or ultrasmall superparamagnetic iron oxide (USPIO), this is virtually a pathognomonic finding for iron deposition.

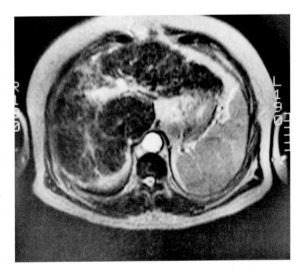

Fig. 2.3. Hemochromatosis. The liver is diffusely hypointense on T2-weighted imaging, secondary to the loss of signal intensity from local field inhomogeneities caused by the iron deposition. This abnormally darkened liver is mimicked only by intravenous iron oxide administration (SPIO or USPIO). There are also associated changes of cirrhosis resulting from the iron deposition

The distinction of parenchymal deposition and reticuloendothelial deposition is also possible by evaluation for signal changes in other involved organs. In hereditary hemochromatosis, similar decreased signal intensity on T2-weighted imaging is also evident in the myocardium, pancreas, and other endocrine glands (STARK et al. 1985; SIEGELMAN et al. 1991).

In addition, MRI permits assessment of portal venous flow and evaluation of secondary development of HCC. Foci of HCC will be seen as areas of bright signal intensity on T2-weighted sequences, contrasted with the low signal intensity background of the iron-laden liver.

2.4
Wilson's Disease

Wilson's disease is an autosomal recessive disorder of copper metabolism, in which copper is deposited along the hepatic sinusoids and in the periportal regions, as well as in the brain and cornea (WALSHE 1982). The hepatic deposition of copper causes an inflammatory reaction which can lead to cirrhosis. The inflammatory reaction is also accompanied by fatty change.

While the deposition of copper results in diffuse increased attenuation of the liver on CT, secondary to the high atomic number of the metal (DIXON and

WALSHE 1984), no corresponding signal intensity changes are seen with MRI, since copper is nonferromagnetic (Fig. 2.4). Thus, CT is the imaging modality of choice for assessment for copper deposition in the liver. Even with CT, however, the findings are nonspecific, since other entities such as iron deposition, gold or amiodarone toxicity, and prior administration of thorium dioxide (Thorotrast) can result in abnormal high attenuation of the liver. Thus, liver biopsy is the diagnostic tool of choice. MRI can be useful, however, for the evaluation of underlying changes of cirrhosis and secondary development of HCC.

2.5
Budd-Chiari Syndrome

Budd-Chiari syndrome is a clinical syndrome which manifests secondary to hepatic venous outflow obstruction (MITCHELL et al. 1982). The venous obstruction results in severe centrilobular congestion, which can lead to hepatocellular necrosis and atrophy. Acute and chronic forms have been described, reflecting the nature of the hepatic venous occlusion. The acute form can be seen as a sequela of hypercoagulable states, such as occur in pregnancy, polycythemia vera, myeloproliferative disorders, sickle cell disease, acute leukemia, and protein S deficiency and with the use of oral contraceptives

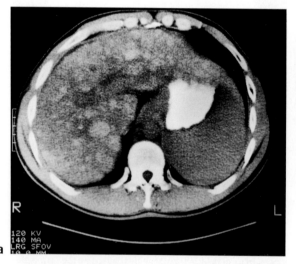
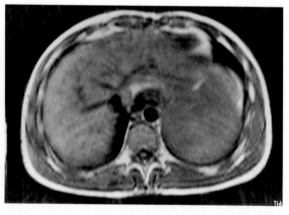

Fig. 2.4 a,b. Wilson's disease. **a** CT appearance. The liver has abnormal high attenuation diffusely. Changes of cirrhosis are also present secondary to hepatic parenchymal insult from the copper deposition. High-attenuation nodules are also present which are secondary to regenerative nodules. **b** MRI appearance of Wilson's disease. No appreciable changes in hepatic signal intensity are noted, since copper is nonferromagnetic

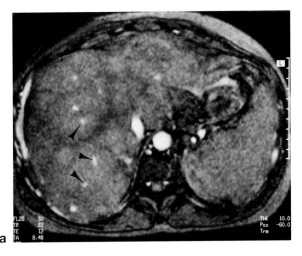

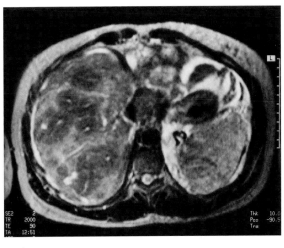

a   b

Fig. 2.5 a,b. Budd-Chiari syndrome: MRI appearance. a Gradient-echo imaging. Multiple intrahepatic collateral vessels are present (*arrowheads*), which form in an attempt to circumvent the hepatic venous obstruction. In this case there is obstruction of the hepatic veins. b T2-weighted imaging. The liver has a very heterogeneous appearance, secondary to the hepatic congestion. The intrahepatic varices are again evident

(MADDREY 1987). It is characterized by thrombosis of the main hepatic veins or of the intrahepatic or suprahepatic inferior vena cava. Thrombosis of the hepatic veins or inferior vena cava can also result from tumor involvement from HCC, renal cell carcinoma, or adrenal carcinoma. Intravascular webs or membranes, and right atrial or vena cava anomalies can cause significant hepatic outflow obstruction, as well, although these are more chronic than acute entities. The chronic form of Budd-Chiari syndrome results in fibrosis of the intrahepatic veins, which is presumably related to inflammation.

Hepatic veno-occlusive disease manifests similarly and is characterized by obliteration of the small sublobular and central hepatic veins (ROLLINS 1986). It can be caused by underlying inflammation of the hepatic veins, which can be caused by drugs or radiation or chemicals, as occurs in Jamaican bush tea disease. Additionally, severe right-sided heart failure can cause hepatic passive congestion, yielding the "nutmeg" appearance of the liver on CT, and may give rise to elevated levels in serum liver function tests.

The MRI appearance of Budd-Chiari syndrome is characteristic. Comma-shaped intrahepatic varices can be seen (Fig. 2.5a), which are formed in an attempt to collateralize the obstructed flow (STARK et al. 1986). Thrombosis, narrowing, or nonvisualization of the hepatic veins and inferior vena cava may also be evident (STARK et al. 1986). One study, which evaluated 22 patients with Budd-Chiari syn-

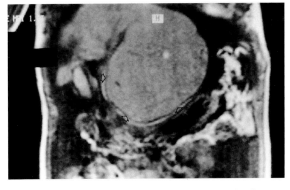

Fig. 2.6. Budd-Chiari syndrome. Coronal T1-weighted imaging shows massive enlargement of the caudate lobe (*open arrows*) of the liver in this child with Budd-Chiari syndrome. The caudate lobe hypertrophies secondary to its separate venous drainage

drome, found heterogeneous signal intensity of the liver on T1- and T2-weighted spin-echo imaging (cf. Fig. 2.5b) in 64% of patients, related to the hepatic congestion (SOYER et al. 1994). Of the three patients who received intravenous contrast material in this study, all had heterogeneous enhancement of the liver, similar to findings described in the CT literature. SOYER et al. also found caudate lobe enlargement in 82% of patients. This occurs as a compensatory measure, since the caudate lobe has a separate venous drainage (Fig. 2.6).

2.6
Schistosomiasis

Schistosoma japonicum and *Schistosoma mansoni* are two species of schistosomes which are known to cause significant hepatic disease. The schistosomes live in the bowel lumen and lay eggs in the mesenteric veins. Some of the eggs within the mesenteric vein will embolize to the portal vein, where they act as a nidus for inflammatory reaction, causing a granulomatous response, eventual fibrosis, and presinusoidal hypertension. The eggs do not survive, and may subsequently calcify.

The periportal and pericapsular calcifications associated with *S. japonicum* infection result in the formation of a characteristic septated appearance of the liver on CT and ultrasound examination, referred to as the "tortoiseshell" appearance (MONZAWA et al. 1993). These characteristic calcifications are not seen with MRI, since calcium appears as a signal void on MRI, and thus MRI plays less of a role for the diagnosis of *S. japonicum* infestation. One report evaluated the use of MRI for assessment of *S. japonicum* infection in 18 patients and found that the fibrous septa, which were often calcified on CT, had abnormally low signal intensity on T1-weighted imaging in nine patients and abnormally high signal intensity in 13 patients with T2-weighted imaging with gradient-moment nulling (MONZAWA et al. 1994).

The hallmark of infection with *S. mansoni* is periportal fibrosis, rather than the typical tortoiseshell calcifications which are seen with *S. japonicum* infection (FATAR et al. 1985). The periportal fibrosis from *S. mansoni* infection is appreciable with MRI, although reports in the literature describing the MRI findings are limited to one case report (WILLEMSEN et al. 1995). In this report the periportal zones were isointense to normal liver on T1-weighted imaging, but brightly enhanced following intravenous injection of gadolinium-DTPA. In addition, these abnormal periportal zones were hyperintense on T2-weighted imaging. This signal intensity change on T2-weighted imaging, a result of periportal edema, was thought to aid in the distinction of periportal inflammation from periportal fibrosis.

Longstanding infections with either *S. japonicum* or *S. mansoni* result in the formation of cirrhosis and subsequent development of hepatocellular carcinoma.

2.7
Sarcoidosis

Sarcoidosis is reported as the most common etiology of hepatic granulomas (KANEL and REYNOLDS 1992). Hepatic involvement with sarcoidosis primarily affects the periportal regions, rather than the hepatic parenchyma. Therefore, the most notable early sequela of hepatic sarcoidosis is the development of portal hypertension. Treatment at this stage of hepatic sarcoidosis is paramount, since steroid therapy can potentially reverse the portal hypertension. In fact, sarcoidosis-related portal hypertension is unique in that it is a potentially reversible disease if properly treated. Without effective treatment, however, periportal fibrosis ensues, leading to cirrhosis and irreversible portal hypertension.

The MRI findings of hepatic sarcoidosis are nonspecific, including hepatomegaly, splenomegaly, and eventually changes of cirrhosis (Fig. 2.7). Sarcoid granulomas in the liver are usually too small to be discerned by MRI and do not result in any appreciable change in the signal intensity of the hepatic parenchyma. One study by KESSLER et al. (1993) used MRI to evaluate ten patients with hepatic sarcoidosis and found the liver to be of normal signal intensity in eight of the patients. Two patients had diffusely abnormally decreased signal intensity in the liver, presumed to be secondary to iron deposi-

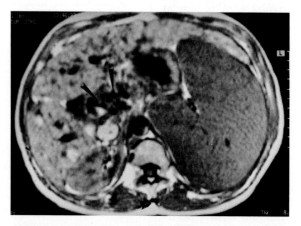

Fig. 2.7. Sarcoidosis. The imaging findings of sarcoidosis are nonspecific, including changes of cirrhosis (in longstanding or severe cases of sarcoidosis) and associated splenomegaly. The actual sarcoid nodules are too small to discern with MRI (or other imaging modalities). In this example, the spleen is massively enlarged and the liver has a cirrhotic appearance. There are extensive periportal collaterals, in addition, which form as a result of the portal hypertension (*arrowheads*)

tion. Periportal increased signal intensity was seen on T2-weighted imaging in seven of the ten patients. Other variable findings included a heterogeneous or nodular hepatic texture and irregularity of the portal and hepatic vein branches.

Thus, while imaging changes can be seen with hepatic sarcoidosis, the findings are variable and nonspecific, and MRI plays little role in the diagnosis of this entity. The diagnosis is instead made by needle biopsy.

2.8
Amyloidosis

Hepatic amyloidosis is characterized by the deposition of protein-mucopolysaccharide complexes along the hepatic sinusoids, within the space of Disse. The liver is the third most common solid abdominal organ to be involved with amyloidosis, with only renal and splenic deposition occurring more frequently (LEVINE 1962). The liver parenchyma may eventually become involved, leading to obscuration of the normal hepatic architecture. Primary and secondary forms of amyloidosis were initially described. The secondary form was distinguished from primary amyloidosis by the presence of a chronic underlying inflammatory disease. Recently, amyloidosis has been reclassified using a system based on the biochemical composition of the amyloid fibrils involved (ROS and SOBIN 1994). This has little radiologic significance, since the hepatic involvement is similar for the different amyloid fibrils. There is some variability, however, in the extent of involvement of the hepatic sinusoids among the different forms.

The MRI appearance of amyloidosis is not well characterized. The most common finding seen on any cross-sectional imaging examination is hepatomegaly, resulting from the massive amyloid deposition. Two reports in the literature which assessed the MRI appearance of amyloidosis showed no characteristic features to distinguish amyloidosis from other diffuse diseases (BENSON et al. 1987; RAFAL et al. 1990). In both reports the signal intensity of the liver was normal on T2-weighted imaging. BENSON et al. (1987) found that the signal intensity was increased on T1-weighted imaging, but unchanged on T2-weighted imaging in an investigation of nine patients with hepatic amyloidosis. This, of course, is nonspecific, since fatty change can cause similar imaging findings. Thus, as with many other inflammatory processes in the liver, MRI does not offer a

clear advantage over other imaging modalities for diagnostic purposes, and adds little to direct histologic evaluation.

2.9
Fatty Change

Fatty change results from increased production or mobilization of fatty acids, or from decreased hepatic clearance of fatty acids, such as occurs with hepatocellular injury. Etiologies include alcohol, obesity, diabetes mellitus, hepatitis, drugs, hyperalimentation, and liver transplantation. The hepatocellular insult may be an isolated acute event, or may be an ongoing process, with repeated episodes of injury leading to fibrosis and cirrhosis.

Fatty change can have a variable distribution, including focal, multifocal, diffuse, and mixed patterns of presentation. Diffuse involvement can be either uniform (Fig. 2.8) or patchy and nonuniform (BAKER et al. 1985; FLOURNOY et al. 1984). Resultant changes in MRI signal intensity are often not dramatic; however, when present, they may be best appreciated on fat suppression sequences. One study evaluated the use of phase-contrast MRI at 1.5 T as a correlate to histologic grading of fatty change and found that some correlation existed (LEVENSON et al. 1991), but this method is not commonly employed in the routine setting to assess fatty change.

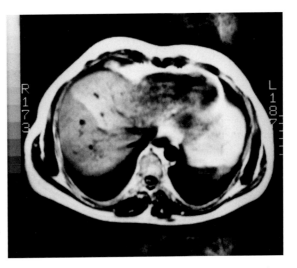

Fig. 2.8. Fatty change. T1-weighted imaging shows involvement of the medial segment of the left hepatic lobe with fatty change. The fatty infiltration results in abnormally high signal intensity of the liver. There is a sharp line of demarcation of fatty liver from the normal right hepatic lobe

2.10
Diffuse Hepatocellular Carcinoma

While hepatocellular carcinoma (HCC) may occur with or without cirrhosis, 80% of patients with HCC in the Western hemisphere have underlying cirrhosis (GORE 1994). HCC can present as a solitary mass, as nodular or multifocal involvement, or as diffuse disease. The diffuse form, also known as the cirrhotomimetic form, is characterized by small foci of malignant cells throughout the liver, giving the liver a nodular appearance mimicking that of cirrhosis. Vascular invasion is also common, with frequent involvement of the portal veins and, to a lesser degree, the hepatic veins.

The cirrhotomimetic form of HCC can give a lobular contour to the liver which mimics that of cirrhosis. The underlying neoplastic infiltration, however, will result in abnormally increased signal intensity on T2-weighted MRI.

Foci of HCC are distinguishable from regenerative nodules or dysplastic nodules, since HCC will have high signal intensity on T2-weighted sequences, while regenerative nodules and dysplastic nodules will be isointense to hypointense on T2-weighted images, as previously discussed. Differentiation of HCC from diffuse metastatic disease is aided by the identification of signs of underlying cirrhosis, since HCC is very common and metastases are distinctly uncommon in the cirrhotic liver.

2.11
Diffuse Metastatic Disease

While metastases are overall the most common malignancy in the noncirrhotic liver, they rarely occur in the cirrhotic liver (MELATO et al. 1989; LISA et al. 1942; GALL 1960; LIEBER 1957; RUEBNER et al. 1961; HAMAYA et al. 1965). Thus, while patients with diffuse metastatic disease to the liver may have an imaging pattern that can mimic that of cirrhosis, such as has been described with treated breast cancer metastases (YOUNG et al. 1994), they will rarely have cirrhosis.

Computed tomography has been the imaging standard for the detection of metastases, with a reported sensitivity of 38%–96% (REINIG et al. 1987; STARK et al. 1987; CHEZMAR et al. 1988; FERRUCCI et al. 1988; HEIKEN et al. 1989). Studies have shown MRI to be at least as sensitive as contrast-enhanced CT for the detection of metastatic involvement, with lesions typically appearing hyperintense on T2-

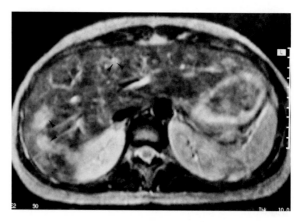

Fig. 2.9. Diffuse metastatic disease to the liver. T2-weighted imaging shows several foci of high signal intensity metastases (*arrowheads*) in this patient with diffuse small cell metastases to the liver. The underlying liver also has abnormally increased signal intensity throughout secondary to the diffuse involvement with metastases

weighted sequences (Fig. 2.9) (REINIG et al. 1987; STARK et al. 1987; CHEZMAR et al. 1988; FERRUCCI et al. 1988; HEIKEN et al. 1989). Diffuse involvement of the liver with metastases can be particularly difficult to identify, with subtle features including architectural and vascular distortion and diffuse parenchymal heterogeneity.

2.12
Lymphoma

Hepatic lymphoma can occur primarily or secondarily. Primary lymphoma of the liver is extremely rare and most often presents as a focal hepatic mass (RYAN et al. 1988). Secondary lymphomatous involvement is much more common, and can be seen with both Hodgkin's and non-Hodgkin's lymphoma. Patterns of involvement include the presence of a focal mass, a diffuse infiltrating form, and a mixed pattern of focal mass with parenchymal infiltration. Between 30% and 40% of patients with lymphomatous involvement of the liver will show either a diffuse infiltrating form or a mixed pattern of focal mass with parenchymal infiltration (WEISSLEDER et al. 1988).

Diffuse lymphomatous involvement of the liver can be difficult to identify with MRI or CT. MRI findings include foci of increased signal intensity on T2-weighted sequences, with relatively decreased signal intensity on T1-weighted sequences. An overall slight increase in signal intensity on T2-weighted sequences may be present with diffuse infiltrating lymphoma (WEISSLEDER et al. 1988; Ros et al. 1993). Significant architectural distortion is generally not present, however. A report by WEISSLEDER et al. (1988) described no overall signal intensity changes in the three patients in their study with diffuse involvement. In the same study, a mixed pattern of involvement was present in two patients, and was evident on MRI as hypointense foci on T1-weighted imaging and hyperintense foci on T2-weighted imaging, with underlying geographic zones of intermediate signal intensity.

2.13
Summary

Magnetic resonance imaging is useful in the evaluation of the cirrhotic liver, and may allow identification of the underlying cause of cirrhosis by demonstration of characteristic signal intensity changes in the liver. Hemochromatosis is an example in which the etiology of cirrhosis can be determined by the recognition of characteristic signal intensity changes, with abnormally decreased signal intensity noted on T2-weighted sequences, secondary to the paramagnetic effect of the deposited iron.

Many diffuse hepatic processes will cause significant signal intensity changes within the liver, predominantly because of resultant changes in T1 and T2 relaxation times. These changes are best appreciated on spin-echo sequences. Cirrhotic livers are particularly amenable to MR evaluation, since differences exist between T2 relaxation times of hepatocellular carcinoma and regenerating nodules and adenomatous hyperplasia, often allowing their distinction. In addition, MRA evaluation of the portal vein provides a noninvasive means of assessment of patency and flow.

Unfortunately, not all diffuse disease results in significant signal intensity changes. Entities in which little or no significant signal intensity change is present include Wilson's disease, amyloidosis, and sarcoidosis. For these processes, hepatic biopsy unquestionably remains the diagnostic procedure of choice. MRI can still be of benefit in the evaluation of hepatic disease in these cases, however, by providing identification of the findings of cirrhosis, and its sequelae.

References

Baker MK, Wenker JC, Cockerill EM, et al. (1985) Focal fatty infiltration of the liver: diagnostic imaging. Radiographics 5:923–939

Benson L, Hemmingsson A, Ericsson A, et al. (1987) Magnetic resonance imaging in primary amyloidosis. Acta Radiol 28:13–15

Brenner DA, Alcorn JM (1992) Pathogenesis of hepatic fibrosis. In: Kaplowitz N (ed) Liver and biliary disease. Williams and Wilkins, Baltimore, pp 118–129

Chezmar JL, Rumancik WM, Megibow AJ, Hulnick DH, Nelson RC, Bernardino ME (1988) Liver and abdominal screening in patients with cancer: CT versus MR imaging. Radiology 168:43–47

Dixon AK, Walshe JM (1984) Computed tomography of the liver in Wilson's disease. J Comput Assist Tomogr 8:46–48

Fatar S, Bassiony H, Satyanath S (1985) CT of hepatic schistosomiasis mansoni. AJR 145:63–66

Ferrucci JT, Freeny PC, Stark DD, et al. (1988) Advances in hepatobiliary radiology. Radiology 168:319–338

Flournoy JG, Pather JL, Sullivan BM, et al. (1984) CT appearance of multifocal hepatic steatosis. J Comput Assist Tomogr 8:1192–1194

Gall E (1960) Primary and metastatic carcinoma of the liver: relationship to hepatic cirrhosis. Arch Pathol 70:753–759

Gore RM (1994) Diffuse liver disease. In: Gore RM, Levine RA, Laufer I (eds) Textbook of gastrointestinal radiology. Saunders, Philadelphia, pp 1968–2017

Hamaya K, Hashimoto H, Maeda Y (1975) Metastatic carcinoma in cirrhotic liver: statistical survey of autopsies in Japan. Acta Pathol Jpn 25:153–159

Harbin WP, Robert NJ, Ferrucci JT (1980) Diagnosis of cirrhosis based on regional changes in hepatic morphology: radiological and pathologic analysis. Radiology 135:273

Heiken JP, Weyman PJ, Lee JK, et al. (1989) Detection of focal hepatic masses: prospective evaluation with CT, delayed CT, CT during portography, and MR imaging. Radiology 171:47–51

Kanel GC, Reynolds TB (1992) Hepatic granulomas. In: Kaplowitz N (ed) Liver and biliary diseases. Williams and Wilkins, Baltimore, pp 406–414

Kessler A, Mitchell DG, Israel HL, Goldberg BB (1993) Hepatic and splenic sarcoidosis: ultrasound and MR imaging. Abdom Imaging 18:159–163

Kraus BB, Sabatelli FN, Abbitt PL, et al. (1993) Comparison of MR imaging, CT, and US in the evaluation of candidates for transjugular intrahepatic portosystemic shunts. Radiology 189(P):253

Levenson H, Greensite F, Hoefs J, et al. (1991) Fatty infiltration of the liver: quantification with phase-contrast MR imaging at 1.5 T vs biopsy. AJR 156:307–312

Levine RA (1962) Amyloid disease of the liver. Am J Med 33:349–357

Lieber M (1957) Rare occurrence of metastatic carcinoma in the cirrhotic liver. Am J Med Sci 233:145–152

Lisa J, Solomon C, Gordon E (1942) Secondary carcinoma in cirrhosis of the liver. Am J Pathol 18:137–140

Maddrey WC (1987) Hepatic vein thrombosis (Budd-Chiari syndrome): possible association with the use of oral contraceptives. Semin Liver Dis 7:32–39

Melato M, Laurino L, Mucli E, Valente M, Okuda K (1989) Relationship between cirrhosis, liver cancer and hepatic metastases; an autopsy study. Cancer 64:455–459

Mitchell MC, Boitnott JK, Kaufman S, et al. (1982) Budd-Chiari syndrome: etiology, diagnosis and management. Medicine 61:199–218

Monzawa S, Vohiyama G, Ohtomo K, Araki T (1993) Schistosomiasis japonicum of the liver: contrast-enhanced CT findings in 113 patients. AJR 161:323–327

Monzawa S, Ohtomo K, Oba H, Nogata Y, Kachi K, Uchiyama G (1994) Septa in the liver of patients with chronic hepatic schistosomiasis japonica: MR appearance. AJR 162:1347–1351

Rafal RB, Jennis R, Kosovsky PA, Marlisz JA (1990) MRI of primary amyloidosis. Gastrointest Radiol 15:199–200

Reinig JW, Dwyer AJ, Miller DL, et al. (1987) Liver metastasis detection: comparative sensitivity of MR imaging and CT scanning. Radiology 162:43–47

Rollins BF (1986) Hepatic veno-occlusive disease. Am J Med 81:297–306

Ros PR, Sobin LH (1994) Amyloidosis: the same cat, with different stripes. Radiology 190:14–15

Ros PR, Ros LH, Stoupis C (1993) Liver: diffuse disease. In: Ros PR, Bidgood WD (eds) Abdominal magnetic resonance imaging. Mosby, St Louis, pp 237–245

Ruebner B, Green R, Miyai K, Caranasos G, Abbey H (1961) The rarity of intrahepatic metastasis in cirrhosis of the liver. Am J Pathol 39:739–746

Ryan J, Straus DJ, Lange C, et al. (1988) Primary lymphoma of the liver. Cancer 61:370–375

Siegelman ES, Mitchell ME, Rubin R, et al. (1991) Parenchymal versus reticuloendothelial iron overload in the liver: distinction with MR imaging. Radiology 179:361–366

Soyer P, Rabenandrasana A, Barge J, et al. (1994) MRI of Budd-Chiari syndrome. Abdom Imaging 19:325–329

Stark DD, Mosely ME, Bacon BR, et al. (1985) Magnetic resonance imaging of hepatic iron overload. Radiology 154:137–142

Stark DD, Hahn PF, Trey C, Clouse ME, Ferrucci JT (1986) MRI of the Budd-Chiari syndrome. AJR 146:1141–1148

Stark DD, Wittenberg J, Butch RJ, Ferrucci JT (1987) Hepatic metastases: controlled comparison of detection with MR imaging and CT. Radiology 165:399–406

Walshe JM (1982) The liver in Wilson's disease (hepatolenticular degeneration). In: Schiff L, Schiff ER (eds) Diseases of the liver. Lippincott, Philadelphia, pp 1037–1050

Weissleder R, Stark DD, Elizondo G, et al. (1988) MRI of hepatic lymphoma. Magn Reson Imaging 6:675–681

Willemsen UF, Pfluger T, Zoller WG, Kueffer G, Hahn K (1995) MRI of hepatic schistosomiasis mansoni. J Comput Assist Tomogr 19:811–813

Young ST, Paulson EK, Washington K, Gulliver DJ, Vredenburgh JJ, Baker ME (1994) CT of the liver in patients with metastatic breast carcinoma treated by chemotherapy: findings simulating cirrhosis. AJR 163:1385–1388

3 Benign Focal Liver Lesions

E.J. Rummeny

CONTENTS

3.1
Introduction

The true prevalence of benign liver tumors is not known. However, autopsy studies indicate that benign liver lesions may occur in more than 50% of adults (KARHUNEN 1986). Against this background, tissue characterization of liver tumors is playing an increasingly important role in diagnostic radiology. Because of its inherent high soft tissue contrast and technical and pharmacologic developments including tissue-specific contrast media, magnetic resonance imaging (MRI) has become an appropriate tool for the diagnosis of focal liver lesions. In this chapter common benign liver tumors, i.e., hemangioma, hepatic adenoma, focal nodular hyperplasia, and cysts, will be discussed.

3.2
Hepatic Hemangiomas

Cavernous hemangioma represents the most common benign neoplasm of the liver. Its incidence in the adult population has been reported to range between 7% and 20%, the highest incidence being reported in an autopsy series by KARHUNEN (1986). The average size of these lesions was 5–10 mm and

E.J. RUMMENY, MD, Institut für Klinische Radiologie, Albert-Schweitzer Straße 33, D-48129 Muenster, Germany

multiple hemangiomas were found in half of the population. Hemangiomas are reported to be more common in women than in men, and are more frequently found in the right lobe of the liver.

The vast majority of hepatic hemangiomas are asymptomatic, and these neoplasms are usually discovered incidentally. Symptoms, when present, are most commonly due to tumor enlargement, and have been noted primarily in patients with lesions exceeding 4 cm in diameter.

Radiologically cavernous hemangiomas represent a particular problem in differential diagnosis from tumor because of their frequent incidental discovery and their potential coexistence with malignant liver lesions in the same patient. About 20% of hemangiomas lack the typical sonographic dense, hyperechoic, through-transmitting appearance (BREE et al. 1983, 1987; WIENER and PARULEKAR 1979). Even bolus-enhanced dynamic CT gives atypical results in many cases if strict criteria are applied (FREENY and MARKS 1986).

Magnetic resonance imaging seems to be the most sensitive modality for detecting hepatic cavernous hemangiomas. Confident MRI diagnosis is based on careful analysis of both the morphologic and the signal intensity characteristics. Because hemangiomas are essentially vascular lakes of slow-flowing, unclotted, oxygenated blood, they demonstrate signal characteristics similar to those of fluid and have T1 and T2 relaxation times which are considerably longer than those of normal liver tissue or solid hepatic tumors. Therefore hemangiomas appear hypointense on T1-weighted images and markedly hyperintense on T2-weighted images (Figs. 3.1, 3.2). If heavily T2-weighted pulse sequences with a repetition time (TR) of ≥2000 ms and an echo time (TE) of ≥100 ms are used, their signal intensity is comparable to that of cerebrospinal fluid, which can serve as an internal standard. Hemangiomas tend to retain their marked signal intensity on heavily T2-weighted multiecho images, accounting for the so-called light bulb sign (WITTENBERG et al. 1988). The high signal intensity of hemangiomas is also

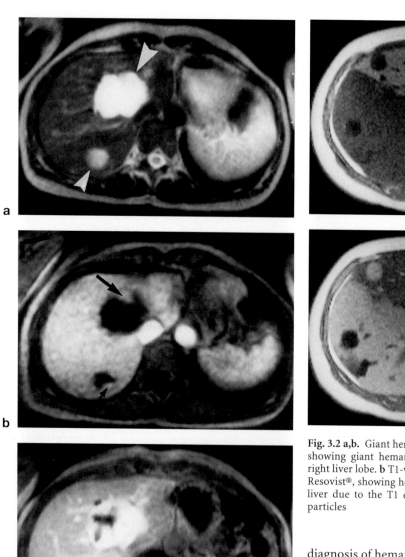

Fig. 3.2 a,b. Giant hemangioma. **a** T1-weighted FLASH image showing giant hemangioma and small hemangioma of the right liver lobe. **b** T1-weighted FLASH image after injection of Resovist®, showing hemangiomas hyperintense in relation to liver due to the T1 effect of superparamagnetic iron oxide particles

Fig. 3.1 a–c. Cavernous hemangioma. **a** Typical (*large arrowhead*) and atypical appearance (*small arrowhead*) on heavily T2-weighted (SE 2500/120) image. **b** T1-weighted turbo-FLASH image (TI, 400 ms; TR, 7 ms; TE, 4 ms; flip angle, 8°) obtained immediately after the initiation of the bolus injection of Gd-DTPA (0.1 mmol/kg). Note the peripheral nodular enhancement (*arrows*). **c** Delayed T1-weighted FLASH image obtained after Gd-DTPA administration, showing complete fill-in of the small hemangioma (*arrow*)

evident on images obtained with other heavily T2-weighted pulse sequences such as fast spin echo (FSE) or ultrafast echoplanar imaging techniques. Several studies indicate that FSE is as reliable in the diagnosis of hemangiomas as conventional SE imaging techniques (GAA et al. 1996; GIOVAGNONI et al. 1996). In general, cavernous hemangiomas exhibit nearly homogeneous signal intensity and sharp margins. Occasionally, however, due to thrombosis, especially in larger hemangiomas (>5 cm), inhomogeneous central areas of lower signal intensity may be present. These low signal intensity clefts and septations have been found to correspond to hypodense regions on dynamic bolus-enhanced computed tomography (CT) scans (CHOI et al. 1989). However, since thrombotic areas and scars may still contain some fluid, scars in hemangiomas may appear bright and isointense to the surrounding hemangioma on heavily T2-weighted scans (RUMMENY et al. 1989a).

Various investigators have utilized additional quantitative criteria in combination with qualitative data in order to characterize hepatic tumors more accurately. Using lesion/liver signal intensity quotients on heavily T2-weighted scans, hemangiomas can be differentiated from malignant lesions in more than 90% of cases (EGGLIN et al. 1990; ITOH et al. 1990; MCFARLAND et al. 1994). However, the light bulb sign and long T2 values are not 100% specific for hemangiomas, as some metastases from hypervascular tumors, such as islet cell tumors, carcinoid, pheochromocytoma, sarcoma, and necrotic or cystic metastases, can exhibit similar morphologic patterns and high T2 signal intensity (WITTENBERG et al. 1988; LOMBARDO et al. 1990; MCNICHOLAS et al. 1996). In an effort to improve diagnostic specificity, MRI contrast agents can be used, at least in difficult cases, to help differentiate hemangiomas from malignant hepatic neoplasms. Fast MRI pulse sequences such as breath-hold T1-weighted gradient echo (GE) or fast GE performed during intravenous bolus injection of gadolinium chelates (Gd-DTPA, Gd-BMA-DTPA, Gd-DOTA), hepatobiliary agents (Gd-BOPTA, Gd-EOB-DTPA), or rapidly injectable superparamagnetic agents, such as Resovist®, can be used to study perfusion patterns of focal liver lesions (HAMM et al. 1990; SEMELKA et al. 1994; REIMER et al. 1997). All these agents have been shown to yield peripheral nodular enhancement on early scans and more or less complete fill-in on delayed scans (HAMM et al. 1990; RUMMENY et al. 1991a). These enhancement patterns are similar to those obtained with dynamic CT.

Although measurements of signal intensities and the use of MR contrast agents have helped to improve the diagnostic specificity of MRI, its overall accuracy in the diagnosis of cavernous hemangiomas is still only about 90%. While the differentiation of hypervascular metastases can be improved by proper use of contrast-enhanced MRI, problem cases remain, particularly when lesions are smaller than 1 cm. These are difficult to diagnose because of volume-averaging effects. Additionally, large hemangiomas with regions of fibrosis may be indistinguishable from metastases in some cases.

3.3
Hepatocellular Adenoma

Hepatocellular adenoma is a rare solid primary liver tumor that is classified as a benign but premalignant neoplasm (CRAIG et al. 1989; ISHAK and RABIN 1975). It is usually discovered accidentally during abdominal imaging studies although patients may present with right upper quadrant discomfort from mass effect or pain following spontaneous intra-abdominal hemorrhage of the tumor. The majority of hepatocellular adenomas are related to the use of oral contraceptives in women and anabolic steroids in men (NIME et al. 1979; KLATSKIN 1977; BAUM et al. 1973): it is estimated that the incidence of hepatocellular adenomas is 4/100 000 users (ROOKS et al. 1979). The premalignant nature of hepatocellular adenoma and its propensity to spontaneous hemorrhage warrant surgical treatment (AMERIKS et al. 1975).

Pathologically most hepatocellular adenomas are large (usually >10 cm) solitary lesions with a smooth thin tumor capsule. These tumors are rich in fat and devoid of portal tracts. Intratumoral hemorrhage can produce areas of infarction and fibrosis.

At MRI, hepatocellular adenomas may mimic malignant liver tumors, with a hypointense appearance on T1-weighted images and slight hyperintensity on T2-weighted images. However, the high fat and/or glycogen content of these tumors can render them isointense or even hyperintense on T1-weighted images (Fig. 3.3) (RUMMENY et al. 1989b; PAULSON et al. 1994; GABATA et al. 1990). When present, a hypointense tumor capsule is best seen on T1-weighted images (the appearance is similar to that of a capsule in well-defined hepatocellular carcinoma). MRI can also demonstrate areas of intratumoral bleeding as hyperintense regions on T1-weighted images and hypointense regions on T2-weighted images. These features reflect the presence of blood degradation products such as methemoglobin, ferritin, and hemosiderin. Areas of fibrosis and intratumoral necrosis may appear hypointense on T1-weighted images, with the latter being hyperintense on T2-weighted images (RUMMENY et al. 1989b). The use of MR contrast agents may provide further diagnostic specificity which may permit differentiation of hepatocellular adenoma from other malignant or benign primary liver tumors. For example, as with dynamic CT, an early arterial blush can be observed during dynamic gadolinium chelate-enhanced MRI using fast scanning techniques (RUMMENY et al. 1991a; MATHIEU et al. 1986; BEERS et al. 1990). With the use of hepatobiliary contrast agents such as Mn-DPDP or Gd-EOB-DTPA, enhancement of these tumors has been noted (Fig. 3.3) (HAMM et al. 1992). However, other benign (focal nodular hyperplasia) and malignant (hepatocellular carcinoma) primary liver tumors may also show enhancement with these hepatobiliary MR contrast agents (HAMM et al. 1992; ROFSKY et al. 1993).

As shown in recent studies, superparamagnetic iron oxide-based contrast agents may be used to

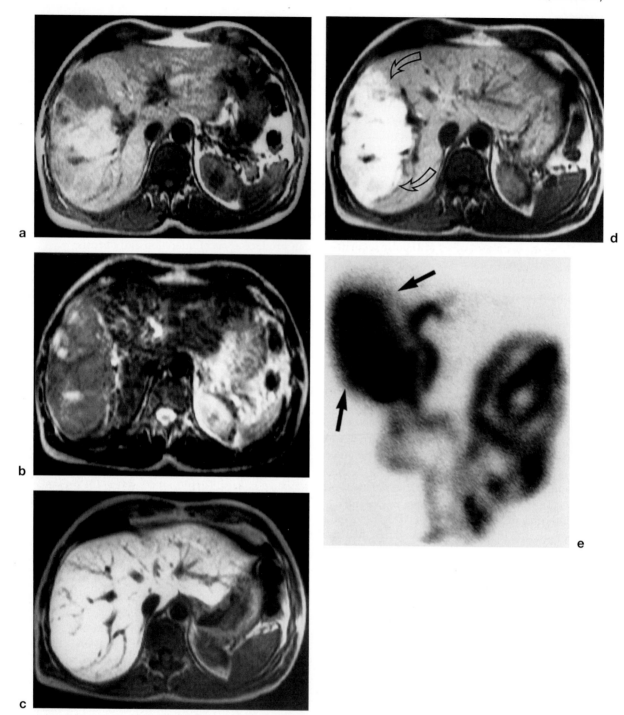

Fig. 3.3 a–e. Hepatocellular adenoma. **a** T1-weighted scan (GE 150/6/60°); the tumor is isointense to slightly hyperintense, except for the anterior necrotic portion, which is hypointense. **b** On this T2-weighted image (SE 2500/90) the tumor is slightly hyperintense relative to normal liver, with some necrotic areas appearing markedly hyperintense. **c** T1-weighted GE image after i.v. injection of Mn-DPDP (20 min p.i.). Liver and tumor are significantly enhanced. **d** On this delayed T1-weighted scan (16 h p.i.), normal liver tissue has returned to normal signal intensity but enhancement of tumor persists (*open arrows*), similar to **e**, a delayed scintigraphic image (*arrows*). (**a–d** from RUMMENY et al. 1993; **e** courtery of Dr. Sciuk)

differentiate hepatic adenomas from malignant hepatocellular carcinomas. As demonstrated by Vogl et al. (1996), hepatic adenomas take up superparamagnetic particles, such as Endorem, leading to a significant reduction in signal intensity on T2-weighted images. This effect may be even stronger in focal nodular hyperplasia and significantly less pronounced in hepatic adenoma, similar to that in hepatocellular carcinoma. However, some overlap is reported in the literature.

When a liver mass is present in a patient at risk for hepatocellular adenoma, multiple imaging tests including radionuclide scintigraphy or angiography may be necessary to make the diagnosis of hepatocellular adenoma. The most specific diagnosis may be achieved with the combination of unenhanced and dynamic bolus CT or MR studies in combination with hepatobiliary enhanced MRI or nuclear scintigraphy. Despite the risk of hemorrhage, hepatocellular adenomas have been biopsied safely and classified on the basis of cytology and histology; nevertheless, the diagnostic utility of percutaneous needle biopsy remains unclear.

3.4
Focal Nodular Hyperplasia

Focal nodular hyperplasia (FNH) is the most common solid benign liver tumor (Craig et al. 1989; Ishak and Rabin 1975). It is usually found incidentally on abdominal imaging studies, although up to one-third of these tumors are discovered because of clinical symptoms. Its etiology is unknown, but there may be a hormonal influence because FNH is more common in women in their 3rd to 5th decades.

Pathologically FNH is a well-circumscribed, usually solitary mass characterized by central scar tissue with surrounding nodules of hyperplastic hepatocytes which are divided into lobules by thin septa that radiate from the central scar (Craig et al. 1989; Casarella et al. 1978; Knowles and Wolff 1976; Kerlin et al. 1983). No normal portal venous structures are present, although bile ducts and arterial vessels course through the tumor and are prominent in the fibrous scar and along the septa that extend from the center to the periphery. The size of FNH varies from less than 1 cm to more than 15 cm, but in most patients these lesions are smaller than 5 cm in diameter. The margin of the lesion is sharp and generally no capsule is present. Hemorrhage, necrosis, and calcification are rare.

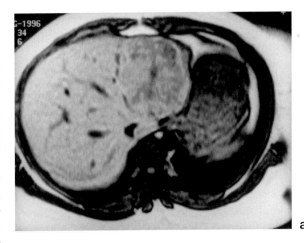

a

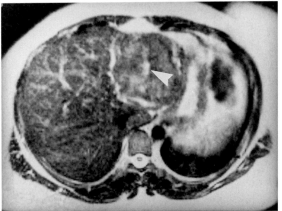

b

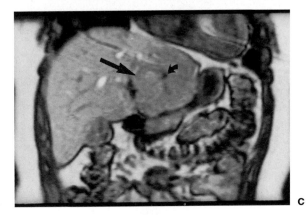

c

Fig. 3.4 a–c. Focal nodular hyperplasia. a Tumor in the left lobe of the liver is slightly hypointense on this T1-weighted GE scan; note the hypointense central scar. b The tumor is only slighly hyperintense on the T2-weighted image (TSE 4600/165); note the characteristic hyperintense appearance of the tumor scar (*arrowhead*). c Coronal T1-weighted FLASH image of the same tumor

Radiographic differentiation of FNH from other primary or secondary hepatic lesions may be difficult (Titelbaum et al. 1988; Wilbur and Gyi 1987; Hamrick-Turner et al. 1994). However, the presence of hepatocellular activity and a central scar with vessels and bile ducts are diagnostic features of FNH.

With MRI the diagnosis of FNH can be suggested if a liver tumor appears isointense on T1- and T2-weighted images and has a central scar (BUTCH et al. 1986; MATTISON et al. 1987). Indeed, in some cases tumors are only detected by their mass effect on normal hepatic vasculature and the presence of the central scar, which is hypointense on T1-weighted and hyperintense on T2-weighted images (BUTCH et al. 1986) (Fig. 3.4). These signal intensity features of tumor and scars reflect the histologic tumor components. Because FNH consists mostly of hyperplastic hepatocytes, it is not surprising that the tumor appears isointense to normal liver. The signal intensity of the scar is based on the multiple vascular channels and bile ductules (RUMMENY et al. 1989a). Unfortunately these signal intensity features of FNH are detectable in only 10%–25% of cases (LEE et al. 1991).

In most cases isointensity is noted on only one of the two (T1- or T2-weighted) pulse sequences. In some cases FNH may mimic other solid liver tumors by being hypointense on T1-weighted images and hyperintense on T2-weighted images. Even hepatic scars are not specific to FNH and have been observed in a variety of benign and malignant liver tumors (RUMMENY et al. 1989a).

For the aforementioned reasons, differentiation of FNH from other malignant or benign solid liver tumors is frequently not possible with plain MRI. Contrast-enhanced MRI, however, has the potential to provide further diagnostic information. Extracellular paramagnetic gadolinium chelates can be used to display the perfusion profile of liver tumors (RUMMENY et al. 1991a). As with contrast-enhanced CT, dynamic T1-weighted MRI of FNH shows dense enhancement in the arterial phase (first 30 s) after bolus injection of Gd-DTPA, followed by rapid washout of the contrast agent leading to isointensity

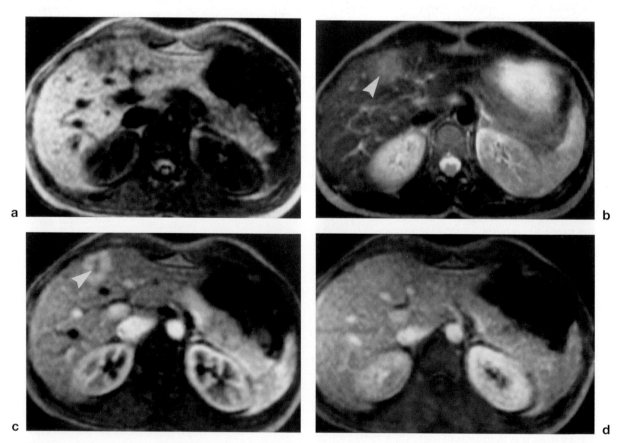

a

b

c

d

Fig. 3.5 a–d. Focal nodular hyperplasia. **a** Unenhanced T1-weighted scan showing the lesion hypointense in relation to surrounding liver and **b** T2-weighted scan showing the tumor as slightly hyperintense (*arrowhead*). **c** Early Gd-DTPA-enhanced T1-weighted image showing tumor blush except for the central scar (*arrowhead*). **d** Delayed Gd-DTPA-enhanced image showing uptake of contrast agent in tumor, scar, and liver to a similar degree, resulting in reduced tumor–liver contrast

of the FNH to normal liver by 60s postinjection (RUMMENY et al. 1991a; LEE et al. 1991) (Fig. 3.5). However, similar lesion enhancement may be seen with hepatocellular carcinoma except that, if present, a capsule associated with the latter will enhance

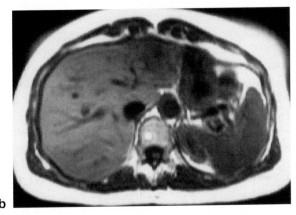

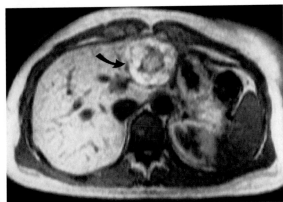

Fig. 3.6 a–c. Focal nodular hyperplasia. **a** T1-weighted GE scan (GE 150/6/60°) before the injection of a hepatobiliary contrast agent; tumor appears slightly hypointense relative to liver. **b** T1-weighted SE scan (SE 500/15) before the injection of Mn-DPDP; tumor appears nearly isointense to liver. **c** Delayed Mn-DPDP-enhanced image (16h p.i.). Note residual enhancement within the tumor

on delayed (5–10min postinjection) images (MATHIEU et al. 1991).

With paramagnetic contrast agents (Mn-DPDP, Gd-EOB-DTPA) which undergo hepatobiliary excretion, FNH enhances after contrast administration and may even appear hyperintense to liver on delayed images (Fig. 3.6). While no secondary liver tumors are known to enhance, several other primary liver tumors such as well-differentiated hepatocellular carcinoma, regenerative nodular hyperplasia, and hepatocellular adenoma also enhance (ROFSKY et al. 1993; RUMMENY et al. 1991b; MURAKAMI et al. 1996). Recently several groups have shown that superparamagnetic iron oxide (SPIO)-enhanced MRI can be helpful in the diagnosis of FNH. Because of RES cells within the tumor, FNH shows uptake of SPIO that parallels uptake of technetium-99m sulfur colloid in nuclear medicine (GRANDIN et al. 1995). Therefore the tumor signal intensity on SPIO-enhanced T2-weighted images is significantly lower than on nonenhanced images (VOGL et al. 1996; GRANDIN et al. 1995). This uptake may increase sensitivity and specificity for the diagnosis of FNH to at least 80% (HAMMERSTINGL et al. 1997).

3.5 Macroregenerative Nodules and Nodular Regenerative Hyperplasia

Macroregenerative nodules occur in approximately 10%–14% of patients with chronic liver disease such as advanced cirrhosis (FURUYA et al. 1988). Macroregenerative nodules may also arise in a setting of severe hepatic injury with extensive hepatic necrosis (STROMEYER and ISHAK 1981). Nodular regenerative hyperplasia (NRH) is a much rarer condition and arises without any hepatic injury or fibrosis; it is associated with a variety of systemic diseases such as rheumatoid arthritis or polyarteritis nodosa, in which vasculitis is an associated event. No specific clinical symptomatology is attributable to these lesions and their discovery usually occurs upon radiologic examination for suspected liver carcinoma.

The pathogenesis of NRH is not known but may be related to occlusion of intrahepatic branches of the portal vein (CRAIG et al. 1989). These nodules vary in size from a few millimeters to 1cm and are usually diffusely scattered throughout the liver.

Radiologic identification of NRH at cross-sectional imaging is often difficult due to the small size of the lesions and the altered gross hepatic morphology that accompanies cirrhosis and macro-regenerative nodules (RABINOWITZ et al. 1974). On MR images, macroregenerative nodules may appear as low signal intensity nodules on T2-weighted images. Pathologic examination suggests that iron deposition and related T2 shortening may be responsible for this imaging appearance (ITAI et al. 1987; MATSUI et al. 1989).

3.6
Hepatic Cysts

Hepatic cysts may be classified as developmental, infectious (e.g., parasitic), or traumatic. In this section only developmental cysts will be reviewed. Hepatic cysts are usually unilocular and can be solitary or multiple. The cyst wall is 1 mm or less in thickness and usually lined by a simple layer of cuboidal epithelium or, less commonly, squamous or columnar epithelium. The adjacent liver tissue is normal, without fibrosis or inflammation (CRAIG et al. 1989). Hepatic cysts are reported to be present in between 5% and 14% of the population, with a higher prevalence in women (CRAIG et al. 1989). Cysts usually occur without any clinical symptoms and are seen as incidental masses at hepatic imaging or surgery. Rarely they can be symptomatic due to infection or bleeding, or produce pain due to a mass effect which may necessitate surgical therapy.

Radiologic differentiation of simple hepatic cysts from other primary or secondary liver tumors is not difficult. When a hepatic cyst is suspected, an ultrasound examination must first be performed. On ultrasonography, hepatic cysts are anechoic (GAINES and SAMPSON 1989). Since they do not attenuate the ultrasound beam, the posterior wall is well seen and there is enhanced through-transmission.

On MR images, hepatic cysts have long T1 and T2 relaxation times. Hence in comparison to normal liver, they appear hypointense on T1-weighted and markedly hyperintense on heavily T2-weighted images and are sharply marginated (WITTENBERG et al. 1988). As with CT, the diagnosis of hepatic cyst by MRI may be complicated by volume averaging, and there may be reduced image quality on T2-weighted images. However, when optimal image quality is achieved, even cysts smaller than 1 cm can be diagnosed. On T2-weighted images their signal intensity is similar to that of cavernous hemangiomas and comparable to that of normal bile and CSF. Hence accurate differentiation between hepatic cysts and cavernous hemangioma may not be possible by MRI

(REINIG 1991). However, this distinction is clinically unimportant and additional information, if needed, can be obtained by ultrasonography.

3.7
Mesenchymal Tumors and Heterotopic Rests

A variety of benign liver tumors can arise from mesenchymal cells in the liver and heterotopic tissue that remains in the liver from a failure in development. Of these, hemangioma is the most common, and its radiologic pattern has been described earlier in this chapter. The prevalence of all remaining benign liver tumors is very low and generally there are no unique radiographic features that permit a tissue-specific diagnosis. The only exception in this respect is tumors that contain fat, including lipoma, angiomyolipoma, and myelolipoma. The nomenclature of these tumors describes the variable degree of fat, myeloid, and vascular cellular components. These tumors have no malignant potential and may occur spontaneously or in a setting of systemic diseases such as tuberous sclerosis.

Combined use of ultrasonography and CT may be sufficient to diagnose hepatic lipomas and to exclude other lipomatous tumors of the liver such as angiomyolipoma and myelolipoma, metastatic dermoid tumors of the ovary (which almost always show calcification), and fatty degenerated hepatocellular carcinoma. Focal fatty infiltration can usually be distinguished from liver lipomas since in most cases it is poorly defined, not well circumscribed, and shows blood vessels traversing through the lesion. At MRI fat-containing tumors also show a characteristic appearance of high signal intensity on T1- and T2-weighted images which is comparable to the signal intensity of subcutaneous or retroperitoneal fat on T1- and T2-weighted images (DOOMS et al. 1985). Chemical shift pulse sequences may allow distinction of purely fatty tumors (lipomas) from tumors with mixed cellularity such as angiomyolipomas, myelolipoma, or focal fatty infiltration.

3.8
Conclusions

The diagnostic evaluation of a liver mass suspected to be a benign tumor will vary depending on the clinical scenario, the availability of equipment, and the imaging experience of the radiologist. The imaging approach must also take into account the pretest probability of whether a patient has a primary tumor.

If MRI is used for differentiation of hepatic lesions, appropriate pulse sequence design and use of one of the various available MR contrast agents are recommended. For the diagnosis of hepatic hemangioma, heavily T2-weighted pulse sequences (TR ≥ 2000, TE ≥ 100) have to be used. The typical light bulb sign and a high signal intensity are specific for hemangiomas and allow correct diagnosis in more than 90% of cases. However, small hemangiomas (≤1 cm) or very large lesions (≥5 cm) may be difficult to diagnose, and need further diagnostic workup using dynamic imaging with gadolinium-based perfusion contrast media or rapidly injectable superparamagnetic iron oxide-based agents. MR images have to be carefully analyzed in patients with known primary hypervascular endocrine neoplasms, since liver metastases from these tumors may also exhibit high signal intensity on T2-weighted images and thus may mimic hemangioma. In these cases additional imaging studies, such as contrast-enhanced MRI, CT, and red blood pool scintigraphy, or even percutaneous needle biopsy, may be performed.

When a liver tumor is present in a patient at risk for hepatocellular adenoma, usually multiple imaging tests are necessary before a specific diagnosis of hepatocellular adenoma can be made (RUMMENY et al. 1993). The most specific diagnosis may be achieved with dynamic contrast-enhanced MRI using gadolinium chelates or MRI using more tissue-specific contrast agents such as hepatobiliary agents (e.g., Mn-DPDP, Gd-EOB-DTPA) or superparamagnetic iron oxides. These agents show uptake within the tumor suggestive of functioning hepatocytes or RES cells in a hepatocellular adenoma and may increase the specificity of MRI. However, in some cases biopsy has to be performed so that the final diagnosis can be made by cytology or histology.

Focal nodular hyperplasia may be diagnosed specifically if only minor differences in signal intensity between tumor and liver are found on unenhanced T1- and T2-weighted images and if a typical central scar, which is hyperintense on T2-weighted images, is visible. However, this appearance is found in only 10%–25% of cases. As the foregoing discussion suggests the use of MR contrast agents may further facilitate the diagnosis of FNH (HAMMERSTINGL et al. 1997). As in hepatocellular adenoma, gadolinium-based perfusion agents or hepatobiliary agents and superparamagnetic RES agents may be of assistance in the diagnosis of FNH, and improve the specificity of MRI to about 80%.

Hepatic cysts can often be diagnosed on the basis of their typical low T1- and high T2-weighted appearance on MRI. Additionally these lesions usually do not take up contrast agents either during the perfusion phase or on delayed MR scans. If exact distinction between cysts and hemangiomas is not possible by their plain MR appearance, dynamic contrast-enhanced imaging or ultrasonography may be added to reach the final diagnosis.

For other benign liver lesions such as macroregenerative nodules or mesenchymal tumors, multiple imaging tests may be required in order to make a specific diagnosis. Furthermore, although the exact diagnosis of these tumors is often of limited clinical relevance, long-term follow-up or biopsy may be needed to achieve the final diagnosis.

References

Ameriks JA, Thompson NW, Frey CF, Appelman HD, Walter JF (1975) Hepatic adenomas, spontaneous liver rupture, and oral contraceptives. Arch Surg 110:548–557

Baum JK, Holtz F, Bookstein JJ, Klein EW (1973) Possible association between benign hepatomas and oral contraceptives. Lancet II:926–929

Beers BV, Demeure R, Pringot J, et al. (1990) Dynamic spin-echo imaging with Gd-DTPA: value in the differentiation of hepatic tumors. AJR 154:515–519

Bree RL, Schwab RE, Neiman HL (1983) Solitary echogenic spot in the liver: is it diagnostic of a hemangioma? AJR 140:41–45

Bree RL, Schwab RE, Glazer GM, Fink-Bennett D (1987) The varied appearances of hepatic cavernous hemangiomas with sonography, computed tomography, magnetic resonance imaging, and scintigraphy. Radiographics 7:1153–1157

Butch RJ, Stark D, Malt RA (1986) MR imaging of hepatic focal nodular hyperplasia. J Comput Assist Tomogr 10:874–877

Casarella WJ, Knowles DM, Wolff M, Johnson PM (1978) Focal nodular hyperplasia and liver cell adenoma: radiologic and pathologic differentiation. AJR 131:393–402

Choi BI, Han MC, Park JH, et al. (1989) Giant hemangioma of the liver: CT and MR imaging in 10 cases. AJR 152:1221–1226

Craig JR, Peters RL, Edmondson HA (1989) Tumors of the liver and intrahepatic bile ducts. Second series, Fascicle 26. AFIP, Washington, DC

Dooms GC, Hricak H, Sollitto RA, Higgins CB (1985) Lipomatous tumors and tumors with fatty component: MR imaging potentials and comparison of MR and CT results. Radiology 157:479–482

Egglin TK, Rummeny E, Stark DD, et al. (1990) Hepatic tumors: quantitative tissue characterization with MR imaging. Radiology 176:107–112

Freeny PC, Marks WM (1986) Hepatic hemangioma: dynamic bolus CT. AJR 147:711–716

Furuya K, Nakamura M, Yamamoto Y, et al. (1988) Macro-regenerative nodule of the liver: a clinicopathologic study in 345 autopsy cases of chronic liver disease. Cancer 61:99–105

Gaa J, Hatabu H, Jenkins RL, Finn JP, Edelman RR (1996) Liver masses: replacement of conventional T2-weighted spin-echo MR imaging with breathhold MR imaging. Radiology 200:459–464

Gabata T, Matsui O, Kodaya M, et al. (1990) MR imaging of hepatic adenoma. AJR 155:1009–1011

Gaines PA, Sampson MA (1989) Prevalance and characterization of simple hepatic cysts by ultrasound examination. Br J Radiol 62:335–337

Giovagnoni A, Paci E, Valeri G, et al. (1996) MRI characterization of focal liver lesions: comparison of T2 weighting by conventional spin-echo and turbo spin-echo sequences. J Magn Reson Imaging 6:589–595

Grandin C, Van Beers BE, Robert A, et al. (1995) Benign hepatocellular tumors: MRI after superparamagnetic iron oxide administration. J Comput Assist Tomogr 19:412–418

Hamm B, Fischer E, Taupitz M (1990) Differentiation of hepatic hemangiomas from hepatic metastases by dynamic contrast-enhanced MR imaging. J Comput Assist Tomogr 14:205–209

Hamm B, Vogl TH, Branding G, Schnell B, Taupitz M, Wolf KJ, Lissner J (1992) Focal liver lesions: MR imaging with Mn-DPDP – initial clinical results in 40 patients. Radiology 182:167–174

Hammerstingl R, Vogl TJ, Schwarz W, et al. (1997) Differentialdiagnose von fokalen Leberläsionen: Intraindividueller Vergleich von Eisenoxid- und Gadolinium-unterstützter MRT mittels ROC-Analyse. Fortschr Röntgenstr 166:85

Hamrick-Turner JE, Shipkey FH, Cranston PE (1994) Fibrolamellar hepatocellular carcinoma: MR appearance mimicking focal nodular hyperplasia. J Comput Assist Tomogr 18:301–304

Ishak KJ, Rabin L (1975) Benign tumors of the liver. Med Clin North Am 59:995–1013

Itai Y, Ohnishi S, Ohtomo K, et al. (1987) Regenerating nodules of liver cirrhosis: MR imaging. Radiology 165:419–423

Itoh K, Saini S, Hahn PF, et al. (1990) Differentiation between small hepatic hemangiomas and metastases on MR images: importance of size-specific quantitative criteria. AJR 155:61–65

Karhunen PJ (1986) Benign hepatic tumors and tumor-like conditions in men. J Clin Pathol 39:183–188

Kerlin P, Davis GL, McGill DB, Weiland LH, Adson MA, Sheedy PF II (1983) Hepatic adenoma and focal nodular hyperplasia: clinical, pathologic and radiologic features. Gastroenterology 84:994–1002

Klatskin J (1977) Hepatic tumors: possible relationship of use of contraceptives. Gastroenterology 73:386–394

Knowles DM II, Wolff M (1976) Focal nodular hyperplasia of the liver – a clinicopathologic study and review of the literature. Hum Pathol 7:533–545

Lee MJ, Saini S, Hamm B, et al. (1991) Focal nodular hyperplasia of the liver: MR findings in 35 proved cases. AJR 56:96–99

Lombardo DM, Baker ME, Spritzer CE, et al. (1990) Hepatic hemangiomas vs metastases: MR differentiation at 1.5 T. AJR 155:55–61

Mathieu D, Bruneton JN, Drouillard J, Pointreau CC, Vasile N (1986) Hepatic adenoma and focal nodular hyperplasia: dynamic CT study. Radiology 160:53–58

Mathieu D, Rahamouni A, Anglade M-C, et al. (1991) Focal nodular hyperplasia of the liver: assessment with contrast-enhanced turboFLASH MR imaging. Radiology 180:25–30

Matsui O, Kadoya M, Kameyama T, et al. (1989) Adenomatous hyperplastic nodules in the cirrhotic liver: differentiation from hepatocellular carcinoma with MR imaging. Radiology 173:123–126

Mattison GR, Glazer GM, Quint LE, Francis IR, Bree RL, Ensminger WB (1987) MR imaging of hepatic focal nodular hyperplasia: characterization and distinction from primary malignant hepatic tumors. AJR 148:711–715

McFarland EG, Mayo-Smith WW, Saini S, Hahn PF, Goldberg MA, Lee MJ (1994) Hepatic hemangiomas and malignant tumors: improved differentiation with heavily T2-weighted conventional spin-echo MR imaging. Radiology 193:43–47

McNicholas MMJ, Saini S, Echeverri J, et al. (1996) T2-relaxation times of hypervascular and non-hypervascular liver lesions: do hypervascular lesions mimic hemangiomas on heavily T2-weighted MR images? Clin Radiol 51:401–405

Murakami T, Baron RL, Federle MP, Peterson MS, Oliver JH III, Davis PL, Confer SR (1996) Cirrhosis of the liver: MR imaging with mangafodipir trisodium (Mn-DPDP). Radiology 198:567–571

Nime F, Pickren JW, Vana J, Aronoff BL, Baker HW, Murphy MP (1979) The histology of liver tumors in oral contraceptive users observed during a national survey by the American College of Surgeons Commission on Cancer. Cancer 44:1481–1489

Paulson EK, McClellan JS, Washington K, et al (1994) Hepatic adenoma: MR characteristics and correlation with pathologic findings: AJR 163:113–117

Rabinowitz JG, Kinbabwala M, Ulerich S (1974) Macro-regenerating nodule in cirrhotic liver: radiologic features and differential diagnosis. AJR 121:401–411

Reimer P, Rummeny EJ, Marx C, et al. (1997) Characterization of focal liver lesions with Resovist as a new SPIO: clinical value of dynamic enhancement with T1- and T2-weighted MRI.European Congress of Radiology, Book of abstracts, 7:293

Reinig JW (1991) Differentiation of hepatic lesions with MR imaging: the last word? Radiology 179:601

Rofsky NM, Weinreb JC, Bernadino ME, Young SW, Lee JKT, Noz ME (1993) Hepatocellular tumors: characterization with Mn-DPDP-enhanced MR imaging. Radiology 188:53–59

Rooks GB, Ory HW, Ishak KG, et al. (1979) Epidemiology of hepatocellular adenoma. The role of oral contraceptive use. JAMA 242:644–648

Rummeny E, Weissleder R, Sironi S, et al. (1989a) Central scar in primary liver tumors: MR features, specificity and pathologic correlation. Radiology 171:323–326

Rummeny E, Weissleder R, Stark D, et al. (1989b) Primary liver tumors: diagnosis by MR imaging. AJR 152:63–72

Rummeny E, Stöber U, Adolph J, Bongartz G, Vestring TH, Fervers J, Peters PE (1991a) Turbo-FLASH MR imaging: perfusion patterns of hepatic tumors. American Roentgen Ray Society, 91st annual meeting, Book of Abstracts, p 203

Rummeny E, Ehrenberg CH, Gehl HB, et al. (1991b) Manganese-DPDP as a hepatobiliary contrast agent in magnetic resonance imaging of the liver – results of clinical phase II trials in Germany including 141 patients. Invest Radiol 26:S142–S145

Rummeny E, Saini S, Compton C (1993) Benign tumors of the liver: hepatocellular adenoma, focal nodular hyperplasia and others. In: Freeny P, Stevenson G (eds) Margulis and

Burhenne's gastrointestinal radiology, 5th edn. Mosby, St. Louis, pp 1645–1661

Semelka RC, Brown ED, Ascher SM, et al. (1994) Hepatic hemangiomas: multi-institutional study of appearance on T2-weighted and serial gadolinium-enhanced gradient-echo MR images. Radiology 192:401–406

Stromeyer FW, Ishak KG (1981) Nodular transformation (nodular "regenerative" hyperplasia) of the liver. Hum Pathol 12:60–71

Titelbaum DS, Burke DR, Meranze SG, Saul SH (1988) Fibrolamellar hepatocellular carcinoma: pitfalls in non-operative diagnosis. Radiology 167:25–30

Vogl TJ, Hammerstingl R, Schwarz W, et al. (1996) Super-paramagnetic iron oxide-enhanced versus gadolinium-enhanced MR imaging for differential diagnosis of focal liver lesions. Radiology 198:881–887

Wiener SN, Parulekar SG (1979) Scintigraphy and ultrasonography of hepatic hemangioma. Radiology 132:149–153

Wilbur AC, Gyi B (1987) Hepatocellular carcinoma: MR appearance mimicking focal nodular hyperplasia. AJR 149: 721–722

Wittenberg J, Stark DD, Forman B, et al. (1988) Differentiation of hepatic metastases from hemangiomas and cysts by MR imaging. AJR 151:79–84

4 Malignant Focal Liver Lesions

R.F. Thoeni

CONTENTS

4.1
Introduction

Computed tomography (CT) and magnetic resonance imaging (MRI) are the preferred imaging methods for focal liver disease, but debate continues as to which should be the modality of choice. Currently, MRI can be considered a complementary method to CT and often is used as a problem-solving modality. CT's high resolution and rapid imaging time coupled with complete and accurate evaluation of the entire abdomen have given CT an increasing role in the diagnosis and management of vascular disorders, particularly vascular invasion by tumor and portal vein thrombosis; however, in equivocal cases, MRI can be diagnostic with one sequence alone. Often, MRI readily distinguishes between bland thrombus and tumor thrombus. Even though the final role of MRI in the armamentarium of imaging techniques for the liver is not completely defined, distinctive MRI features for characterization of malignant liver lesions have been recognized. Gadolinium enhancement often adds to the characterization of focal liver lesions which are based on T1- and T2-weighted sequences. More recently, liver-specific contrast agents have been introduced

R.F. Thoeni, MD, Professor of Radiology, Department of Radiology, Box 0628, University of California, San Francisco, CA 94143-0628, USA

which promise to further improve results with MRI.

In the following sections, typical MRI features of metastatic and primary hepatic lesions will be described and the role of MRI for evaluating patients with malignant focal liver lesions will be assessed.

4.2
Hepatic Metastases

Evaluation for metastatic disease is still the most common indication for liver imaging. In the United States, ultrasonography (US) is not used for this purpose because of its low sensitivity and low specificity. US results may improve with the introduction of contrast agents such as microbubbles (KUDO et al. 1992) and then US may become the front runner as a fast and cost-effective imaging technique for evaluating patients with suspected metastatic disease. Currently, both MRI and CT are used in assessing these patients and often the choice of modality depends on the user's experience and preference.

4.2.1
MRI Features

Generally, at low, mid, and high magnetic field strengths, focal metastatic liver lesions appear as low signal intensity areas on T1-weighted spin ech. (SE) sequences (THOENI 1991a) and as high signal intensity structures on T2-weighted SE sequences. On T2-weighted SE sequences, metastases are often heterogeneous with areas of higher and lower increased signal intensity (Fig. 4.1). Metastases occasionally appear as bright lesions on T1-weighted SE sequences due to hemorrhage, melanin-like material, or high protein (mucin) content. For medium and low field strengths, a heavily T1-weighted SE sequence usually is the imaging sequence of choice for the detection of liver metastases. In the high field, unless an inversion recovery sequence with its inherent heavy T1

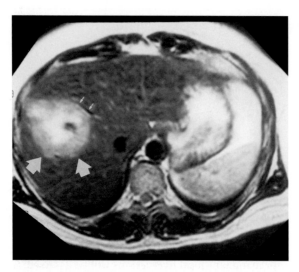

Fig. 4.1. A T2-weighted fast spin-echo sequence shows the typical appearance of a malignant lesion with heterogeneous signal intensity (*large arrows*). Note that the middle hepatic vein (*small arrows*) is displaced but not invaded by this metastasis from a gastric adenocarcinoma

weighting is used, T2-weighted sequences show a higher sensitivity for lesion detection than T1-weighted images, particularly if a fat suppression technique is employed. T1-weighted sequences show no specific differences between hepatocellular carcinoma (HCC), metastases (except for fatty metamorphosis), and benign lesions, including cysts and hemangiomas, but T2-weighted sequences can be used to distinguish these various masses. It is therefore necessary to use both T1- and T2-weighted sequences to screen patients suspected of suffering from malignant liver tumors.

Several features can be used to distinguish between malignant and benign tumors (EGGLIN et al. 1990). On a T2-weighted image, a peripheral halo or a wedge-shaped area of bright signal intensity surrounding a metastasis may be seen in approximately 25% of metastatic liver lesions and in approximately 21% of HCC and is thought to be due to peritumoral "edema" or compression of normal liver parenchyma by the focal lesion (GIOVAGNONI et al. 1994). This feature is seen much less often (12%) in benign lesions, such as hemangiomas or abscess. This peritumoral "edema" is responsible for the increase in size of the lesion on T2-weighted images and usually assumes a wedge or pyramidal configuration. If heavily T2-weighted sequences are used (TR 2000–2500 ms; TE 160 ms), hypovascular metastases (which constitute the majority of metastatic lesions to the liver) demonstrate a gradual loss of hyper-

intensity and sharpness of the margins that is due to decreasing signal-to-noise ratios and motion artifacts related to long scanning times. This is in contradistinction to benign lesions such as cysts and hemangiomas which show persistence of high signal intensity on these heavily T2-weighted sequences (WITTENBERG et al. 1988; LI et al. 1988). For an unequivocal diagnosis, T2-weighted sequences with an echo delay of at least 120 ms (CHOI et al. 1990) and no fat suppression should be used. However, highly vascularized or cystic metastases, such as those from endocrine tumors (islet cell), pheochromocytomas, carcinoids, sarcomas and carcinoma, also show persistence of high signal intensity on delayed echo images. Usually, metastases have slightly irregular margins which distinguish them from the mostly sharp margins of cysts or small hemangiomas. On T2-weighted sequences, malignant lesions tend to appear heterogeneous, but large hemangiomas can mimic this appearance (ROS et al. 1987). Hepatic metastases also can assume the appearance of target lesions consisting of ring-like areas of high and low signal intensities (Fig. 4.2).

Gadolinium enhancement can improve detection of lesions in some instances (WARD et al. 1995) and further help to define the histologic nature of a tumor (VAN BEERS et al. 1990). If multiple lesions are present which show slightly irregular margins, have completely enhanced rims when a good bolus of contrast material is used, and have slightly heterogeneous centers, the diagnosis of metastatic disease is very likely. However, partial volume artifacts and poor bolus technique can render results equivocal. Gradient-echo sequences obtained immediately following administration of the gadolinium bolus (sinusoid phase) appear to have the highest sensitivity for detecting hypervascular lesions (LARSON et al. 1994), similar to results with helical CT where the early arterial phase is used for diagnosing hypervascular metastases. Some hypervascular metastases may mimic the enhancement pattern of a hemangioma if they are small, but in general, hypervascular metastases can be distinguished from hemangiomas based on the presence of a completely enhanced nodular ring in the periphery and a heterogeneous enhancement pattern within the lesion (Fig. 4.3).

A cyst is a sharply defined lesion of low signal intensity on a T1-weighted sequence and of persistently high signal intensity on a T2-weighted sequence, and it demonstrates no peripheral or central enhancement during or after enhancement with gadolinium. These lesions retain their low signal

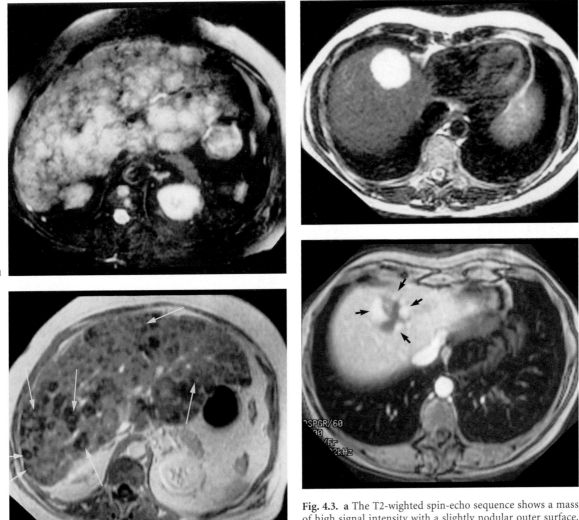

Fig. 4.2. **a** A T2-weighted spin-echo sequence with fat suppression shows multiple nodular areas of high signal intensity throughout the liver. **b** The corresponding gadolinium-enhanced gradient-echo sequence demonstrates multiple target lesions (*arrows*) indicative of diffuse metastatic disease from a sarcoma

Fig. 4.3. **a** The T2-wighted spin-echo sequence shows a mass of high signal intensity with a slightly nodular outer surface. Hypervascular metastasis or hemangioma should be considered. **b** The gadolinium-enhanced gradient-echo sequence establishes unequivocally the presence of a hemangioma based on the nodular incomplete rim of enhancement (*arrows*) in the early phase (1 min)

intensity on delayed scans because they are filled with fluid which does not communicate with the vascular space. If a cyst becomes very large, it may compress liver tissue, which may appear as an enhancing rim. Gadolinium-enhanced gradient-echo sequences are particularly useful for characterizing lesions as cystic or solid even if they measure only between 5 and 15 mm in diameter (SEMELKA et al. 1992a). Complex cysts may demonstrate higher signal intensity values on T1-weighted sequences (spin-echo as well as gradient-echo sequences) because they contain

debris, blood, or infectious material. An unequivocal diagnosis of a cyst only can be made with US. In many cases, US may help exclude cysts or hemangiomas.

Typical MRI features of hemangioma include a sharply defined lesion with a nodular enhanced incomplete rim on early gadolinium-enhanced scans, gradual fill-in of the lesion by intravenous contrast material over time, and complete homogeneous enhancement on delayed scans (delay of 10–20 min). Large hemangiomas or very small hemangiomas often do not exhibit the typical features for an unequivocal diagnosis. Small hemangiomas may appear as completely enhanced areas in the early phase, and large hemangiomas may never demonstrate the complete fill-in or suffer from heterogeneous contrast enhancement. Scintigraphy with blood pool imaging should be used for equivocal cases and provides excellent results in patients with lesions 3 cm and larger in diameter and, if single-photon emission computed tomography (SPECT) is used, in patients with even smaller lesions (>2.5 cm). If a lesion measures less than 3 cm for planar or 2.5 cm for SPECT scintigraphy or if a lesion is close to the heart or major vessels (large vascular pools), scintigraphy should not be used.

The use of gadopentetate dimeglumine carries the disadvantage of a very narrow imaging window which requires optimal conditions such as good venous access and rapid scanning capabilities. New contrast agents which are commercially available in the United States promise better results by means of a wide imaging window. These contrast agents include iron oxide particles (SAINI et al. 1995) and manganese dipyridoxaldiphosphate (Mn-DPDP) (HAMM et al. 1992). Imaging windows of up to 1 h are reported for these agents. Mn-DPDP also has been shown to make possible the distinction between tumors of hepatic and nonhepatic origin (see Sect. 4.3.1). Obviously such an approach creates logistic problems if images before and after administration of contrast agent are needed. Many of these techniques, with and without intravenous contrast

agent, remain in flux pending results from larger series. In one small series (BIRNBAUM et al. 1994), the investigators detected more lesions on the Mn-DPDP-enhanced MRI images than on the contrast-enhanced CT scans, but overall the results with CT and MRI depended on the expertise of the individual reader with each technique. However, gadolinium can be used freely and its only limitation is the observation of increased creatinine levels. In patients with increased creatinine, and particularly those in whom values are rising, administration of gadolinium should be used with caution and may be contraindicated, but there appears to exist a larger tolerance for gadolinium than for iodinated contrast agents.

4.2.2
Results and Role of MRI

For the detection of metastases, MRI has been shown to have an overall sensitivity of 78%–83% and a specificity of 89% for resectability (SOYER et al. 1996; NELSON et al. 1988; KUHLMAN et al. 1994; URHAHN et al. 1996). The sensitivity for CT reaches as high as 89% (URHAHN et al. 1996), and overall results for CT have improved with helical CT because the speed with which the liver can be scanned eliminates breathing artifacts, and better bolus techniques and reconstruction at smaller slice increments than were scanned improve lesion conspicuity (URBAN et al. 1993; ZEMAN et al. 1993).

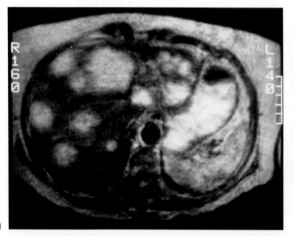

a

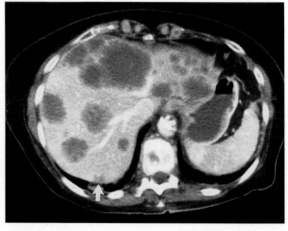

b

Fig. 4.4. a A T2-weighted spin-echo sequence reveals multiple metastatic lesions from a colon carcinoma. b CTAP of the same patient obtained on the same day demonstrates one additional small lesion (*arrow*) and there were other small lesions on lower sections, none of which were identified by MRI

Currently, no large series has been published on the sensitivity and specificity of helical CT for metastatic disease. For CT with arterial portography (CTAP), sensitivities between 77% and 94% have been reported (MATSUI et al. 1987; HEIKEN et al. 1989; SOYER et al. 1993a) and are higher than those for delayed CT, which consists of a repeat study 4–6 h following administration of 60 g of iodine. On a delayed study, normal hepatocytes contain iodine and appear bright whereas abnormal hepatocytes such as in metastases do not enhance. The sensitivity of CTAP decreases if a significant amount of contrast material is used during the preliminary angiography because seepage of contrast agent into the tumor results in diminished liver–tumor contrast. The results with CTAP also can be improved by using helical CT (NAPEL et al. 1992; FREENY et al. 1995). Overall, CTAP is slightly more accurate than MRI for detecting the total number of lesions, and particularly lesions less than 1 cm in diameter (Fig. 4.4), but it is a costly and invasive procedure and should be used only for those patients requiring a decision on whether to resect liver lesions or to place a chemoperfusion pump.

At present, if only the liver needs to be evaluated, MRI appears to be of equal value to CT, but some of the lesions measuring less than 1 cm may be missed by MRI. These MRI results most likely will be improved once a liver-specific intravenous contrast material such as Mn-DPDP becomes universally available and fast imaging techniques are used. In most institutions in the United States, CT is the initial method to search for liver metastases. However, gadolinium-enhanced MRI often can distinguish more readily between benign and malignant disease than CT can, based on signal intensity and other morphologic features unique to MRI which disclose the internal architecture of a lesion (HAMM et al. 1994). Therefore, either CT or MRI can be used for assessing the liver, but presently, CT is preferable because it is faster and can provide information for the entire abdomen which is of superior resolution to that obtained with MRI, particularly for the gastrointestinal tract. In a young patient and/or in a patient without a known or suspected primary tumor, no further workup is needed if multiple hepatic lesions are found which appear to be hemangiomas or cysts. In patients with a known primary tumor and lesions in the liver that might be resectable, CTAP (NELSON et al. 1989) should be used because it provides the highest sensitivity for detection and assessment of vascular involvement. One study (PAULSON et al. 1994) comparing short

tau inversion recovery (STIR) MRI and CTAP found no significant difference between the methods except for the medial segment, where CTAP detected more lesions than STIR MRI. Whether positron emission tomography will change the approach in patients with suspected metastatic disease of the liver remains to be seen, and results with large series of patients are eagerly awaited.

4.3
Primary Malignant Lesions

The most important primary tumors of the liver are epithelial tumors [HCC (75%), fibrolamellar hepatocellular carcinoma (FLHCC), hepatoblastoma (7%), cholangiocarcinoma (6%)], mesenchymal tumors of the blood vessels (angiosarcoma and hemangioendothelioma), other mesenchymal tumors (embryonal sarcoma and fibrosarcoma), tumors of muscle tissue (leiomyosarcoma and rhabdomyosarcoma), and other miscellaneous tumors (particularly primary lymphoma and teratomas). We will discuss HCC, FLHCC, cholangiocarcinoma, angiosarcoma, and lymphoma. In patients with liver cirrhosis and suspected HCC, MRI should be considered the primary imaging technique whereas for most of the other primary tumors, the role of MRI is complementary or equal to the role of CT.

4.3.1
Hepatocellular Carcinoma

In most of the industrialized world, HCC has an incidence of 0.2%–0.8%, a peak age in the 6th and 7th decades, and a male-to-female ratio of 2.5:1. The average survival time after diagnosis is 6 months. In Southeast Asia, Africa, and Japan, the incidence is 5%–20%, the peak age is in the 3rd and 4th decades, and the male-to-female ratio is 5:1. The 5-year survival is less than 30%, the resectability rate is 17%, and the average survival time after diagnosis is 6 months. HCC develops in 12% of patients with chronic hepatitis B or C and in only 5% of patients with alcoholic liver cirrhosis. The FLHCC subtype of HCC has a 5-year survival rate of 63%, a resectability rate of 48%, and an average survival time after diagnosis of 32 months. Treatment consists of resection if possible and/or chemotherapy, with remission of up to 3 years being achieved in more than 40% of patients.

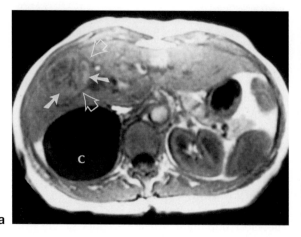

a

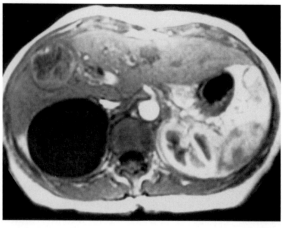

b

Fig. 4.5. a A precontrast T1-weighted gradient-echo sequence (fast multiplanar spoiled grass gradient-echo) demonstrates a low signal intensity peripheral rim representing the capsule (*open arrows*), higher signal intensity in the periphery (*solid arrows*), and irregular lower signal intensity in the center as compared with the surrounding cirrhotic liver. *C*, Renal cyst. **b** A postcontrast T1-weighted gradient-echo sequence (fast multiplanar spoiled grass gradient-echo) demonstrates these features more readily and visualizes viable tumor as enhancing areas

4.3.1.1
MRI Features of Hepatocellular Carcinoma

The MRI diagnosis of HCC is based on the presence of steatosis, hemorrhage, a capsule, and/or vascular invasion (EBARA et al. 1986). In 10%–47% of all MRI cases of HCC, the lesion may appear on T1-weighted sequences as a bright spot rather than a dark area due to central steatosis or hemorrhage (ITOH et al. 1987) (Fig. 4.5). Occasionally, some steatosis is present in adenomas or even focal nodular hyperplasia (FNH) (NOKES et al. 1988). In approximately 24%–42% of HCC cases, a dark peripheral rim or capsule may be seen on T1-weighted sequences, which is thought to be due to a fibrous pseudocapsule or peripheral venous-lake formation (Fig. 4.5). The higher percentage is seen in the Asian population. A typical feature of HCC is the presence of daughter nodules immediately adjacent to the main lesion, which can be seen on T1- and T2-weighted sequences.

On T2-weighted sequences, a mosaic pattern is seen, closely reflecting the pattern seen on sections through a gross specimen (ROSENTHAL and DAVIS 1992) (Fig. 4.6). Low signal intensity within the lesion represents a collagenous scar, old hemorrhage (hemosiderin), or tumor necrosis. Occasionally, such a scar may contain edema and appear hyperintense on T2-weighted images, but such an appearance is rare and, when seen together with homogeneity, should suggest FNH. A scar is a nonspecific finding and can

also be found in a large hemangioma (where it tends to assume a crescent shape) and in hepatic adenoma with old hemorrhage. In these cases, the history and absence of an elevated α-fetoprotein should be helpful. In 21% of HCCs, similar to metastases, peritumoral edema may be seen which represents compressed hepatic tissue rather than true edema (GIOVAGNONI et al. 1994). Extension beyond the liver capsule also may be visible as partial tumor projection into the surrounding area and satellite nodules (IMAEDA et al. 1994). These features are often better demonstrated by MRI than by CT. Overall, MRI is superior to CT in detecting small HCC (less than 20 mm in diameter), its sensitivity being 81.6% as compared with only 53.8% for CT (HIRAI et al. 1991).

On spin-echo sequences, one of the most important features of HCC is the detection of high signal intensity within the inferior vena cava (IVC), portal vein and/or hepatic venous channels. This high signal intensity in the venous structures represents (tumor) thrombus (Fig. 4.6) which may extend to the right atrium, but flow phenomena must be excluded. Such thrombus was present in 29% of the series of that of RUMMENY et al. (1989a). The incidence of portal vein invasion can reach 33% and that of hepatic vein invasion, 15%. Involvement of the IVC is seen in only 5%–7%, but is more frequent when the tumor is close to the IVC or central hepatic veins. Phase images can be used to distinguish among simple thrombus, tumor thrombus, and normal

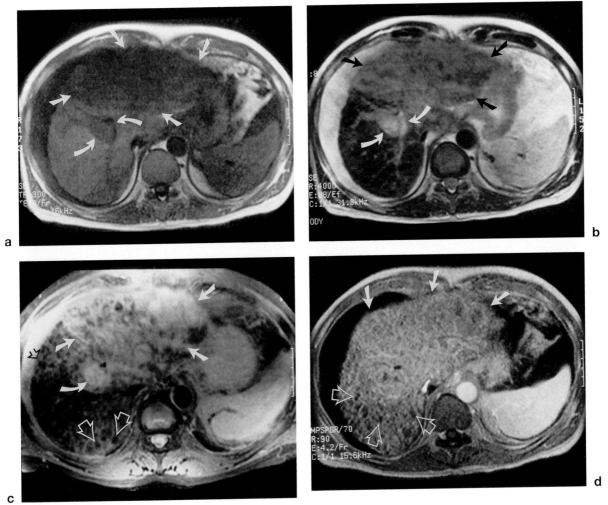

Fig. 4.6. a A T1-weighted sequence demonstrates liver cirrhosis and a low signal intensity lesion in the left lobe representing an HCC (*straight arrows*). Also note the high signal intensity in the right portal vein representing thrombus (*curved arrows*). **b** The T2-weighted fast spin-echo sequence clearly shows the mixed signal intensity of the lesion in the left lobe (*straight arrows*) and the high signal intensity thrombus in the right portal vein (*curved arrows*), which is markedly distended by tumor mass. **c** The T2-weighted conventional spin-echo sequence shows high signal intensity in the left lobe (*straight arrows*), the thrombus in the right portal vein (*curved arrow*), and multiple low signal intensity areas representing regenerating nodules throughout the cirrhotic liver (*open arrows*). **d** A gadolinium-enhanced gradient-echo sequence shows the enhanced HCC (*straight arrows*) and the low signal intensity nodules (*open arrows*) to great advantage

flowing blood. Also, gradient-echo sequences with small flip angles or gradient-echo sequences with larger flip angles (60°–70°) and gadolinium enhancement can help determine the presence or absence of portal and/or hepatic vein thrombosis.

In patients with liver cirrhosis, regenerating nodules (≤1 cm in diameter) which contain iron (hemosiderin) are of low signal intensity on both T1- and T2-weighted sequences and are best demonstrated on gradient-echo sequences with and without gadolinium enhancement (OHTOMO et al. 1990). Vascular fibrous septa surrounding these nodules also can help demonstrate these lesions. However, the appearance of regenerating nodules generally is quite variable, and some are isointense on both sequences and some are hyperintense on T1 and isointense on T2-weighted images (KOSLOW et al. 1991). Hyperplastic adenomatous nodules (macro-regenerative nodules or nodular adenomatous hyperplasia) are larger than 1 cm in diameter and usually are isointense or hyperintense compared with the remaining liver parenchyma on T1-weighted sequences and hypointense on T2-weighted sequences (Fig. 4.7). When hyperplastic adenomatous nodules become

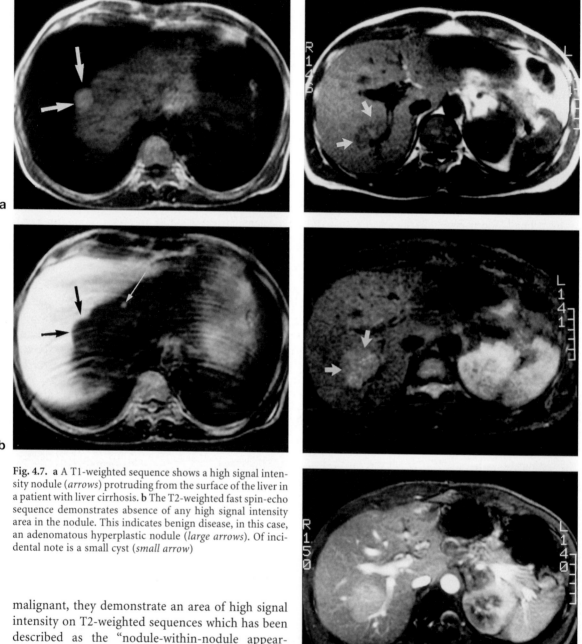

Fig. 4.7. a A T1-weighted sequence shows a high signal intensity nodule (*arrows*) protruding from the surface of the liver in a patient with liver cirrhosis. **b** The T2-weighted fast spin-echo sequence demonstrates absence of any high signal intensity area in the nodule. This indicates benign disease, in this case, an adenomatous hyperplastic nodule (*large arrows*). Of incidental note is a small cyst (*small arrow*)

malignant, they demonstrate an area of high signal intensity on T2-weighted sequences which has been described as the "nodule-within-nodule appearance"; this indicates the presence of a small HCC or carcinoma in situ within a low signal intensity nodule full of iron (hemosiderin) (MITCHELL et al. 1991).

Similar to CT, on precontrast gradient-echo studies, HCC appears as a hypointense to isointense mass often associated with a circumferential, well-defined circular zone of lower density (capsule) (Fig. 4.5). On postgadolinium MRI studies, intense, transient heterogeneous enhancement (mosaic pattern) is present. Homogeneous enhancement suggests benign disease unless the lesion is very small (Fig. 4.8). Extension beyond the liver capsule also may be vis-

Fig. 4.8. a A T1-weighted sequence shows an ill-defined area of low signal intensity (*arrows*). **b** The T2-weighted sequence demonstrates a high signal intensity mass (*arrows*). Based on the T1- and T2-weighted spin-echo sequences, benign disease cannot be distinguished from malignant focal liver disease. **c** The gadolinium-enhanced gradient-echo sequence (2 min delay) strongly suggests that the lesion represents FNH based on the homogeneous and intense enhancement of a hypervascular lesion

ible. On delayed scans, a capsule again may be seen, and large vascular channels and scattered areas of low attenuation may extend to the peripheral zone. Careful analysis of the vascular structures often reveals a tumor thrombus. As a general rule, gadolinium rarely enhances the lesion to such an even degree that it completely disappears, as may be the case with CT. T2 values based on T2-weighted spin-echo sequences with long echo delays and delayed gadolinium-enhanced gradient-echo sequences further help distinguish between hypervascular HCC and hemangioma (OHTOMO et al. 1989).

Dual liver helical CT has been helpful in diagnosing even small lesions, based on the hypervascularity of HCC. In the arterial phase of contrast enhancement (immediate and 1-min scan series), the tumor is often clearly shown through enhancement of the hypervascular areas, but it may disappear completely in the portal-venous phase, particularly if the lesion is small. This enhancement effect is related to the fact that HCC is a hypervascular tumor and, as with hypervascular metastases, the dual liver protocol can take advantage of these enhancement features. If the patient is scanned with a significant delay following the bolus of contrast material, a hypervascular lesion may become isodense and be missed altogether.

More recently, it has been shown that Mn-DPDP can distinguish between HCC and other focal liver masses of nonhepatic origin. In the study by HAMM et al. (1992), FNH and regenerative nodules also enhanced with Mn-DPDP, but cholangiocarcinoma, lymphoma, and metastases did not demonstrate any uptake of the contrast agent. In another study of Mn-DPDP (ROFSKY et al. 1993), MRI permitted distinction between hepatocellular and nonhepatocellular tumors based on the presence of enhancement and the enhancement pattern of a lesion, with a sensitivity of 100%, a specificity of 92%, and an accuracy of 93.6%. A small liver MRI study (LIOU et al. 1994) using Mn-DPDP and comparing enhancement of the normal liver parenchyma with that of focal liver lesions also found that HCC showed significant enhancement and thus conspicuity of this malignant focal lesion was decreased; by contrast other focal hepatic lesions which were not of hepatocellular origin demonstrated no uptake and conspicuity of these lesions was increased. It therefore appears that Mn-DPDP might be helpful in distinguishing between metastatic disease to the liver and primary tumor of the liver.

4.3.1.2
MRI Features of Fibrolamellar Hepatocellular Carcinoma

Although FLHCC is a rare liver tumor, its recognition is important because its prognosis is much better and curative resection is frequently possible, even when the tumor is large. This tumor is seen in young patients (5–35 years of age) and occurs with equal frequency in women and men. Patients with FLHCC do not have cirrhosis associated with the tumor and the α-fetoprotein levels are normal. The tumor tends to calcify more often than HCC (40%) and is often well circumscribed. The 5-year survival rate is 63%. Fibrolamellar carcinomas are often at an advanced stage at the time of diagnosis. Metastatic disease may be present in up to 70% at the time of initial diagnosis (STEVENS et al. 1995), but the tumor is considered resectable in 48% of cases. Recurrence after resection with intent to cure is common, and early and frequent follow-up imaging is necessary for optimizing surgical management in patients with this neoplasm.

Both MRI and CT show features of FLHCC similar to those of HCC with the exception of vascular invasion, which is less common in FLHCC. The nonenhancing central stellate scar is a typical feature of FLHCC (RUMMENY et al. 1989b) and distinguishes it from HCC (Fig. 4.9). When it is present (in approximately 50%), this scar can be easily detected by MRI because it remains dark on T2-weighted images and does not enhance with gadolinium, and on helical CT the stellate scar is very conspicuous within the contrast-enhanced lesion.

4.3.1.3
Results and Role of MRI

Either CT or US is often the initial test for the detection of HCC. On conventional CT and helical CT with a single helix, HCC appears as a vascular mass, often with central necrosis, but if optimal bolus timing is not used, small lesions can be missed altogether. Dual helical CT increase the ability to detect even small lesions (1 cm) because in the early or arterial phase, this tumor is enhanced by tumor vessels fed by the hepatic artery and tumor enhancement can be seen. On the delayed or portal-venous phase, however, HCC may become isointense. Even with this major improvement in the CT technique and a reported overall sensitivity of 84% (UEDA et al. 1995), perfusion artifacts due to fibrosis remain a diagnostic dilemma as many of these patients also suffer

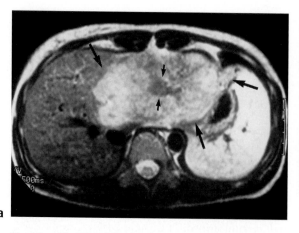

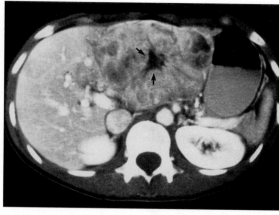

a   b

Fig. 4.9. a The T2-weighted sequence shows a mixed high–low signal intensity mass (*large arrows*) with a central low signal intensity area (*small arrows*) in this patient with an FLHCC. **b** Helical CT in the same patient shows a heterogeneously enhanced mass with a central stellate nonenhancing scar (*arrows*). Because of the long scanning time for the T2-weighted sequence, the stellate appearance is not as easily seen as on CT with breath-holding

from moderate to severe liver cirrhosis. Results with MRI are not influenced by uneven perfusion of liver parenchyma due to fibrosis and frequently can provide accurate information on the presence or absence of HCC. CT with Lipiodol has reached a sensitivity of up to 92% (DE SANTIS et al. 1992), but this technique is not used in the United States in routine clinical practice. Therefore, MRI should be the initial test in patients with liver cirrhosis who are at risk for developing this tumor or in patients with elevated α-fetoprotein. In these patients, MRI is superior for detecting tumor and distinguishing between metastatic disease and HCC. CTAP is most sensitive for determining whether the tumor consists of a single lesion or represents the multifocal manifestation, but in patients with severe cirrhosis, perfusion artifacts also can cause diagnostic dilemmas. The final diagnosis often must be made by biopsy.

Magnetic resonance imaging easily reveals tumor in patients with liver cirrhosis and distinguishes focal hyperplastic or macro-regenerative nodules without malignant focus from those which contain a malignant focus (early HCC). A study on serial MRI in patients with a nodule-in-nodule appearance (MITCHELL et al. 1991) showed a volume doubling time of 9.5 weeks and a diameter doubling time of 29 weeks (SADEK et al. 1995). This rapid growth rate must be taken into consideration when treatment or follow-up studies are planned. MRI is sensitive for detecting the presence of tumor (82%), but it often does not detect all lesions if the tumor is multifocal (THOENI et al. 1991b). Because of this lack of sensitivity for true extent of tumor, the decision on resec-

tion of this tumor cannot be based on MRI. Both MRI and US can be used to assess venous involvement in the liver.

Overall, MRI has a reported sensitivity of 62%–82% for detecting HCC (BARTOLOZZI et al. 1996; UEDA et al. 1995; DE SANTIS et al. 1992; THOENI et al. 1991b). At present, no data from a large series have been published which assess the sensitivity of MRI using Mn-DPDP. Both helical CT and MRI can detect vascular invasion with great ease and US is often a cost-effective means of assessing the presence of venous occlusion in these patients if CT or MRI provides equivocal results (SHIMAMOTO et al. 1992). Overall, because of the absence of confusing enhancement patterns, MRI is the method of choice in patients with liver cirrhosis and suspected HCC. MRI and CT provide similar results in patients with suspected HCC but without liver cirrhosis.

4.3.2
Cholangiocarcinoma

Intrahepatic cholangiocarcinoma is the second most common primary hepatic neoplasm, but only 8%–13% of all cholangiocarcinomas occur in the liver alone. Intrahepatic cholangiocarcinoma can be classified into peripheral cholangiocarcinoma, which originates from an interlobular biliary duct, and hilar cholangiocarcinoma, which is also called Klatskin tumor and is more common (SOYER et al. 1995b). Most of these lesions develop in the extrahepatic biliary system. The average age of patients is 50–60

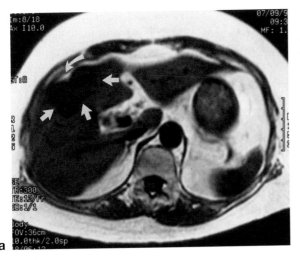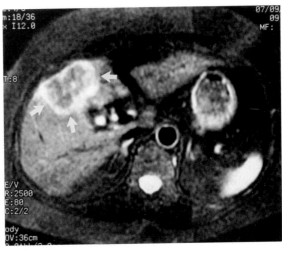

a

b

Fig. 4.10. a A T1-weighted spin-echo sequence shows a low signal intensity mass (*straight arrows*) with retraction of the capsule (*curved arrow*) which suggests but is not diagnostic of a desmoplastic cholangiocarcinoma. **b** A T2-weighted spin-echo sequence with fat suppression shows a high signal intensity lesion with a peripheral zone of higher signal intensity and a central zone of mixed high and low signal intensity (*arrows*)

years and the male-to-female ratio is 3:2. Less than 20% of cholangiocarcinomas are considered resectable and the 5-year survival rate is 30%.

4.3.2.1
MRI Features

On gross pathology specimens, cholangiocarcinoma appears as a firm, hypovascular mass with a significant amount of fibrous stroma. In contradistinction to HCC, cholangiocarcinoma demonstrates encasement but not invasion of large vessels. Desmoplastic reaction may be prominent and small foci of necrosis or hemorrhage may be present. Occasionally, a combination of HCC and cholangiocarcinoma can be encountered, in which case features of both tumors are present and an unequivocal diagnosis is close to impossible.

Involvement of the liver by a cholangiocarcinoma may be difficult to diagnose because some of these tumors are quite small, particularly if they extend as narrow tumor sheaths along the portal triad. A radiographic feature which has been described in the literature for the diagnosis of a cholangiocarcinoma in the liver consists of detection of shrinkage of liver parenchyma and retraction of the capsule in a segment involved by this tumor (SOYER 1994). This feature is more frequently observed in the left lobe of the liver (Fig. 4.10), but it also can be seen with other tumors, most frequently with the rare epithelioid hemangioendothelioma. Also, scans obtained with a delay of 7–10 min following an intravenous bolus of contrast material demonstrate delayed enhancement of the tumor which is diagositc for the detection of this tumor mass and helps to guide biopsy needles into the neoplastic area. This feature can be observed with CT and MRI.

On T1-weighted spin-echo sequences, cholangiocarcinoma appears as a homogeneous mass of low signal intensity, but occasionally it is isointense (CHOI et al. 1995). On T2-weighted MRI spin-echo sequences, the mass becomes hyperintense, often with associated central areas of low signal intensity representing fibrosis. The higher signal intensity in the periphery is indicative of viable tumor tissue. Also, areas of high signal intensity extending along the portal triad can represent evidence of a cholangiocarcinoma. Cholangiocarcinomas tend to produce biliary dilatation more often than does HCC, a feature which can be readily demonstrated by MRI and CT. Usually there is no evidence of tumor thrombus, but large vessels such as the portal vein or IVC may be encased (POWERS et al. 1994; SOYER et al. 1995a). The enhancement pattern consists of progressive concentric enhancement, usually without opacification of the central area of fibrosis. As with CT, the delayed enhancement with gadolinium serves as a reliable indicator of the presence of a cholangiocarcinoma. Delayed gadolinium-enhanced sequences demonstrate this feature as prolonged central enhancement with a peripheral rim of congestive liver parenchyma and dilated sinusoids with greater enhancement in the late phase than in the early phase (MURAKAMI et al. 1995).

4.3.2.2
Results and Role of MRI

The sensitivities of MRI and CT in detecting cholangiocarcinoma are similar, but most published series are either small or were not obtained with helical CT for state-of-the-art comparison of the two modalities. For both techniques, a reliable diagnosis can only be made if delayed contrast-enhanced images are obtained. Because a biopsy is often needed for a histologic diagnosis, the preferred imaging method is CT.

4.3.3
Angiosarcoma

Angiosarcoma is the most common sarcoma of the liver and is encountered more frequently than leiomyosarcoma, fibrosarcoma, or malignant fibrohistiocytoma. However, angiosarcoma is a rare neoplasm of the liver (<2% of all primary live neoplasms) which has been found more frequently in patients with previous and long-standing exposure to radiation from Thorotrast (7%–10% of all angiosarcomas, latent period 15–24 years), or in patients who have worked with arsenic or polyvinyl products (latent period 4–28 years) (POWERS et al. 1994). The peak incidence is in the 6th and 7th decades. It also may be encountered in patients with von Recklinghausen's disease and in hemochromatosis. Most of these patients develop a neoplasm, usually angiosarcoma, within 20 years after initial administration of the contrast agent or toxic agent. Hemorrhagic ascites is common in these patients and percutaneous biopsies of this lesion may lead to massive bleeding. Therefore, it behoves the radiologist to recommend an open biopsy. The median survival is only 6 months, which can be prolonged to about 1 year with chemotherapy. At the time of initial diagnosis, as many as 60% of patients have metastatic disease to lung or spleen.

Hepatic angiosarcoma consists of multiple foci of poorly organized vessels lined with malignant cells. The tumor cells also may grow along preexisting vascular channels, especially the sinusoids. If the tumor is caused by Thorotrast, the liver surface shows a significant amount of fibrosis because of the peripheral accumulation of the Thorotrast. The tumor grows in two patterns: multifocal or multinodular (approximately 70%) and as a large solitary mass.

Thorotrast is an obsolete contrast material which was used for angiography and liver scanning. This contrast agent emits α-particles. Following injection of Thorotrast, the contrast material is stored in the reticuloendothelial system, particularly in the liver, spleen, and bone marrow. The contrast agent tends to accumulate as a linear network of opacities in the liver, spleen, and local lymph nodes. Plain films of the abdomen typically reveal calcifications in the liver and usually more intense opacities in the spleen and lymph nodes. The liver and particularly the spleen are often shrunken. Initially, the liver is densely opacified, but the degree of liver opacification diminishes over time while that of the spleen increases.

4.3.3.1
MRI Features

On CT, circumferential displacement of Thorotrast is suggestive of angiosarcoma of the liver. Depending on the degree of hyalinization and sclerosis, areas of hyper- and hypovascularity can be seen. On MRI, angiosarcoma appears as a very large, vascular mass with calcifications, heterogeneous signal intensities (BUETOW et al. 1994), and hypointense bands representing fibrotic septations or as multiple nodules that coalesce into larger masses over time. Large feeding vessels or collaterals often can be identified.

Compensatory hypertrophy of the uninvolved liver is present with large tumor masses. On T1-weighted sequences, the lesion is predominantly hypointense with areas of high signal intensity if hemorrhage is present. On T2-weighted sequences, the lesion is hyperintense with heterogeneity throughout its mass. Often, the MRI appearance of an angiosarcoma is similar to that of a large cavernous hemangioma consisting of a hyperintense mass interlaced with multiple linear hypointense fibrous septa (OHTOMO et al. 1992) (Fig. 4.11). Large areas of necrosis also may be seen. Calcifications may be difficult to identify on MRI but are readily detected by CT.

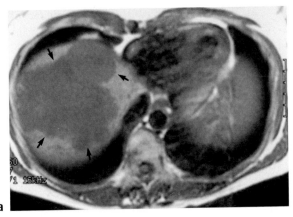

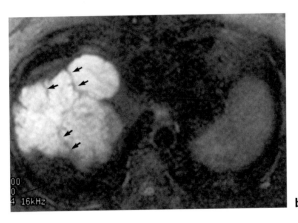

a

b

Fig. 4.11. **a** A T1-weighted spin-echo sequence shows a large irregular low signal intensity mass (*arrows*). **b** A T2-weighted spin-echo sequence with fat suppression shows that the same mass has overall high signal intensity with multiple low signal intensity bands traversing it (*arrows*). The patient suffered from an angiosarcoma, but a very large hemangioma can assume a similar appearance

At times, on gadolinium-enhanced gradient-echo sequences of the mulitifocal variety of angiosarcoma, target lesions can be seen representing areas of vascular tumor and central areas of myxoid and hyalinized stroma. If a large solitary mass is present, initial rim enhancement may be present followed by persistent heterogeneous opacification of the lesion. Compression of noninvolved adjacent liver tissue may show high signal intensity on T2-weighted images due to vascular congestion. Such an appearance can mimic tumor extension. CT is not as sensitive to such congestion and, therefore, may be more accurate in predicting the true tumor extent, which allows appropriate treatment planning.

4.3.3.2
Results and Role of MRI

Computed tomography and MRI demonstrate angiosarcoma of the liver equally well and may be interchangeable methods. If surgery is contemplated, caution must be exercised in interpreting the overall extent of tumor by MRI as compression of normal liver tissue by the large tumor mass may lead to overstaging.

4.3.4
Lymphoma

Primary lymphoma of the liver is a rare disease and is usually a non-Hodgkin's lymphoma. Most primary lymphomas of the liver occur as a single, well-defined lesion. Secondary hepatic lymphoma is more common; it occurs in 60% of patients with Hodgkin's lymphoma and in 50% with non-Hodgkin's lymphoma, and usually presents as multiple or diffusely infiltrating lesions (GAZELLE et al. 1994). Often no alteration in the hepatic architecture can be detected. If the liver is diffusely infiltrated by lymphoma, the tumor mass can be missed.

4.3.4.1
MRI Features

On T1-weighted sequences, lymphomatous lesions appear as hypointense, isointense, or slightly hyperintense to the liver, whereas on T2-weighted sequences, the lesions are hyperintense and homogeneous or slightly heterogeneous (SOYER et al. 1993b; FUKUYA et al. 1993). Portal vein branches may be identified within the tumor, which would be an unusual finding in other malignant neoplasms. If gadolinium and gradient-echo sequences are employed, the mass(es) may demonstrate marked and heterogeneous enhancement (Fig. 4.12).

In patients with hematologic malignancies and in immunodepressed patients with transplants or neoplasms, hepatosplenic candidiasis can mimic lymphoproliferative disease and only biopsies can distinguish reliably between the two pathologic findings. Often, renal candidiasis also can be seen. Under appropriate antifungal chemotherapy, these lesions get smaller and may disappear completely if treatment is successful. In diffuse hepatic and/or splenic candidiasis, the lesions tend to be of equal and often small size, are diffusely distributed throughout the parenchyma, and tend to have an

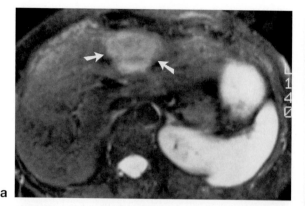

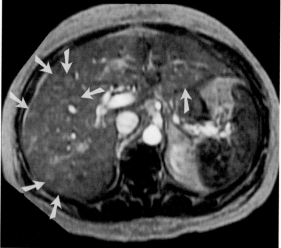

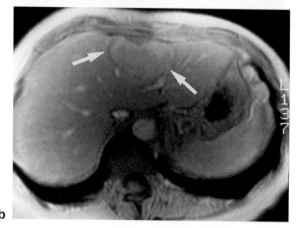

a

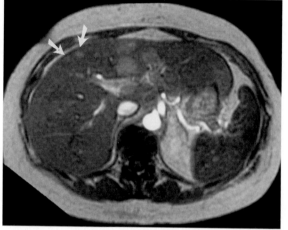

b

Fig. 4.12. a The T2-weighted spin-echo sequence shows a slightly heterogeneous lesion in the medial segment of the left lobe of the liver (*arrows*) in a patient with a histologically proven hepatic lymphoma. **b** The gadolinium-enhanced gradient-echo sequence reveals a densely but heterogeneously opacified lesion (*arrows*)

Fig. 4.13. a In a patient with known acute myelogenous leukemia and candida infection of the mouth and throat, multiple small high signal intensity foci (*arrows*) of similar size are seen throughout the liver. These lesions demonstrated some enhancement after gadolinium injection. Lymphoproliferative disease can present in a similar fashion. **b** Ten days after antifungal therapy, the liver shows only two lesions. While the appearance in **a** is not diagnostic of candida alone, the follow-up examination which reveals disappearance of most lesions is strong evidence of an infectious process, in this case hepatic candidiasis

enhancing rim with gadolinium enhancement. On T1-weighted spin-echo sequences, parenchymal candidiasis usually is poorly demonstrated, but on T2-weighted sequences it is readily identified as hyperintense lesions (Fig. 4.13). In patients with candidiasis or lymphoproliferative disease, iron oxide particles can help visualize even small lesions (5–10 mm). One study comparing CT and MRI (SEMELKA et al. 1992b) demonstrated that MRI can visualize hepatosplenic candidiasis more consistently.

disease, or hepatosplenic candidiasis. Except for candidiasis in the liver and/or spleen, where MRI has the edge, CT and MRI appear to provide similar results.

4.3.4.2
Results and Role of MRI

No data on large series are currently available which define the exact role or sensitivities of CT and MRI for detecting lymphoma, lymphoproliferative

4.4
Summary of the Role of MRI

While the debate as to which method is best for evaluating patients with suspected malignant liver lesions is ongoing, some recommendations can be made for the diagnostic workup. For metastases, MRI is slightly less accurate than helical CT, and for patients who are candidates for partial liver resection, CTAP should be used. In patients with cirrhosis and suspected HCC, MRI is the modality of choice as it does not suffer from perfusion artifacts, which can be prominent on CT and mimic the appearance of a tumor. In patients with angiosarcoma, cholangiocarcinoma, and lymphoma, MRI and CT are often equally accurate, but when a biopsy of a potential lesion is planned and/or indicated, CT is preferred. For hepatosplenic candidiasis, MRI may demonstrate lesions which are difficult to see with CT or US.

In the United States, because of its overall poor sensitivity and specificity (especially for lesions less than 10 mm in diameter), US is not used as the screening method for suspected focal liver lesions, but it is the primary screening method in patients with jaundice or with high clinical suspicion for gallbladder disease. CT provides fast scanning, volume acquisition, high resolution, easy reconstruction in multiple planes or 3D, and higher diagnostic confidence, all of which are obvious advantages for patient comfort and throughput and improved diagnoses. The advantages can justify the purchase of a CT unit even under current restrictions on health care costs.

While MR angiography has enjoyed great success in many vascular applications, its role has been challenged not only by color Doppler US but also by CT angiography. For the assessment of the liver, CT traditionally has been used as the primary technique because of its high sensitivity if performed in a state-of-the-art manner and because of its excellent evaluation of the remainder of the abdomen, particularly of neighboring structures and retroperitoneum. Its popularity has further increased with the introduction of helical CT, which has opened the door for many new applications such as CT arteriography, faithful 3D reconstruction, and improved monitoring of interventional procedures. With its ability to depict vascular structures in great detail, helical CT offers an alternative to the traditional role of US for the assessment of vascular pathology, although US continues to have the advantages that it does not need an intravenous contrast agent, does not use ionizing radiation, and is less costly. In addition, the lengthy reconstruction times for 3D CT angiography must to be considered.

With wider clinical use of liver-specific contrast agents, it is possible that MRI will become the primary modality for the diagnosis of malignant focal liver disease, particularly if faster sequences with echo planar MRI are employed.

References

Bartolozzi C, Lencioni R, Caramella D, Palla A, Bassi AM, Di Candio G (1996) Small hepatocellular carcinoma. Detection with US, CT, MR imaging, DSA, and Lipiodol-CT. Acta Radiol 37:69–74

Birnbaum BA, Weinreb JC, Fernandez MP, Brown JJ, Rofsky NM, Young SW (1994) Comparison of contrast enhanced CT and Mn-DPDP enhanced MRI for detection of focal hepatic lesions. Initial findings. Clin Imaging 18:21–27

Buetow PC, Buck JL, Ros PR, Goodman ZD (1994) Malignant vascular tumors of the liver: radiologic-pathologic correlation. Radiographics 14:153–166

Choi BI, Han MC, Kim CW (1990) Small hepatocellular carcinoma versus small cavernous hemangioma: differentiation with MR imaging at 2.0 T. Radiology 176:103–106

Choi BI, Han JK, Shin YM, Baek SY, Han MC (1995) Peripheral cholangiocarcinoma: comparison of MRI with CT. Abdom Imaging 20:357–360

De Santis M, Cristani A, Cioni G, Casolo A, Canossi G, Ventura E, Romagnoli R (1992) The magnetic resonance of small hepatocarcinoma. A comparison with echography, computed tomography, digital angiography and computed tomography with lipiodol. Radiologia Medica 84:587–595

Ebara M, Ohto M, Watanabe Y, et al. (1986) Diagnosis of small hepatocellular carcinoma: correlation of MR imaging and tumor histologic studies. Radiology 159:371–377

Egglin TK, Rummeny E, Stark DD, et al. (1990) Hepatic tumors: quantitative tissue characterization with MR imaging. Radiology 176:107–110

Freeny PC, Marks WM (1986) Patterns of contrast enhancement of benign and malignant hepatic neoplasms during bolus dynamic and delayed CT. Radiology 160:613–618

Freeny PC, Nghiem HV, Winter TC (1995) Helical CT during arterial portography: optimization of contrast enhancement and scanning parameters. Radiology 194:83–90

Fukuya T, Honda H, Murata S, et al. (1993) MRI of primary lymphoma of the liver. J Comput Assist Tomogr 17:596–598

Gazelle GS, Lee MJ, Hahn PF, Goldberg MA, Rafaat N, Mueller PR (1994) US, CT, and MRI of primary and secondary liver lymphoma. J Comput Assist Tomogr 18:412–415

Giovagnoni A, Terilli F, Ercolani P, Paci E, Piga A (1994) MR imaging of hepatic masses: diagnostic significance of wedge-shaped areas of increased signal intensity surrounding the lesion. Am J Roentgenol 163:1093–1097

Hamm B, Vogl TJ, Branding G, Schnell B, Taupitz M, Wolf KJ, Lissner J (1992) Focal liver lesions: MR imaging with Mn-DPDP-initial clinical results in 40 patients. Radiology 182:167–174

Hamm B, Thoeni RF, Gould RG, et al. (1994) Focal liver lesions: characterization with nonenhanced and dynamic contrast material-enhanced MR imaging. Radiology 190:417–423

Heiken JP, Weyman PJ, Lee JKT, Balfe DM, Picus D, Brunt EM, Flye MW (1989) Detection of focal hepatic masses: prospective evaluation with CT, delayed CT, CT during arterial portography, and MR imaging. Radiology 171:47–51

Hirai K, Aoki Y, Abe H, Nakashima O, Kojiro M, Tanikawa K (1991) Magnetic resonance imaging of small hepatocellular carcinoma. Am J Gastroenterol 86:205–209

Imaeda T, Kanematsu M, Mochizuki R, Goto H, Saji S, Shimokawa K (1994) Extracapsular invasion of small hepatocellular carcinoma: MR and CT findings. J Comput Assist Tomogr 18:755–760

Itoh K, Nishimura K, Togashi K, et al. (1987) Hepatocellular carcinoma: MR imaging. Radiology 164:21–25

Koslow SA, Davis PL, DeMarino GB, Peel RL, Baron RL, Van Thiel DH (1991) Hyperintense cirrhotic nodules on MRI. Gastrointest Radiol 16:339–341

Kudo M, Tomita S, Tochio H, et al. (1992) Small hepatocellular carcinoma: diagnosis with US angiography with intra-arterial CO_2 microbubbles. Radiology 182:155–160

Kuhlman J, Romanchuk K, Steinberg E, Fishman E (1994) Determination of hepatic resectability: a comparison of CT during arterial portography and MR. Do differences in test performance impact on surgical decision making? Annu Meet Int Soc Tech Assess Health Care 17:Abstract No. 050

Larson RE, Semelka RC, Bagley AS, Molina PL, Brown ED, Lee JK (1994) Hypervascular malignant liver lesions: comparison of various MR imaging pulse sequences and dynamic CT. Radiology 192:393–399

Li KC, Glazer GM, Quint LE, et al. (1988) Distinction of hepatic cavernous hemangioma from hepatic metastases with MR imaging. Radiology 169:409–415

Liou J, Lee JK, Borrello JA, Brown JJ (1994) Differentiation of hepatomas from nonbepatomatous masses: use of MnDPDP-enhanced MR images. Magn Reson Imaging 12:71–79

Matsui O, Takashima T, Kadoya M, et al. (1987) Liver metastases from colorectal cancers: detection with CT during arterial portography. Radiology 165:65–69

Mitchell DG, Rubin R, Siegelman ES, Burk DL Jr, Rifkin MD (1991) Hepatocellular carcinoma within siderotic regenerative nodules: appearance as a nodule within a nodule on MR images. Radiology 178:101–103

Murakami T, Nakamura H, Tsuda K, et al. (1995) Contrast-enhanced MR imaging of intrahepatic cholangio-carcinoma: pathologic correlation study. J Magn Reson Imaging 5:165–170

Napel S, Marks NP, Rubin GD, et al. (1992) CT angiography with spiral CT and maximum intensity projection. Radiology 185:607–610

Nelson RC, Chezmar JL, Steinberg HV, Torres WE, Baumgartner BR, Gedgaudas-McClees RK, Bernadino ME (1988) Focal hepatic lesions: detection by dynamic and delayed computed tomography versus short TE/TR spin echo and fast field echo magnetic resonance imaging. Gastrointest Radiol 13:115–122

Nelson RC, Chezmar JL, Sugarbaker PH, Bernardino ME (1989) Hepatic tumors: comparison of CT during arterial portography, delayed CT, and MR imaging for preoperative evaluation. Radiology 172:27–34

Nokes SR, Baker ME, Spritzer CE, et al. (1988) Hepatic adenoma: MR appearance mimicking focal nodular hyperplasia. J Comput Assist Tomogr 12:885–887

Ohtomo K, Itai Y, Yoshida H, et al. (1989) MR differentiation of hepatocellular carcinoma from cavernous hemangioma: complementary roles of FLASH and T2 values. Am J Roentgenol 152:505–507

Ohtomo K, Itai Y, Ohtomo Y, Shiga J, Iio M (1990) Regenerating nodules of liver cirrhosis: MR imaging with pathologic correlation. Am J Roentgenol 154:505–507

Ohtomo K, Araki T, Itai Y, et al. (1992) MR imaging of malignant mesenchymal tumors of the liver. Gastrointest Radiol 17:58–62

Paulson EK, Baker ME, Paine SS, Spritzer CE, Meyers WC (1994) Detection of focal hepatic masses: STIR MR vs. CT during arterial portography. J Comput Assist Tomogr 18:581–587

Powers C, Ros PR, Stoupis C, Johnson WK, Segel KH (1994) Primary liver neoplasms: MR imaging with pathologic correlation. Radiographics 14:459–482

Rofsky NM, Weinreb JC, Bernardino ME, Young SW, Lee JK, Noz ME (1993) Hepatocellular tumors: characterization with Mn-DPDP-enhanced MR imaging. Radiology 188:53–59

Ros PR, Lubbers PR, Olmstead WW, Morillo G (1987) Hemangioma of the liver: heterogeneous appearance on T2-wighted images. Am J Roentgenol 149:1167–1170

Rosenthal RE, Davis PL (1992) MR imaging of hepatocellular carcinoma at 1.5 Tesla. Gastrointest Radiol 17:49–52

Rummeny E, Weissleder R, Stark DD, et al. (1989a) Primary liver tumors: diagnosis by MR imaging. Am J Roentgenol 152:63–72

Rummeny E, Weissleder R, Sironi S, et al. (1989b) Central scars in primary liver tumors: MR features, specificity, and pathologic correlation. Radiology 171:323–326

Sadek AG, Mitchell DG, Siegelman ES, Outwater EK, Matteucci T, Hann HW (1995) Early hepatocellular carcinoma that develops within macroregenerative nodules: growth rate depicted at serial MR imaging. Radiology 195:753–756

Saini S, Edelman RR, Sharma P, et al. (1995) Blood-pool MR contrast material for detection and characterization of focal hepatic lesions: initial clinical experience with ultrasmall superparamagnetic iron oxide (AMI-227). Am J Roentgenol 164:1147–1152

Semelka RC, Shoenut JP, Kroeker MA, et al. (1992a) Focal liver disease: comparison of dynamic contrast-enhanced CT and T2-weighted fat-suppressed, FLASH, and dynamic gadolinium-enhanced MR imaging at 1.5 T. Radiology 184:687–694

Semelka RC, Shoenut JP, Greenberg HM, Bow EJ (1992b) Detection of acute and treated lesions of hepatos-plenic candidiasis: comparison of dynamic contrast-enhanced CT and MR imaging. J Magn Reson Imaging 2:341–345

Shimamoto K, Sakuma S, Ishigaki T, et al. (1992) Hepatocellular carcinoma: evaluation with color Doppler US and MR imaging. Radiology 182:149–154

Soyer P (1994) Capsular retraction of the liver in malignant tumor of the biliary tract MRI findings. Clin Imaging 18:255–257

Soyer P, Levesque M, Caudron C, Elias D, Zeitoun G, Roche A (1993a) MRI of liver metastases from colorectal cancer vs. CT during arteria portography. J Comput Assist Tomogr 17:67–74

Soyer P, Van Beers B, Grandin C, Pringot J, Levesque M (1993b) Primary lymphoma of the liver: MR findings. Eur J Rodiol 16:209–212

Soyer P, Bluemke DA, Sibert A, Laissy JP (1995a) MR imaging of intrahepatic cholangiocarcinoma. Abdom Imaging 20:126–130

Soyer P, Bluemke DA, Reichle R, Calhoun PS, Bliss DF, Scherrer A, Fishman EK (1995b) Imaging of intrahepatic cholangiocarcinoma. 2. Hilar cholangiocarcinoma. Am J Roentgenol 165:1433–1436

Soyer P, de Givry SC, Gueye C, Lenormand S, Somveille E, Scherrer A (1996) Detection of focal hepatic lesions with MR imaging: prospective comparison of T2-weighted fast spin-echo with and without fat suppression, T2-weighted breath-hold fast spin-echo, and gadolinium chelate-enhanced 3D gradient-recalled imaging. Am J Roentgenol 166:1115–1121

Stevens WR, Johnson CD, Stephens DH, Nagorney DM (1995) Fibrolamellar hepatocellular carcinoma: stage at presentation and results of aggressive surgical management. Am J Roentgenol 164:1153–1158

Thoeni RF (1991a) Clinical applications of magnetic resonance of the liver. Invest Radiol 26:266–273

Thoeni RF, Sica G, Shyn P (1991b) MR imaging: Detection of hepatocellular carcinoma in patients with liver cirrhosis. Radiology 181(P):290

Ueda K, Kitagawa K, Kadoya M, Matsui O, Takashima T, Yomahana T (1995) Detection of hypervascular hepatocellular carcinoma by using spiral volumetric CT: comparison of US and MR imaging. Abdom Imaging 20:547–553

Urban BA, Fishman EK, Kuhlman JE, et al. (1993) Detection of focal hepatic lesions with spiral CT: comparison of 4- and 8-mm interscan spacing. Am J Roentgenol 160:783–785

Urhahn R, Adam G, Keulers P, Kilbinger M, Gunther RW (1996) Detectability of focal liver lesions: comparison of MRI at 1.5 T and dynamic spiral CT. Rofo Fortschr Geb Rontgenstr Neuen Bildgeb Verfahr 164:301–307

Van Beers B, Demeure R, Pringot J, et al. (1990) Dynamic spin-echo imaging with Gd-DTPA: value in the differentiation of hepatic tumors. Am J Roentgenol 154:515–519

Ward J, Baudouin CJ, Ridgway JP, Robinson PJ (1995) Magnetic resonance imaging in the detection of focal liver lesions: comparison of dynamic contrast-enhanced TurboFLASH and T2 weighted spin echo images. Br J Radiol 68:463–470

Wittenberg J, Ferrucci JT, Stark DD, et al. (1988) Differentiation of hepatic metastases from hepatic cysts and hemangiomas by using MR imaging. Am J Roentgenol 151:79–84

Zeman RK, Fox SH, Silverman PM, et al. (1993) Helical (spiral) CT of the abdomen. Am J Roentgenol 160:719–725

5 Spleen

R.C. Semelka and H.B. Marcos

CONTENTS

5.1
Magnetic Resonance Imaging Techniques

Most splenic lesions are hypointense on T1-weighted images and hyperintense on T2-weighted images. This appearance tends to parallel the signal intensity of the spleen, rendering detection of splenic lesions difficult. Breath-hold spoiled gradient echo (SGE) acquired immediately after administration of gadolinium DTPA is an effective technique in the evaluation of the spleen. The majority of splenic lesions enhance less than background spleen on these images, which improves their conspicuity.

Normal spleen enhances in a serpiginous or arciform pattern within 1 min postcontrast (Fig. 5.1). This appearance correlates with the anatomic structure of the spleen with division into fast and slow channels. Blood traversing through filtration process in splenic cords is termed open circulation or slow channels and appears as bands of lower signal on immediate postgadolinium images. Blood traversing

through capillaries in the splenic sinuses into splenic veins is termed closed circulation or fast channels and appears as bands of higher signal on immediate postgadolinium images. Arciform enhancement is the pattern of enhancement of normal spleen in nondiseased patients and in some patients with inflammatory or neoplastic diseases. Uniform high signal intensity is seen in patients with inflammatory or malignant diseases or patients who have undergone chemotherapy (Hamed et al. 1992; Mirowitz et al. 1991; Semelka et al. 1992b; Weiss 1983). Diffuse low signal intensity of the spleen on immediate postgadolinium images is seen in all patients who have had multiple blood transfusions within 1 year, due to T2* effect of hemosiderin (Siegelman et al. 1991, 1996).

5.2
Splenomegaly

Splenomegaly is observed in a number of disease states such as portal hypertension, connective tissue disease, leukemia, lymphoma, metastases, and various infections. The commonest cause of splenomegaly is portal hypertension.

Arciform or uniform high signal intensity enhancement on immediate postgadolinium images is an important observation that is consistent with portal hypertension and excludes the presence of malignant disease (Fig. 5.2).

5.3
Trauma

The spleen is the most commonly ruptured abdominal organ in the setting of trauma. Splenic injury may take several forms such as subcapsular hematoma, contusion or laceration, and infarction. Subcapsular hematoma or intraparenchymal hematoma secondary to contusion or laceration demonstrates a time course of changes in signal intensity due to the

R.C. Semelka, MD, Director of MR Services and Associate Professor of Radiology, Deparment of Radiology, University of North Carolina, Chapel Hill, NC 27599-7510, USA
H.B. Marcos, MD, Clinical Research Fellow in MR Services, Department of Radiology, University of North Carolina, Chapel Hill, NC 27599-7510, USA

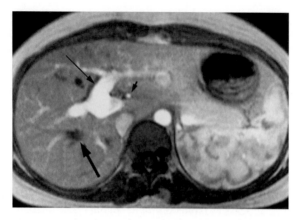

Fig. 5.1. Arciform enhancement in the normal spleen. Note the serpiginous, tubular band of low signal intensity throughout the splenic parenchyma. The presence of contrast in the portal vein (*long arrow*) and hepatic arteries (*small arrow*) and the lack of contrast in hepatic veins (*large arrow*) define the capillary phase of enhancement. The portal vein is prominent, which is an incidental finding

paramagnetic properties of the degradation products of hemoglobin. Subacute hemorrhage demonstrates a high signal intensity on T1- and T2-weighted images (Fig. 5.3). Traumatic injury of the spleen, especially devascularization, is well seen on immediate postgadolinium SGE images. Areas of devascularization are near signal void compared with the high signal intensity of the normal vascularized tissue.

5.4
Infection

The most common viruses involving the spleen are Epstein-Barr virus, varicella, and cytomegalovirus. Viral infection may be associated with splenomegaly. Nonviral infections that involve the spleen in patients with a normal immune status include

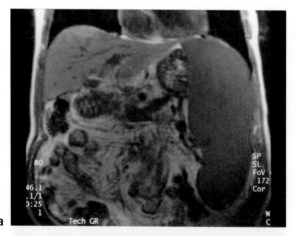

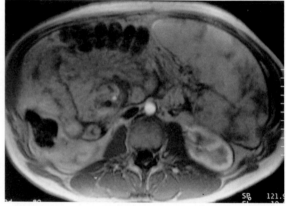

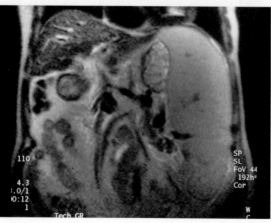

Fig. 5.2 a–c. Splenomegaly secondary to portal hypertension. Coronal T1-weighted SGE (**a**), immediate postgadolinium T1-weighted SGE (**b**), and coronal T2-weighted HASTE (**c**) images. Massive splenomegaly is demonstrated on all MR images. The presence of arciform enhancement on the immediate postgadolinium SGE image (**b**) excludes the presence of malignant disease

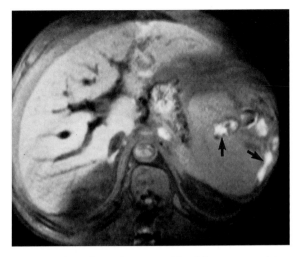

Fig. 5.3. Splenic laceration. T1-weighted fat-suppressed image demonstrating high signal intensity fluid in an intraparenchymal and subcapsular location in the spleen, consistent with subacute blood (*arrows*)

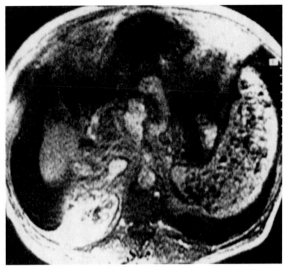

Fig. 5.4. Focal iron deposition in the spleen (Gamna-Gandy bodies). Postgadolinium T1- weighted SGE image. Multiple small signal void foci are present in the spleen and result in susceptibility artifact

histoplasmosis, tuberculosis, and echinococcosis. In immunocompromised patients the most common hepatosplenic infection is fungal infection with *Candida albicans*. Acute lesions are generally more apparent in the spleen than in the liver, while the reverse is true for subacute treated and chronic healed lesions. Magnetic resonance images can demonstrate lesions in the acute phase, the subacute treated phase, and the chronic healed phase (SEMELKA et al. 1992a). In the acute phase, hepatosplenic candidiasis results in well-defined small abscesses in the spleen and liver. These lesions are well shown on T2-weighted fat-suppressed images as high signal intensity foci. They may also be visible on postgadolinium images, but usually are not visualized on precontrast SGE images. Magnetic resonance imaging should be used routinely in the investigation of hepatosplenic candidiasis.

5.5
Gamna-Gandy Bodies

Gamna-Gandy bodies are commonly seen in patients with liver cirrhosis and portal hypertension. Gamna-Gandy bodies are foci of iron deposition in splenic parenchyma due to intraparenchymal hemorrhage (Fig. 5.4).

The lesions are of low signal intensity or signal void in all T1- and T2-weighted images and result in

susceptibility artifact that is well shown on gradient-echo images.

5.6
Malignant Lesions

5.6.1
Lymphoma

The most common malignancy affecting the spleen is lymphoma, which can be either of the Hodgkin's or the non-Hodgkin's type. The spleen is usually enlarged; however, lymphoma may also involve normal-sized spleens.

Lymphoma may also appear as a large mass in the left upper quadrant involving the spleen, stomach, pancreas, and adrenal glands (BRAGG et al. 1986; CASTELLINO 1986). Conventional unenhanced spin-echo magnetic resonance imaging has had only limited success in imaging lymphomatous involvement of the spleen. Immediate postgadolinium SGE images, however, surpass computed tomography for evaluation of lymphoma. Immediate postgadolinium images show large irregularly enhancing regions of high and low signal intensity representing diffuse infiltration (Fig. 5.5) or focal low signal intensity mass lesions scattered throughout the spleen. The signal intensity of lymphomatous lesions rapidly equilibrates with background spleen and by 1–

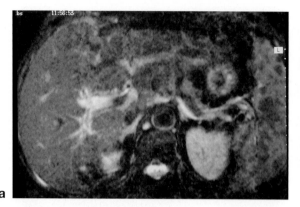

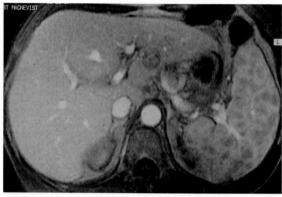

Fig. 5.5 a,b. Diffuse infiltration with lymphoma. T2-weighted fat-suppressed turbo spin-echo (**a**) and immediate postgadolinium SGE (**b**) images. Large irregular regions of low signal intensity on the T2-weighted image are identified in the spleen (**a**), and enhance minimally on the postgadolinium image (**b**)

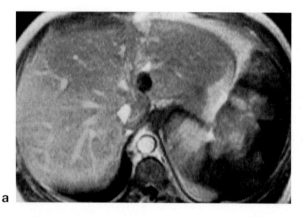

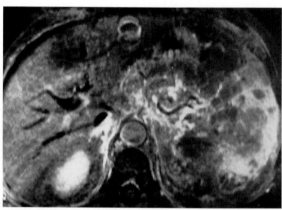

Fig. 5.6 a,b. Diffuse lymphoma. Immediate postgadolinium SGE image (**a**) and interstitial phase gadolinium-enhanced fat-suppressed spin-echo (**b**) image in a second patient. Large irregular regions of increased or diminished enhancement are present in the spleen, consistent with diffuse infiltration

2 min postcontrast they approach isointensity. On T1-weighted images, lymphomatous lesions are usually minimally hypointense to isointense. On T2-weighted images, masses are usually isointense to mildly hyperintense. Occasionally masses are hypointense on T2-weighted images (Fig. 5.6) which may be a distinguishing feature between focal lymphomatous deposits and metastases, since the latter are usually isointense to hyperintense.

Superparamagnetic particles can also improve the accuracy of diagnosis of splenic lymphoma. This contrast agent is selectively taken up by reticuloendothelial system (RES) cells, and not by malignant cells, improving tumor – spleen contrast. Normal spleen is rendered low in signal intensity on T2-weighted images while the signal intensity of mass lesions is unchanged, resulting in a relatively high signal intensity of lesions (WEISSLEDER et al. 1989).

5.6.2
Metastases

Splenic metastases occur most often in the setting of advanced malignant disease. Metastases appear as discrete nodules or aggregate masses of tumor that have a propensity to disrupt the normal splenic architecture. Primary tumors most likely to involve the spleen are malignant melanoma, breast cancer, lung

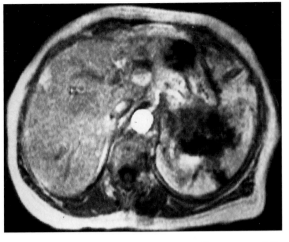

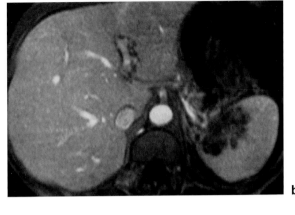

Fig. 5.7 a,b. Splenic metastases. Immediate postgadolinium SGE image (a) in a patient with splenic metastases from macrocystic adenocarcinoma of the pancreas. Multiple low signal intensity metastatic lesions are seen in the spleen. An interstitial phase postgadolinium fat-suppressed SGE image (b) in a second patient with ovarian cancer demonstrates a heterogeneous, minimally enhanced mass in the splenic hilum

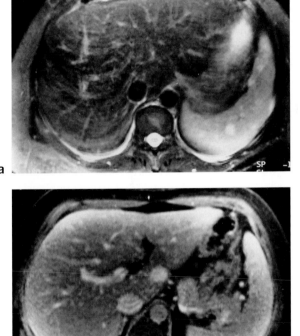

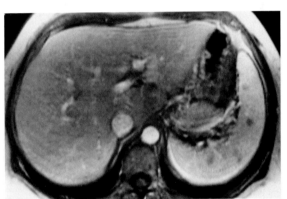

Fig. 5.8 a–c. Splenic hemangiomas. T2-weighted fat-suppressed spin-echo (a), immediate postgadolinium SGE (b), and 90-s fat-suppressed SGE (c) images. Multiple small moderately hyperintense lesions are present on the T2-weighted fat-suppressed image (a). Peripheral enhancement is seen on the immediate postgadolinium image (b), and enhancement progresses to uniform fill-in on the 90-s postcontrast image (c)

cancer, and islet cell tumor (FREEMAN and TONKIN 1976; PIEKARSKI et al. 1980).

On T1-weighted images metastases are usually minimally hypointense to isointense with spleen. If metastases are hemorrhagic or result in hemorrhage then they may appear hyperintense on T1-weighted images. Metastases are isointense to mildly hyperintense on T2-weighted images. On immediate postgadolinium SGE images, metastases appear low in signal intensity (Fig. 5.7). Metastases rapidly equilibrate with splenic parenchyma and may become isointense by 1 min postcontrast.

Superparamagnetic iron oxide particles render metastases higher in signal intensity than background spleen, reflecting uptake by the RES system and lack of uptake by metastatic deposits (WEISSLEDER et al. 1988, 1989).

5.7
Benign Lesions

5.7.1
Hemangiomas

Hemangiomas are the most common benign splenic lesions, although they are uncommon (DISLER and CHEW 1991). Splenic hemangiomas usually are small, <2 cm in diameter. Splenic hemangiomas are mildly hypointense to isointense on T1-weighted images and mildly to moderately hyperintense on T2-weighted images. Hemangiomas are likely similar in signal intensity to hepatic hemangiomas; however, their signal intensity differences are less due to the similar signal intensity of the background organ.

Three patterns of contrast enhancement are observed for splenic hemangiomas (RAMANI et al. 1995): (a) immediate homogeneous persistent enhancement, (b) peripheral enhancement with progression to uniform enhancement on delayed images, and (c) peripheral enhancement with centripetal progression and persistence of a central scar. These patterns of enhancement are similar to those observed with hepatic hemangiomas. Peripheral enhancement in splenic hemangiomas usually does not appear as well-defined nodules of contrast (Fig. 5.8), as is seen with hepatic hemangiomas.

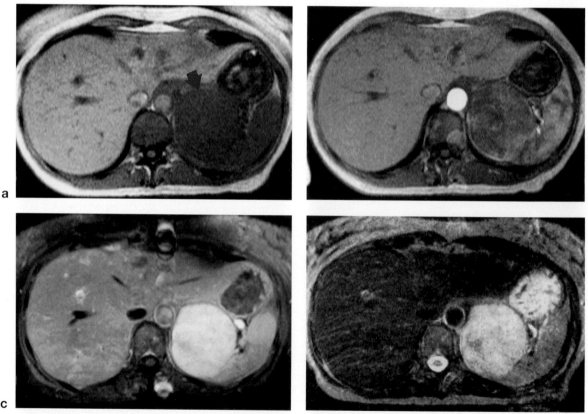

Fig. 5.9 a–d. Hamartoma. T1-weighted SGE (**a**), immediate postgadolinium SGE (**b**), interstitial phase gadolinium-enhanced fat-suppressed spin-echo (**c**), and T2-weighted fat-suppressed (**d**) images. A large mass lesion (*arrow*, **a**) arises from the posterior aspect of the mid portion of the spleen. The mass is low in signal intensity on the T1-weighted image (**a**), demonstrates diffuse heterogeneous enhancement on the immediate postgadolinium SGE image (**b**), and is moderately high in signal intensity on the interstitial phase gadolinium-enhanced T1-weighted fat-suppressed image (**c**). The tumor is also high in signal intensity on the T2-weighted fat-suppressed image (**d**)

5.7.2
Hamartomas

Splenic hamartomas are rare benign lesions. Hamartomas tend to be large, measuring >4 cm in diameter. They have intermediate signal intensity on T1-weighted images and moderately high signal intensity on T2-weighted images.

On immediate postgadolinium SGE images, hamartomas enhance in a relatively intense diffuse heterogeneous fashion (Fig. 5.9) (PINTO et al. 1995; OHTOMO et al. 1992). Enhancement becomes progressively more uniform on more delayed images.

5.7.3
Cysts

Cysts are relatively common benign splenic lesions (URRUTIN et al. 1996). Three types of splenic cysts occur: (a) posttraumatic (pseudocyst), (b) epidermoid cyst, and (c) hydatid cyst. Pseudocysts are the most common type of cyst (DACHMAN et al. 1986) .

Cysts are moderately to mildly hypointense on T1-weighted images and moderately hyperintense on T2-weighted images. Cysts that are complicated by protein or hemorrhage may have regions of high signal intensity on T1-weighted images or regions of mixed signal intensity on T2-weighted images. Cysts do not enhance after contrast administration (SHIRKHODA et al. 1995). The observation that lesions do not enhance on serial postcontrast images and do not change in size or shape between early and late images confirms that they represent cysts (Fig. 5.10).

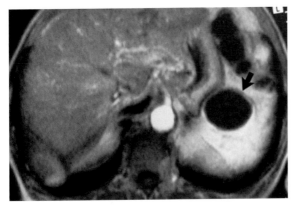

Fig. 5.10. Splenic cyst. Immediate postgadolinium SGE image demonstrates a signal-void cystic lesion (*arrow*). The cyst is sharply demarcated following contrast administration

5.8
Summary

Magnetic resonance imaging detects and characterizes a wide range of splenic lesions. Serial postgadolinium SGE images are useful, and the images acquired immediately following gadolinium administration constitute the most important set of postgadolinium images. Iron oxide particles improve lesion detection and may have a future role in the detection of splenic involvement by lymphoma and metastatic disease.

References

Bragg DG, Colby TV, Ward JH (1986) New concepts in the non-Hodgkin lymphoma: radiologic implications. Radiology 159:289–304

Castellino RA (1986) Hodgkin disease: practical concepts for the diagnostic radiologist. Radiology 159:305–310

Dachman AH, Ros PR, Murari PJ, Olmsted WW, Lichtenstein JE (1986) Nonparasitic splenic cysts: a report of 52 cases with radiologic-pathologic correlation. AJR 147:537–542

Disler DG, Chew FS (1991) Splenic hemangioma. AJR 157:44

Freeman MH, Tonkin AK (1976) Focal splenic defects. Radiology 121:689–692

Hamed MM, Hamm B, Ibrahim ME, Taupitz M, Mahfour AE (1992) Dynamic MR imaging of the abdomen with gadopentetate dimeglumine: normal enhancement patterns of the liver, spleen, stomach, and pancreas. AJR 158:303–307

Mirowitz SA, Brown JJ, Lee JKT, Heiken JP (1991) Dynamic gadolinium-enhanced MR imaging of the normal spleen: normal enhancement patterns and evaluation of splenic lesions. Radiology 179:681–686

Ohtomo K, Fukudo H, Mori K, et al. (1992) CT and MR appearances of splenic hamartoma. J Comput Assist Tomogr 16:425–428

Piekarski J, Federle MP, Moss AA, London SS (1980) CT of the spleen. Radiology 135:683–689

Pinto PD, Avidago P, Garcia H, Aves FC, Marques C (1995) Splenic hamartoma: a case report. Eur Radiol 5:93–95

Ramani M, Reinhold C, Semelka RC, Siegelman ES, Liang L, Ascher SM, Brown JJ, Eisen RN, Bret PM (1997) Splenic hemangiomas and hamartomas: MR imaging characteristics of 28 lesions. Radiology 202:166–172

Semelka RC, Shoenut JP, Greenberg HM, Bow EJ (1992a) Detection of acute and treated lesions of hepatosplenic candidiasis: comparison of dynamic contrast-enhanced CT and MR imaging. J Magn Reson 2:341–345

Semelka RC, Shoenut JP, Lawrence PH, Greenberg HM, Madden TP, Kroeker MA (1992b) Spleen: dynamic enhancement patterns on gradient-echo MR images enhanced with gadopentetate dimeglumine. Radiology 185:479–482

Shirkhoda A, Freeman J, Armin AR, Cacciarelli AA, Morden R (1995) Imaging features of splenic epidermoid cyst with pathologic correlation. Abdom Imaging 20:449–451

Siegelman ES, Mitchell DG, Rubin R, et al. (1991) Parenchymal versus reticuloendothelial iron overload in the liver: distinction with MR imaging. Radiology 179:361–366

Siegelman ES, Mitchell DG, Semelka RC (1996) Abdominal iron deposition metabolism, MR findings, and clinical importance. Radiology 199:13–22

Urrutin M, Mergo PJ, Ros LH, Torres GM, Ros PR (1996) Cystic masses of the spleen: radiologic-pathologic correlation. Radiographics 16:107–129

Weiss L (1983) The red pulp of the spleen: structural basis of blood flow. Clin Haematol 12:375–395

Weissleder R, Hahn PF, Stark DD, et al. (1988) Superparamagnetic iron oxide: enhanced detection of focal splenic tumors with MR imaging. Radiology 169:399–403

Weissleder R, Elizondo G, Stark DD, et al. (1989) The diagnosis of splenic lymphoma by MR imaging: value of superparamagnetic iron oxide. AJR 153:175–180

6 Biliary System

N. Holzknecht and T. Helmberger

6.1 Introduction

Screening for diseases of the biliary system demands examination modalities with high sensitivity and tolerable specificity combined with wide availability and low costs. Magnetic resonance imaging (MRI) examinations are expensive compared with most other diagnostic tests and are not widely available. Therefore MRI should only be used in conjunction with positive screening tests like laboratory findings and ultrasonography (US). For economic reasons, US is definitely the first choice in noninvasive diagnostics of the biliary system. When US findings are unclear, computed tomography (CT) is used additionally as a noninvasive test.

In the past, it was important to recognize additional biliary pathology on MRI scans that were obtained for other reasons. The advent of fast and ultrafast imaging techniques has led to a significant improvement in image quality, especially in the upper abdomen. Therefore, familiarity with the faster imaging techniques and contrast manipulation options is important for the radiologist, permitting the recognition and solution of diagnostic problems less well addressed by other modalities.

Well-known advantages of MRI over CT are the excellent soft tissue contrast and the multiplanar imaging capability. However, MRI does have limitations: spatial and time resolution are lower than with CT, and cost per examination is higher. "Conventional" spin-echo (SE) techniques allow for T1- and T2-weighted scans of the upper abdomen with acquisition times ranging from 5 to 20 min. These scan times result in motion artifacts arising from respiration, cardiovascular pulsation, and bowel movement. This is especially true in the upper abdomen (CHEZMAR 1991). The improved hardware and software of current MR systems have allowed for the implementation of fast and ultrafast imaging sequences such as echo planar imaging (EPI) and echo planar hybrid imaging (fast SE, RARE, HASTE). The combination of fast imaging techniques and contrast manipulation has led to an armamentarium of imaging sequences which have mostly been developed for specific applications like MR angiography or MR cholangiography or for other well-defined purposes.

Against this background, there is no general application for MRI in the diagnosis of biliary disease. Regarding the staging of biliary diseases, multiplanar imaging, for example, might be appropriate in selected cases in which MRI might be superior to CT, but in general CT remains the staging modality of choice. MR cholangiography, as a new and very promising technique, has to be compared with other established tests such as endoscopic retrograde cholangiopancreatography (ERCP) and percutaneous transhepatic cholangiography (PTC). Other diagnostic modalities, e.g., functional tests of the biliary system, might be enhanced by the

N. Holzknecht, MD, Department of Diagnostic Radiology, Klinikum Großhadern, Ludwig-Maximilians University, Marchioninistrasse 15, D-81377 München, Germany
T. Helmberger, MD, Department of Diagnostic Radiology, Klinikum Großhadern, Ludwig-Maximilians University, Marchioninistrasse 15, D-81377 Munich, Germany

introduction of biliary targeted contrast agents, which are currently under clinical investigation.

The aim of this chapter is to discuss specific applications of biliary MRI, and in particular MR cholangiography, and to present the MR appearance of biliary variants and pathologic processes.

6.2
MRI Techniques and Contrast Agents

The selection of a suitable imaging sequence depends on the available scanner hardware and software, but even more on the diagnostic task. Solid biliary processes such as cholangiocarcinoma have moderately prolonged T1- and T2 relaxation times. Therefore, sequences with moderate T1 and T2 weighting provide sufficient differentiation of these processes from normal tissue. The sequences for the delineation and differentiation of solid biliary lesions do not differ from those suitable for other abdominal processes. Consequently these sequences are discussed only briefly.

In contrast, imaging of biliary fluid (MR cholangiography) relies on the use of heavily T2-weighted sequences emphasizing the high water content of the bile. A broad spectrum of imaging sequences are employed for MR cholangiography, and their advantages and drawbacks will be discussed in more detail below. A short discussion of

biliary contrast media, currently undergoing clinical trials for hepatic imaging, is also included.

6.2.1
T1-Weighted Sequences

T1-weighted SE sequences typically obtain a 2D imaging volume in a scan time of 3–5 min. Shortening of the measurement time is restricted mainly by technical limitations in respect of shortening the echo time (TE) and the number of slices that can be obtained with a given repetition time (TR) using the multislice technique. Therefore, this sequence type always results in a certain incidence of motion artifacts, caused by respiratory, cardiac, and bowel movement (Fig. 6.1a). When using the multislice technique, fast or turbo SE techniques are not a very adequate way of accelerating the acquisition process, because increasing the echo train length will decrease the number of slices available at a specific T1-weighted repetition time.

Gradient-echo (GRE) techniques like FLASH (fast low angle shot) use gradients to refocus the MR signal, which is produced with lower angle excitation pulses. The result is an effective shortening of TE and TR, leading to significantly shorter acquisition times. Spoiler pulses are necessary between excitations to eliminate T2* contrast resulting from remaining transverse magnetization, an important characteris-

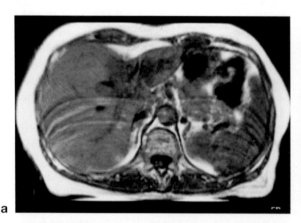

a

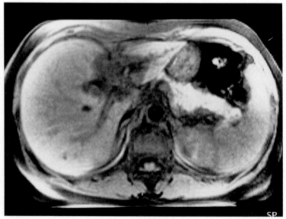

b

Fig. 6.1 a,b. Fifty-two year old female with a central cholangiocellular carcinoma. **a** T1-weighted SE sequence (TR 440 ms; TE 12 ms; 4 acquisitions; imaging time for 20 slices with 8 mm slice thickness, 4.17 min) following administration of 0.1 mmol Gd-DTPA. The central cholangiocellular carcinoma is delineated with lower signal intensity, and surrounding slightly dilated biliary ducts are seen. The relatively long acquisition time causes motion artifacts, which spread along the phase-encoding direction (anterior-posterior). **b** T1-weighted FLASH (spoiled GRE) sequence (TR 140 ms; TE 4.8 ms; flip angle 70°; 1 acquisition; imaging time for 18 slices with 8 mm slice thickness, 20 s during breath-hold). There are clearly less motion artifacts and enhanced sensitivity to contrast medium. The cholangiocellular carcinoma is delineated with low signal intensity, and dilated biliary ducts can be better seen, accompanied by portal venous vessels

tic of FLASH (or spoiled GRE). When this technique is used with one excitation and the scanner system allows for echo times <5 ms, acquisition covering the upper abdomen can be done within one breath-hold. We typically use FLASH with TR 140 ms, TE 4.8 ms, flip angle 70°, and 5–8 mm slice thickness, and acquire 18 slices in a 20-s breath-hold (Fig. 6.1b) on a 1.5-T scanner system (Magnetom Vision, Siemens, Erlangen). In uncooperative or severely ill patients, acquisition can be further shortened to 10 s with nine slices and a TR of 70 ms. Using this sequence type for T1-weighted imaging in combination with a flexible phase array body coil (four segments), image noise can be reduced by 300% and image quality is additionally enhanced due to increased signal- and contrast-to-noise ratios (GAUGER et al. 1996).

Faster gradient-echo imaging sequences like turbo FLASH (snapshot GRE) use even shorter TR/TE times. For optimal signal reception, flip angles of 5–10° have to be used. This results in a proton density weighting and necessitates signal preparation techniques. T1-weighted preparation pulses using an inversion technique make possible T1-weighted contrast. Generally, this sequence type has a different contrast behavior and a lower signal-to-noise ratio compared with FLASH. It has a role in fast contrast-enhanced dynamic imaging (one to two images per second) and in uncooperative patients.

6.2.2
Moderately and Heavily T2-Weighted (MRC) Sequences

T2-weighted SE sequences have a typical acquisition time of 5–10 min (Fig. 6.2a). This usually results in a significant rate of motion artifacts, especially in less cooperative patients.

The refocusing of multiple echoes from every excitation pulse is an effective way to reduce acquisition time [fast spin-echo (FSE) or turbo spin echo (TSE)]. The so-called echo train is represented by the number of echoes collected after each excitation. T2-weighted imaging with an echo train length (ETL) of five to nine echoes can be achieved within 2 min (Fig. 6.2b), while longer echo trains of up to 29 enable breath-hold acquisition in less than 20 s (Fig. 6.2c). The collection of all echoes following a single excitation was first introduced by HENNIG et al. (1986) and termed "rapid acquisition with relaxation enhancement" (RARE). The combination of RARE with read-

ing only half of the k-space (half-Fourier imaging) halves the scan time and was introduced as the half-Fourier single-shot turbo spin-echo (HASTE) technique (Fig. 6.2d) (LAUB et al. 1995; SANANES et al. 1995).

Due to artifact reduction and ease of use, breath-hold T2-weighted imaging (e.g., TSE with ETL 29, TR 3300 ms, TE 105 ms, flip angle 180°, 11 slices in 17 s breath-hold at 5–8 mm slice thickness) or snapshot HASTE (ETL 72, echo spacing 4.3 ms, effective TE 60 ms, flip angle 140°, 1.4 s per slice, typically 17 slices in 19 s) should be preferred for imaging of solid processes adjacent to the biliary system. The application of these techniques is determined by the shortest echo time available on the scanner system, because longer echo times prevent the collection of late echoes with a sufficient signal. Due to both the high sensitivity to susceptibility effects and the low spatial resolution, ultrafast EPI sequences are not routinely used for imaging of the upper abdomen.

The concept of MR cholangiopancreatography (MRCP) is based on the use of heavily T2-weighted pulse sequences emphasizing structures with very long T2 relaxation times such as bile fluid. Fat (intermediate T2 relaxation time) and solid organs such as the liver and pancreas (short T2 relaxation times) present with very low signal intensities on these strongly T2-weighted imaging sequences. Additional contrast of the bile fluid can be obtained by spectral or inversion fat suppression techniques. Furthermore, flowing blood and rapidly flowing cerebrospinal fluid are not displayed due to flow void phenomena. Thus, the portal and hepatic veins present a signal void, which facilitates differentiation between the biliary system and vascular structures. Some smaller peripheral branches of the hepatic and portal veins are depicted with intermediate signal intensity, if excited blood does not leave the imaging plane before readout of the signal.

The different sequence types and variants that are used for MRCP reflect the variety of available soft- and hardware. There are reports of adequate results with many techniques; thus MRCP can be implemented on almost every currently available scanner. However, there are also clear differences between these techniques.

6.2.2.1
Gradient-Echo Techniques

Wallner, Schumacher, and co-workers were the first to apply a steady state free precession (SSFP) GRE

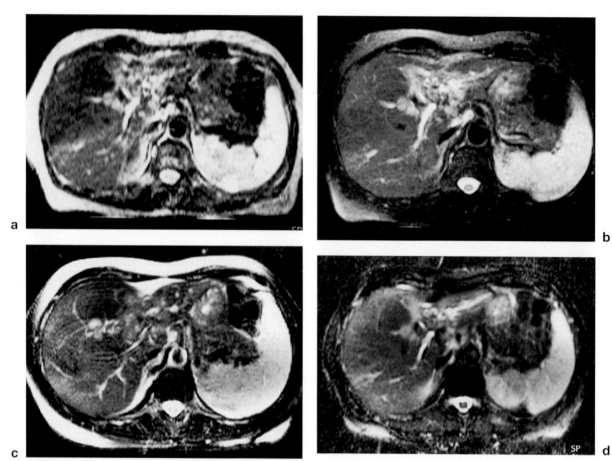

Fig. 6.2 a–d. Fifty-two year old female with a central cholangiocellular carcinoma. **a** T2-weighted SE sequence (TR 2200 ms; TE 90 ms; 2 acquisitions; imaging time for 20 slices with 8 mm slice thickness, 7.06 min). Respiratory motion during acquisition results in diffuse elevation of liver signal intensity, which reduces the quality of visualization of peripheral blood vessels and biliary ducts. **b** T2-weighted TSE sequence acquired without breath-hold (TR 4000 ms; TE 90 ms; 2 acquisitions; imaging time for 20 slices with 8 mm slice thickness, 4.09 min). Using this TSE sequence, the acquisition time can be clearly shortened, but still no intrahepatic ducts of second order are adequately visualized. **c** T2-weighted breath-hold TSE sequence (TR 2400 ms; TE 138 ms; 1 acquisition; imaging time for 11 slices with 8 mm slice thickness, 11 s during breath-hold). The ETL of 29 allows for clear reduction of imaging time. Breath-hold acquisition permits elimination of motion artifacts, but contrast of the tumor is inferior to that achieved with non-breath-hold techniques. **d** T2-weighted breath-hold HASTE sequence (TR 8000 ms; TE 82 ms; 1 acquisition; imaging time for 20 slices with 8 mm slice thickness, 16 s during breath-hold). Snapshot HASTE allows for acquisition of single slices in approximately 1 s, thus eliminating motion artifacts effectively. Contrast is comparable to that with non-breath-hold techniques; peripheral bile ducts are visualized

technique for the evaluation of the biliary tree (SCHUMACHER et al. 1991; WALLNER et al. 1991). They investigated five volunteers and 13 patients with obstructive jaundice with this technique within a breath-hold of 12 s. Unlike in a normal SSFP sequence, they used a time inverted variant with TE = 2 TR, which produces a refocused and therefore T2-weighted echo; this GRE sequence type is named CE-FAST (contrast-enhanced fast acquisition in steady state) or PSIF (time inverted FISP = fast imaging in steady state precession). The authors reported effective detection of bile duct dilatation and assessment of the level of obstruction; however, parts of the biliary system below the obstruction and most normal ducts in volunteers could not be visualized. Limited resolution, partial volume effects, and flow effects were discussed as possible reasons for these limitations.

MORIMOTO et al. (1992) compared a 3D version of CE-FAST (or PSIF) and direct cholangiography (PTC) in 12 patients with malignancy-related obstructive jaundice. 3D acquisition allows for lower slice thickness with adequate signal-to-noise ratios compared with 2D CE-FAST. Morimoto et al.

reported a good correlation between 3D maximum intensity reconstructions (MIP) of MR images and percutaneous transhepatic cholangiography (PTC) with regard to dilatation and level of obstruction.

In several other studies this GRE technique has been used for MR cholangiography (HALL-CRAGGS et al. 1993; Low et al. 1994). All such studies have stressed the high sensitivity of the segmented GRE technique to motion artifacts when the patient is unable to achieve long breath-hold times. More importantly, there is a lack of visualization of nondilated parts of the biliary system, e.g., distal to an obstruction. This makes the determination of the length of stenosis or obstruction difficult. Although WALLNER et al. (1991) interpreted the signal loss from slowly flowing bile to be a possible reason for this effect, the limited spatial resolution of the CE-FAST sequence seems a more plausible explanation. Because CE-FAST images already have low signal-to-noise ratios, slice thickness cannot be further reduced.

Recently, EPI was tested for use as an MRCP technique (WIELOPOLSKI et al. 1995). The relatively low resolution with matrix sizes of 128^2 and the extreme sensitivity to susceptibility artifacts resulted in inferior image quality compared with newer breath-hold TSE variants. For these reasons, EPI currently does not seem suitable for the diagnosis of biliary diseases, but using concepts of EPI for further acceleration of TSE techniques may be an efficient way to develop even faster MRC sequences (WIELOPOLSKI et al. 1995).

6.2.2.2
Fast Spin-Echo Techniques

The use of FSE or TSE (RARE and HASTE) sequences with extremely short echo times permits acceptable breath-hold times. Like CE-FAST and PSIF, heavily T2-weighted FSE sequences depict bile fluid with high signal intensity while solid organs and flowing blood are depicted with low signal intensities.

Fast SE sequences offer several advantages compared with the GRE techniques. The increased signal intensities acquired by these sequences result in a higher contrast-to-noise ratio, allowing for thinner slice thickness in comparison to CE-FAST/PSIF (both 3D and 2D variants). FSE techniques are less sensitive to motion artifacts and flow effects than GRE techniques. Additionally, the signal is a more exact measurement of T2 relaxivity than with CE-

FAST (T2/T2*). Promising initial results were reported by GUIBAUD et al. (1994, 1995) and TAKEHARA et al. (1994). The comparison of 2D FSE and 3D CE-FAST by REINHOLD et al. (1995) showed significantly better results for 2D FSE techniques with regard to dilated and nondilated biliary ducts and the pancreatic duct.

A limitation of the available 2D FSE techniques is the minimum slice thickness of 2–3mm due to the current gradient restrictions. Recently 3D FSE sequences have become available, allowing for a slice thickness below 1mm. BARISH et al. (1995) and SOTO et al. (1995, 1996) used a T2-weighted 3D multislab FSE sequence with respiratory triggering. Using parameters of 5000/240 (TR/TE), an echo train of 31, and a matrix size of 256 × 192 with one signal acquisition, they were able to image a volume of 10cm in approximately 15min. Because FSE sequences are less sensitive to motion artifacts than GRE sequences, this technique should be preferred over 2D FSE, when the patient is not able to hold his breath during 2D FSE acquisition.

Recent technical advances have improved the image quality of MRC. Gradient moment nulling implemented in FSE significantly reduces the motion artifacts resulting from periodic motion such as respiration and vessel pulsation. These artifacts normally degrade image quality in the phase-encoding direction.

In general, the signal-to-noise ratio and consequently also the contrast-to-noise ratio, of MRC images is enhanced using a surface coil; however, the field of view may be limited [a flexible shoulder coil is used for MRP (TAKEHARA et al. 1994)]. If a multichannel acquisition and a phased array multicoil are available, the advantages of a surface coil are combined with a sufficient field of view covering the upper abdomen.

Spectral or inversion fat saturation has become routine because of the improved conspicuity of the bile ducts due to suppression of surrounding fatty tissue. Furthermore, motion artifacts arising from subcutaneous fat are reduced.

6.2.2.3
Techniques During Breath-hold

Theoretically, acquisition during breath-hold should completely eliminate respiratory artifacts, which are a problem for all non-breath-hold MRC protocols. TAKEHARA et al. (1994) reported the use of a flexible shoulder coil and a breath-hold FSE in patients with chronic pancreatitis. To minimize acquisition time, they used an ETL of 32, one signal acquisition, and a matrix size of 128 × 256. The acquisition was segmented in three or four periods of 18–22 s of breath-hold. However, not all patients are able to perform this type of breath-holding and most scanners do not permit this type of segmented acquisition. Additionally, the technique is not able to cover the necessary volume for biliary imaging.

Following this first report of breath-hold MRP, several investigators reported modifications of the FSE and coil technique to cover a larger volume in a shorter acquisition time. LAUBENBERGER et al. (1995) studied 30 patients using a single-shot RARE sequence. This sequence can be used as a single-slice technique with an acquisition time of 4 s per slice. When applied without slice selection, a 4-s ac-

quisition of the entire volume is possible, allowing for immediate availability of projection images of the biliary and pancreatic duct system. However, because of the lack of slice selection, individual tomographic sections cannot be examined, and the ability of this technique to detect small stones surrounded by high signal intensity has not yet been evaluated. In addition, to date no comparisons of RARE with other MRC techniques have been made.

Further modifications of RARE include the development of 3D-RARE (WIELOPOLSKI et al. 1995) and half-Fourier RARE (or TSE sequences), with HASTE (half-Fourier single-shot turbo spin-echo) as an acronym. During a breath-hold of 18–25 s, thin single slices can be obtained. HASTE MRCP, first presented by SANANES et al. (1995), allows for T2-weighted

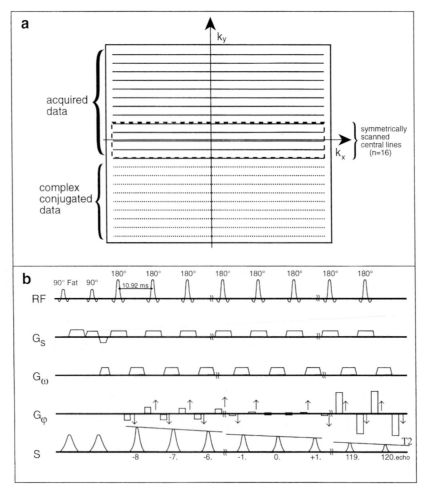

Fig. 6.3 a,b. HASTE k-space and sequence design. **a** Raw-data/k-space sampling pattern. For a 240 × 256 matrix in the half-Fourier technique, 128 echoes are acquired. The 16 central ones are used for phase correction. **b** HASTE pulse sequence diagram. *RF*, radiofrequency; G_s, slice selection gradient; G_ω, read-gradient; G_ψ, phase-encoding gradient; *S*, signal. For details see text

single-shot acquisition of tomographic slices with 2–5 mm thickness within 1.4 s per slice. An important technical restriction is the collection of an echo train of 240 (RARE) or 128 echoes (HASTE), which demands a high gradient strength and/or a phased-array coil to receive a sufficient signal. With less strong gradient systems, slice thickness might be limited to 5 mm and therefore not be adequate for MRCP.

We use a 1.5-T Magnetom "Vision" whole-body scanner (Siemens Medical Systems, Erlangen, Germany) and a body phased-array coil with four elements for signal reception. In the HASTE sequence, after a single spin excitation with a selective 90° RF pulse a train of 128 spin echoes is generated by an equal number of selective 180° pulses, in analogy to a Carr-Purcell-Meiboom-Gill sequence (MEIBOOM and GILL 1958). Each of the echoes is differently phase encoded. For this purpose a phase-encoding gradient is applied before each echo to create the correct signal phase corresponding to each measured Fourier line. In order to avoid phase artifacts, a so-called rewinder phase-encoding gradient follows the echo to force the phase shift to zero before the next phase-encoding gradient is applied, as shown in Fig. 6.3b. With the half-Fourier technique only slightly more than half of the Fourier space is sampled (FEINBERG et al. 1986; MARGOSIAN 1986). The HASTE pulse sequence on our scanner for MRCP begins with eight lines off center, scanning through the center until the upper part of the k-space. Consequently 128 Fourier lines have to be

measured to achieve a 240 × 256 matrix (Fig. 6.3a). The contrast of the image is determined by the delay between the 90° RF pulse and the echoes corresponding to the central Fourier lines, which is 8 times the echo spacing (time between two 180° RF pulses) of 10.9 ms, i.e., 87 ms. The acquisition time per slice is 1.4 s.

Magnetic resonance cholangiography studies are performed with a 3- to 4-mm slice thickness. A field of view of 280–320 mm provides 1.17–1.33 × 1.09–1.25 mm in-plane resolution. Thirteen slices can be acquired within a single breath-hold of 26 s. In dyspneic patients the number of slices can be reduced to nine or five with an 18 or 10 s breath-hold time, respectively. We use 15° oblique coronal planes adjusted for the optimal depiction of the intra- and extrahepatic bile ducts.

6.2.3
Contrast Agents for Biliary Imaging

Recently, several lipophilic contrast agents with a hepatobiliary pathway such as gadolinium-gadoxetic acid disodium (Gd-EOB-DTPA; HAMM et al. 1995), gadolinium-benzylopropionictetraacetate (Gd BOPTA; VOGL et al. 1992), and mangafodipir trisodium (Mn-DPDP; HAMM et al. 1992) have

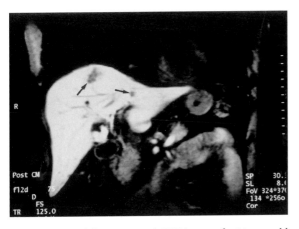

Fig. 6.4. Coronal fat-suppressed GRE image of a 54-year-old male with colon cancer 40 min following administration of Gd-EOB. Two hypointense metastatic lesions (*arrows*) are visible in the liver surrounded by hyperintense normal liver. The biliary ducts and gallbladder are also enhancing, and Gd-EOB is visible in the duodenum and proximal jejunum

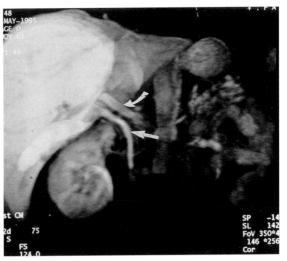

Fig. 6.5. MIP calculation of ten coronal fat-suppressed GRE images 40 min after administration of Gd-BOPTA in a 67-year-old patient. The hyperintense liver prevents the complete visualization of intrahepatic bile ducts with MIP, but can be evaluated using the source images. Note excellent delineation of extrahepatic bile ducts (*arrow*) and also weak visualization of the main portal stem (*curved arrow*) as a sign of a remaining intravascular component

become available for clinical trials. Currently the focus of the use of these contrast agents is the detection and differentiation of focal hepatic lesions, but their biliary excretion route also provides an interesting alternative technique for MRC. These contrast agents show significant enhancement of liver tissue in T1-weighted sequences like SE or FLASH (GRE) because of uptake by hepatocytes. Biliary secretion follows with ductal and duodenal enhancement (Fig. 6.4, Gd-EOB). Because biliary enhancement is paralleled by hepatocyte enhancement, projection images with the maximum intensity projection (MIP) do not display the same quality as images obtained with T2-weighted MR cholangiography (Fig. 6.5, Gd-BOPTA). However, T1-weighted MRC techniques using these contrast agents may be an effective modality for the diagnosis of biliary leakage and cholecystitis, and may replace scintigraphic tests like ^{99m}Tc-IDA. Currently, however, only single case reports are available regarding these indications.

6.3
Normal Anatomy

The biliary duct system is an arborized tree, in which the bile ducts of the portal triad join subsegmental and then segmental branches to form the right and left biliary main ducts. Generally, the bile ducts follow the segmental hepatic anatomy. A left medial and a left lateral segmental duct usually join to form the left hepatic bile duct. The left hepatic duct has a longer extrahepatic portion than the right hepatic duct, and it therefore tends to dilate more than the right hepatic duct in the case of obstruction. In approximately 60% of patients, a dorsocaudal branch drains the posterior segments (segments 6 + 7) and a ventrocranial branch drains the anterior segments (segments 5 + 8) of the right lobe of the liver. The drainage of the caudate lobe is very variable and can be via the left or the right hepatic duct. The right and left hepatic ducts join at the porta hepatis to form the 3- to 4-cm-long common hepatic duct. The common hepatic duct lies anteriorly to the portal vein and laterally to the hepatic artery in the hepatoduodenal ligament. This duct joins the cystic duct at a variable level in a suprapancreatic position to form the common bile duct. The common bile duct is usually 6–7 cm in length and is divided into suprapancreatic, intrapancreatic, and ampullary segments. In approximately 30% of patients the common bile duct courses on the posterior surface of the pancreas without a true intrapancreatic portion. The common bile duct enters the posterior medial aspect of the duodenum through a 1- to 2-cm-long intramural tunnel terminating at the papilla of Vater. The union with the pancreatic duct varies; in most cases the ducts join within the duodenal wall to form a short common channel. Variations include a missing common channel with separate orifices and an extramural union with a long common channel. The common channel is surrounded by the sphincter of Oddi, and the distal common bile duct is surrounded by the sphincter of Boyden.

For the visualization of the nondilated biliary system, as in volunteers, only data regarding the visibility criteria have been published. Using a GRE technique (CE-FAST), Wallner and Schumacher examined five volunteers as controls for their patient study (SCHUMACHER et al. 1991; WALLNER et al. 1991). In only two of these five volunteers could MRC delineate the right and left hepatic ducts and some portions of the common bile duct. The diameter of these structures was determined by ultrasound to be less than 5 mm. Peripheral parts of the intrahepatic biliary tree could not be seen with either US or MRC. Therefore, compared with other reported techniques, GRE techniques do not seem to be suitable for depiction of the normal biliary anatomy.

In contrast to the results obtained with GRE techniques, REINHOLD et al. (1996) demonstrated the nondilated biliary system and even anatomic variants using the non-breath-hold 2D FSE technique. The normal extrahepatic bile ducts were visualized in nearly 100% of patients. Using the breath-hold RARE technique, LAUBENBERGER et al. (1995) could delineate all intrahepatic and extrahepatic biliary ducts in 30 volunteers. Using the HASTE sequence, MIYAZAKI et al. (1996) were able to delineate the extrahepatic ducts with good or excellent quality in 35 (88%) of 40 volunteers. The intrahepatic ducts up to third-order branches were seen with good quality or better in more than 90%.

We examined 20 healthy volunteers with both RARE and HASTE sequences. Three radiologists independently evaluated the RARE and HASTE images, including MIP reconstructions, with a five-step grading system for the anatomic visualization and rated motion artifacts, vessel visualization, and overall image quality. HASTE (Fig. 6.6) had significantly higher SNR and CNR values compared with RARE (Fig. 7) projections ($P < 0.01$) because of lower background noise and higher signal intensity of bile.

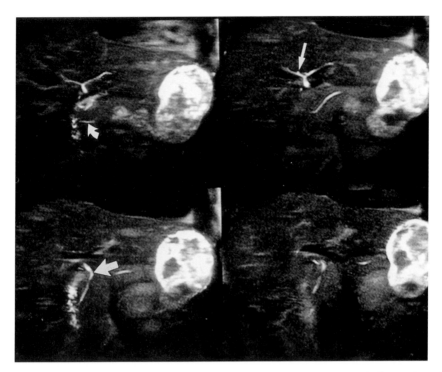

Fig. 6.6. Four of 23 coronal HASTE single slices of a 32-year-old healthy volunteer. The left and right hepatic ducts, second-order ducts (*thin arrow*), the common hepatic duct, and the common bile duct (*thick arrow*) can be delineated. Note also delineation of the main pancreatic duct and duct of Santorini (*small curved arrow*)

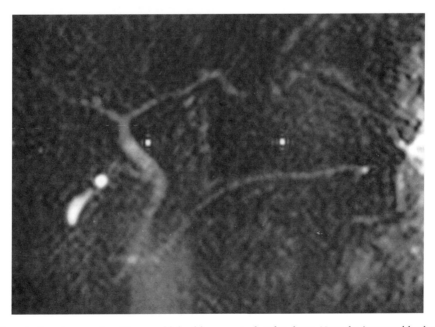

Fig. 6.7. RARE projection image of a 32-year-old healthy volunteer acquired with a coronal oriented 60-mm slab. The same structures as in Fig. 6.6 are delineated, except for second-order ducts. Note the increased background noise of RARE and the contracted gallbladder after the volunteer had a meal

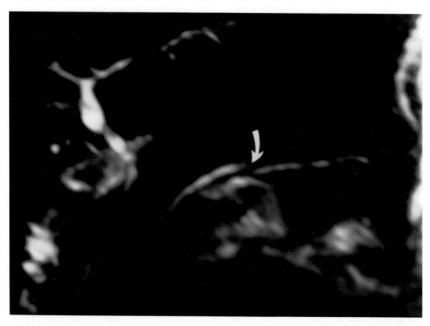

Fig. 6.8. Maximum intensity projection (MIP) image calculated from all 23 coronal HASTE slices (Fig. 6.6) of a 32-year-old volunteer. Biliary ducts seen on the different HASTE images are calculated in a single projection image, similar to ERC. Note the vertical step in the pancreatic duct (*curved arrow*) resulting from patient movement between slices

The rating of vessel visualization for both HASTE and RARE was low with regard to the hepatic artery, portal vein, and vena cava because excited blood spins left the imaging plane before the readout time. Only for intrahepatic portal vein branches was there intermediate signal intensity in some volunteers as a result of slow blood flow. In no volunteer were blood vessels imaged with high signal intensity; therefore interference with the visualization of high signal bile duct fluid was not seen. Because both HASTE (1.4 s/image) and RARE (5 s/projection) are fast snapshot techniques, motion artifacts were only rarely seen (Fig. 6.8).

First- (2.4 ± 0.5 mm diameter) and second- (1.8 ± 0.6 mm) order intrahepatic bile branches were routinely visualized in all volunteers, while third-order branches (1.2 ± 0.5 mm) were seen in a few cases and fourth-order branches in only one case. The common hepatic bile duct, common bile duct, and gallbladder were visualized in all volunteers. The cystic duct was identified in 85% of volunteers. The visualization of the common hepatic duct, first-order branches, and lower common bile duct was significantly ($P \leq 0.05$) better rated for HASTE than for RARE. The duct of Wirsung, which is helpful for anatomic orientation in the intrapancreatic portion of the common bile duct, was also seen significantly better ($P < 0.001$) with HASTE.

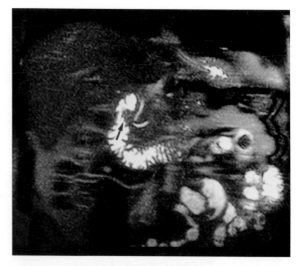

Fig. 6.9. Coronal HASTE image of a 45-year-old volunteer depicting the papillary region and duodenum. Fluid in the duodenum allows for exact delineation of the duodenal folds and the papillary region (*arrow*). The distal common bile duct and duct of Wirsung are depicted as linear high-signal intensities

The results of our volunteer study demonstrated excellent visualization of the biliary system up to first-order branches, while higher-order branches were visualized only in part. We found RARE to be inferior to HASTE in the depiction of the intra-pancreatic portion of the common bile duct, the proximal part of the duct of Wirsung, and first- and second-order intrahepatic branches. HASTE and to a lesser degree RARE are therefore suitable for imaging of the nondilated biliary system, which might be important for the detection of anatomic anomalies. When the duodenum contains some fluid during the examination, the papillary region is also visualized in detail (Fig. 6.9).

6.4
Anatomic and Congenital Variations

Anatomic variations and anomalies of the biliary system are common findings. Although most variants have no pathologic significance, understanding of them is important for the radiologic diagnosis. In almost 5% of cases an aberrant right hepatic duct enters the common hepatic duct or cystic duct at any one of a variety of possible locations. In addition, in almost 2% of cases an accessory right hepatic duct joins the common hepatic duct at different locations. Congenital anomalies like an unusually high or low insertion of the cystic duct may become a significant finding in patients undergoing biliary surgery, especially when surgery is done using a laparoscopic route. These variants place the patient at higher risk of bile duct injury at surgery.

Against this background, numerous reports emphasize the importance of identifying these bile duct variants using intraoperative cholangiography. But there are also reports that a significant number of bile duct injuries occur even before the preparation of the cystic duct and the performance of intraoperative cholangiography. Also, in most institutions intraoperative cholangiography is restricted to cases of suspected residual common bile duct stones because it is time consuming. While US and CT do not identify these variants, intravenous cholangiography displays the biliary anatomy sufficiently, but has the limitations of con-trast-related side-effects and dependence on liver function.

In contrast, MRC has been shown to be very accurate in identifying these variants of biliary anatomy (TAOUREL et al. 1996) when non-breath-hold 2D FSE sequences are used. In our patient group, too, we identified anatomic variants such as low (Fig. 6.10) or high (Fig. 6.11) cystic duct junction with the common hepatic duct without difficulties. However,

the practical relevance of MRC for the identification of variants before surgery has not yet been evaluated. The use of MRC before every laparoscopic cholecystectomy may not be cost-effective.

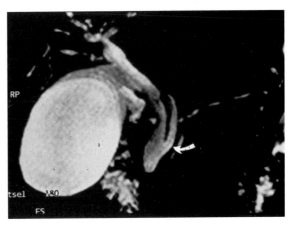

Fig. 6.10. Seventy-one year-old female before cholecystectomy because of cholecystolithiasis (not seen on this MIP calculation). MIP of HASTE slices shows an extremely distal junction of the cystic and common hepatic duct (*curved arrow*), almost in an intrapancreatic position. This is an important finding for the planning of gallbladder surgery

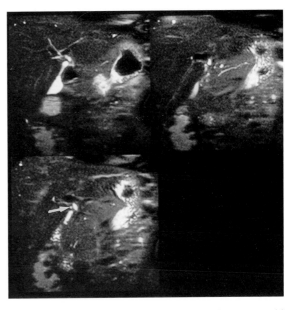

Fig. 6.11. Three of 23 coronal HASTE slices of a 26-year-old volunteer. In contrast to Fig. 6.10, the cystic duct joins the common hepatic duct in a normal proximal location (*arrow*)

6.5
Bile Duct Dilatation, Stenosis, and Obstruction

Both CT and US are highly accurate in the diagnosis of biliary obstruction and proximal bile duct dilatation. Cholangiography should therefore primarily be used to determine the precise position and cause of an obstruction. For patients with obstructive jaundice, scintigraphy and intravenous cholangiography have in the past been the only noninvasive methods to obtain a projection image of the biliary system. However, neither modality is effective in the presence of severe jaundice, and image quality may be inadequate for the planning of drainage or surgery. In contrast, MRC, as a completely noninvasive technique, is totally independent from the serum bilirubin level and allows delineation even of biliary duct components not visualized with other cholangiographic techniques.

HALL-CRAGGS et al. (1993) detected the presence of obstruction in 97% and the correct location of the

obstruction in 89% of 40 patients using a GRE technique. However, the biliary duct system distal to the obstruction was seen in only 28%. LAUBENBERGER et al. (1995) correctly detected the presence and location of obstruction in all 25 of their cases using a breath-hold RARE sequence. The biliary ducts distal to the obstruction were also seen in all cases. Similar data, published for non-breath-hold 3D FSE and HASTE (MIYAZAKI et al. 1996; REINHOLD et al. 1995), support the conclusion that the length of a duct occlusion can be better determined using FSE techniques.

In our patient group, 34 of 61 patients presented with bile duct dilatation due to obstruction (Figs. 6.12, 6.13). Bile duct dilatation was correctly diagnosed by MRC in 94.1%, while minor dilatation in two patients was not diagnosed by MRC. There was a high correlation with the results of ERC. Bile duct dilatation was correctly excluded in 25 patients. Discrepancies between MRC and ERC were only found in cases of minor dilatation of the ductal system, and resulted from different reader opinions. Increase in injection pressure at ERC may result in dilatation of the biliary duct system, and therefore false-negative MRC results may indeed represent false-positive ERC results. Despite these facts, snapshot MRC proved highly effective in the detection of bile duct dilatation.

Regardless of the technical variant used, MRC has inferior spatial resolution compared with direct cholangiography (PTC) and ERC, but presents a

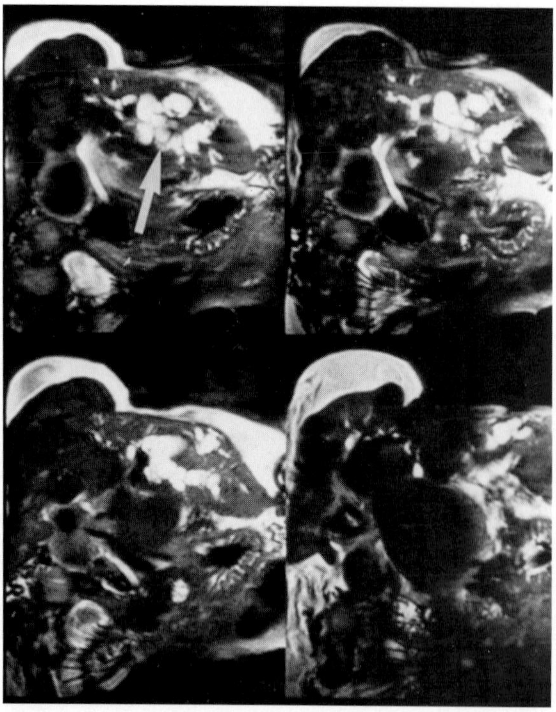

Fig. 6.12. Four consecutive coronal HASTE images in a 32-year-old female patient 10 weeks postpartum and with live failure. HASTE demonstrates ascites, clear dilatation of the left hepatic duct, and side branches without obstruction (*arrow*). Follow-up of this patient revealed no change of this finding, which was assumed to be congenital in nature

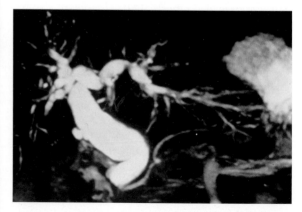

Fig. 6.13. Fifty-four year old patient with diabetes following combined pancreas and kidney transplantation, who developed cholestasis. US findings were unclear because of air superposition. Unenhanced CT demonstrated an enlarged pancreatic head. MIP calculation of HASTE demonstrates severe biliary dilatation; unenhanced GRE demonstrated retropancreatic immunocytoma (not shown)

comparable image quality. The information obtainable with MRC regarding biliary dilatation is therefore comparable to or even better than (prestenotic segments) that acquired with invasive imaging techniques.

The excellent spatial resolution of the plain film usually allows for detailed analysis of the morphology of a biliary duct stricture in ERCP. Length, symmetry, wall contour, tapering, and other morphologic features can be accurately analyzed. The injection of contrast medium allows additional evaluation of the possible distention of a stricture during injection. Therefore, distinction between benign and malignant strictures of the biliary system is possible in most cases. Studies using GRE techniques (MORIMOTO et al. 1992; WALLNER et al. 1991) show poor delineation of poststenotic nondilated duct segments; therefore, the length of a stenosis cannot be accurately determined. Also, differentiation of the cause of obstruction has proved impossible using GRE techniques (ISHIZAKI et al. 1993). Recently, better results were reported with 2D and 3D FSE techniques: Malignant bile obstruction was diagnosed with a sensitivity of 86% and a specificity of 98% (14/79 patients) in a study reported by GUIBAUD et al. (1995). SOTO et al. (1995) diagnosed nine of ten cases of stenosis (90%) using non-breath-hold FSE. Several other reports support these results with non-breath-hold FSE and faster MRC techniques like RARE and HASTE.

In our patient group, ERC demonstrated 36 stenoses in 33 patients, comprising 15 malignant stenoses due to pancreatic or cholangiocellular carcinoma and 21 benign stenoses (Figs. 6.14, 6.15) due to different causes. MRC diagnosed 32 stenoses correctly, but failed to diagnose four stenoses in three patients. These stenoses were located in the hepatic bile duct (two cases), in the lower common bile duct (one case), and in the left hepatic bile duct (one case). In all cases of missed stenoses there was no prestenotic dilatation, while in 27 of the 32 diagnosed stenoses (84.4%) there was prestenotic dilatation. There were three false-positive diagnoses with MRC. Two of these cases were in the common hepatic duct near the intrahepatic bifurcation and one was in the right hepatic duct. In all false-positive diagnoses, there was no prestenotic dilatation. Snapshot MRC diagnosed biliary stenosis with a sensitivity of 88.9% and a specificity of 84% in our patient group. We correctly diagnosed all 15 cases of malignant stenoses, while there were three false-positive low-grade stenoses. Two of these were caused by a collapsed common hepatic duct, which was misin-

terpreted on MRC as possible stenosis. There were four cases of low-grade stenoses in the common hepatic duct and upper common bile duct which were not seen by MRC.

The slightly worse MRC results for the diagnosis of biliary stenoses may result from the fact that MRC delineates the physiologic situation with partially

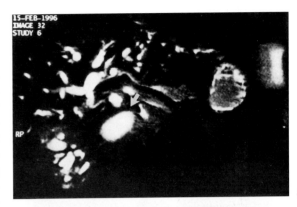

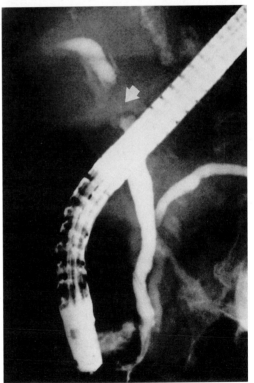

Fig. 6.14 a,b. Eighty-four year old female with a high-grade stenosis of the proximal common bile duct following multiple episodes of cholangitis. a Coronal HASTE shows no connection of high signal intensity bile in the common bile duct and medium-grade intraheptic duct dilatation. This results in the diagnosis of a high-grade stenosis of the common bile duct (*arrow*). b ERC on the next day demonstrates the high-grade stricture of the common bile duct (*arrow*)

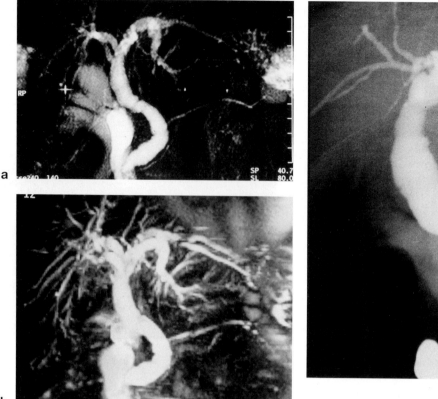

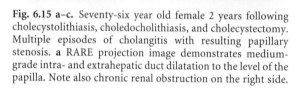

Fig. 6.15 a–c. Seventy-six year old female 2 years following cholecystolithiasis, choledocholithiasis, and cholecystectomy. Multiple episodes of cholangitis with resulting papillary stenosis. **a** RARE projection image demonstrates medium-grade intra- and extrahepatic duct dilatation to the level of the papilla. Note also chronic renal obstruction on the right side.

b MIP of coronal HASTE slices demonstrates the same findings with some movement of the patient during acquisition. **c** ERC shows the findings of papillary stenosis. Note incomplete filling of the intrahepatic ducts because of the risk of cholangitis due to ERC

collapsed duct areas while ERC causes low-grade distention by injection of contrast medium. Therefore, ERC seems more accurate for the exclusion of low-grade strictures without dilatation. In cases of total occlusion of segments of the biliary tract, MRC is able to delineate the dilated duct portion proximal to the occlusion while ERC allows for the detection of the occlusion only. A clear advantage of MRC is the visualization of the surrounding parenchyma, which allows for exclusion of mass lesions infiltrating ducts (Fig. 6.16). This is even better appreciated on the parenchymal imaging sequences, which are additionally used in most MRC examinations. For intrahepatic duct stenoses, MRC diagnosed advanced sclerosing cholangitis in one patient and one benign stenosis following cholangitis. So far, MRC seems to be effective in the diagnosis of malignant stenoses but the efficiency in the diagnosis of low-grade benign stenoses, like in early sclerosing cholangitis, has to be further evaluated.

6.6
Cholangiolithiasis

The incidence of gallstones increases with age, obesity, rapid weight reduction, and ileal disease or resection. Women are twice as likely as men to develop gallstones. Between 1% and 2% of asymptomatic patients per year will develop symptoms, and the risk of development of complications such as acute cholecystitis is also 1%–2%. Ultrasonography is highly specific in the diagnosis of cholecystolithiasis and cholangiolithiasis, but only sensitive enough in the region of the gallbladder because air often prevents the accurate visualization of the common bile duct (LAING et al. 1984). CT has a reported specificity exceeding 95%, but its sensitivity in detecting cholangiolithiasis remains low, at 23%–85% (BARON 1987; PANASEN et al. 1992), despite recent technical advances. Therefore, invasive tests like ERC and PTC are often used for the diagnosis of cholangiolithiasis.

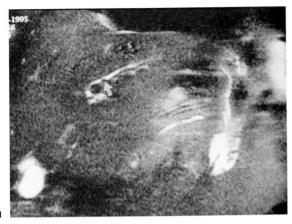

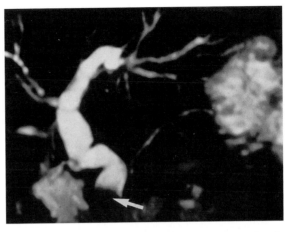

Fig. 6.17. MIP image of HASTE slices in a 55-year-old male presenting with cholestasis. ERC was not done because of difficult anatomy following stomach surgery. MRC demonstrates mild duct dilatation, typical pronouncement of left hepatic dilatation, and a lower common bile duct stone as the cause of obstruction (*large arrow*, stone with low signal)

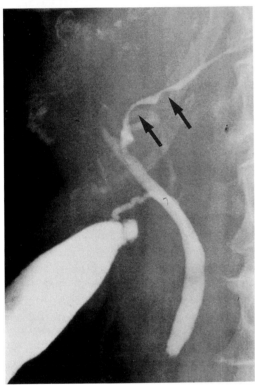

Fig. 6.16 a,b. Sixty-four year old female with intermittent signs of cholestasis. **a** Coronal HASTE demonstrates an irregular course of the left hepatic duct (*arrows*). On MRC there are no signs of a mass that could be responsible for the impression of the duct. **b** ERC shows the same irregular course of the proximal left hepatic duct. Because ERC does not image extraductal parenchyma, there was uncertainty about a possible mass responsible for this finding (*arrows*)

However, diagnostic ERC is technically unsuccessful in approximately 4% of cases (BILBAO et al. 1976) and carries a 0.6%–5.0% risk of procedure-related complications like pancreatitis, cholangitis, and even death (BILBAO et al. 1976; SEIFERT 1977; ZIMMON et al. 1975). Therefore, a noninvasive diagnostic test which allows reliable and detailed visualization of the biliary system even in patients who provide limited cooperation is highly desirable.

Conventional MRI seems superior to conventional CT in detecting common duct stones because T2-weighted sequences provide a higher contrast between a signal-void stone and high signal intensity bile. Because all reported MRC techniques allow for higher resolution compared with conventional SE techniques, MRC should also be more accurate than CT for the detection of cholangiolithiasis. Currently, no report is available comparing the accuracy of CT and MRC. Few data exist on the accuracy of MRC in respect of cholangiolithiasis. Using a GRE technique, ISHIZAKI et al. (1993) correctly diagnosed all six cases of choledocholithiasis among 20 patients who underwent MRC. GUIBAUD et al. (1994) delineated all ten cases of known choledocholithiasis in a retrospective study with 2D FSE sequences. PAVONE et al. (1996) reported a sensitivity of 91.7%, a specificity of 100%, and a diagnostic accuracy of 96.8% for non-breath-hold 3D FSE in the diagnosis of choledocholithiasis.

In our patient group ($n = 61$), the correlation between MRC and ERC results was excellent. Cholangiolithiasis (Figs. 6.17, 6.18) was diagnosed by MRC with a sensitivity of 92.3% and a specificity of 95.8% compared with ERC. The positive predictive value was 85.7% and the negative predictive value, 97.8%. The diameter of stones ranged from 3 to 30 mm (9.4 ± 7.5 mm). While most stones were diagnosed without difficulty, in one patient a stone was

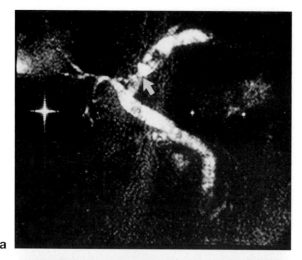

a

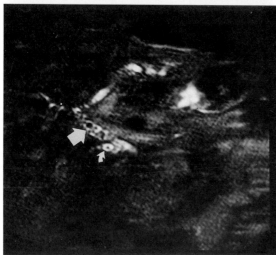

b

Fig. 6.18 a,b. Forty-seven year old male with known stenosis of the proximal left hepatic duct following cholangitis. **a** The signal intensity of the common hepatic duct, common bile duct, and left hepatic duct is inhomogeneous in the RARE projection image, but single concrements cannot be delineated. There is stenosis of the left hepatic duct (*arrow*). **b** Coronal HASTE image shows multiple oval areas of low signal intensity filling the common hepatic duct (*large arrow*) and even the cystic duct (*curved arrow*). Additional stones were seen in the left hepatic duct and common bile duct. ERC removed numerous stones 2–5 mm in diameter

not diagnosed due to observer error. In two patients, low-intensity flow voids in the intrapancreatic portion of the common bile duct caused the false-positive diagnosis of choledocholithiasis. Bile duct stones were correctly excluded in 46 patients.

These results are similar to those reported for ERCP and represent continuous improvement of the reported MRC techniques. The most important differential diagnostic problems with MRC are pneumobilia and flow artifacts, both of which result in

signal voids surrounded by bile and can be misinterpreted as bile duct stones. In two patients we saw flow voids in the center of the lower portion of the common bile duct, always surrounded by high signal bile. US and CT seem not to be sufficient to exclude the presence of cholangiolithiasis reliably. Because these tests are highly specific, no further imaging test is necessary in the presence of a positive finding.

Magnetic resonance cholangiography seems to be very accurate for the diagnosis of choledocholithiasis but biliary gas and flow voids may result in false-positive findings. On the other hand, ERC may fail to delineate all intrahepatic biliary segments, or this is avoided to prevent deterioration of cholestasis as in sclerosing cholangitis (BEUERS et al. 1992). In such cases, MRC is a helpful adjunct to incomplete ERC (Fig. 6.19).

6.7
Cholecystitis and Cholangitis

Acute cholecystitis is caused by stone impaction in the cystic duct in approximately 95% of cases. Local inflammation, worsening cystic duct obstruction, secondary ischemia, and transmural necrosis are the consequences of this obstructive process. Generally, when pain lasts for at least 24 h, it is more likely to be associated with acute inflammation without spontaneous resolution. Imaging can reduce the number of patients explored for diseases that mimic acute cholecystitis and detect major complications like emphysematous cholecystitis and perforation. Usually, US and cholescintigraphy are the main imaging methods in acute cholecystitis. While cholescintigraphy can diagnose cystic duct obstruction with moderate specificity and high sensitivity, US can image morphologic features like cholelithiasis, gallbladder wall thickening, pain over the gallbladder, and intramural edema.

Computed tomography and MRI play little role in the initial evaluation of patients with suspected acute cholecystitis (Fig. 6.20). The normal gallbladder concentrates bile with resorption of fluids and electrolytes, while in acute cholecystitis the gallbladder may actually secrete fluid into its lumen. Therefore, hypointense gallbladder bile relative to liver in a fasting patient suspected to have acute cholecystitis is an indicator for disease. McCARTHY et al. (1986) found a sensitivity of 75% and a specificity of 100% for hypointense bile in the diagnosis of cholecystitis. WEISSLEDER et al. (1988) emphasized the combined use of this sign with morphologic indicators like

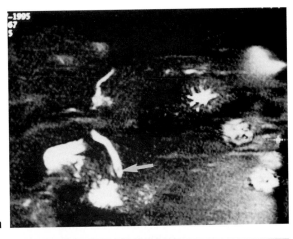

a

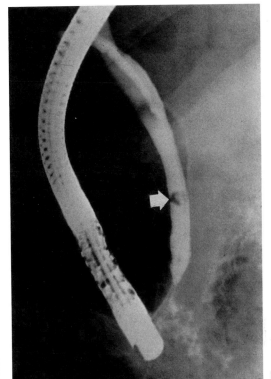

b

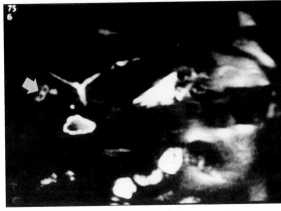

c

Fig. 6.19 a–c. Sixty-seven year old male with intermittent signs of cholestasis. **a** Coronal HASTE image demonstrates a 5-mm signal void in the lower common bile duct (*arrow*). **b** ERC demonstrates the 5-mm stone in a slightly superior position in the common bile duct, due to pressure of contrast medium injection. The stone was removed by ERC without complications. **c** Coronal HASTE demonstrates two additional stones in the duct of segment 5/6 (*arrow*). There were not seen by ERC because contrast injection failed to fill this duct area. There stones were confirmed by follow-up US

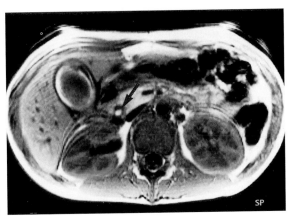

a

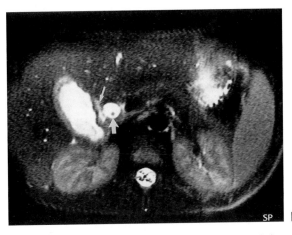

b

Fig. 6.20 a,b. Thirteen year old boy with acalculous cholecystitis 2 months following perforating appendicitis and peritonitis. **a** T1-weighted gradient-echo breath-hold sequence demonstrates thickened gallbladder wall and hyperintense wall representing diffuse hemorrhage at surgery. The hypointensity of the gallbladder bile reflects the impaired concentrating function of the gallbladder. The common bile duct is enlarged with a hyperintense concrement (*arrow*) due to cholesterol. **b** T2-weighted HASTE image demonstrates gallbladder thickening with moderate hyperintensity due to edema with hyperintense foci of abscess formation. Pericholecystic fluid (*small arrow*) and multiple concrements in the common bile duct (*large arrow*) and cystic duct were further findings

thickening of the gallbladder wall, intramural abscess, pericholecystic fluid, and the presence of gallstones, which may be more specific. MATSUI et al. (1989) reported a high sensitivity of godolinium-enhanced fat-suppressed T1-weighted imaging, which may improve delineation of inflammatory hyperemia and intramural abscess.

Chronic cholecystitis presents with a small, irregularly shaped gallbladder with increased wall thickening. The differentiation of acute and chronic cholecystitis depends on the degree of mural enhancement, which seems to reflect the severity of the inflammation.

Infectious cholangitis is the result of ascending infection from the gastrointestinal tract. Thickening of the ductal wall, dilatation, and substantial enhancement of the ductal walls are the principal imaging features. The formation of intrahepatic abscesses may further complicate this disease. MRI diagnosis should be made on the basis of gadolinium-enhanced T1-weighted sequences, and the use of fat suppression improves the conspicuity of ductal wall enhancement. Segmental cholangitis can result in diffuse edematous infiltration of liver parenchyma and mimic hepatic tumor. Edema presents with

hypodensity on CT, and with T1-weighted hypointensity and T2-weighted hyperintensity on MRI. Liver-specific contrast agents can help to differentiate inflammatory process and tumor (Fig. 6.21). This is especially useful in sclerosing cholangitis, where cholangitis and cholangiocellular carcinoma are two frequent complications.

Primary sclerosing cholangitis is combined with inflammatory bowel disease (typically ulcerative colitis) in 70% of patients. It is characterized by alternating segments of narrowed and dilated ducts, resulting in a beaded or stenotic appearance of the ductal system (Fig. 6.22). The bile duct wall is moderately thickened to 3–4 mm (TEEFEY et al. 1988); thickening exceeding 5 mm is a feature of developing cholangiocarcinoma (SCHULTE et al. 1990). T1-weighted gadolinium-enhanced fat-suppressed MRI is successful in the demonstration of bile duct wall thickening, substantial enhancement is not present because of only moderate inflammation in primary sclerosing cholangitis. The future use of cholangiographic contrast media such as Gd-EOB, Gd-BOPTA, or Mn-DPDP may have an important impact on imaging of the bile duct wall and detection of pathologic thickening. MRC may play an increas-

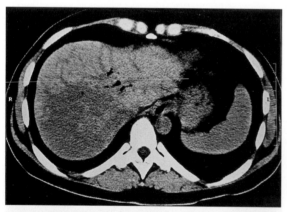

a

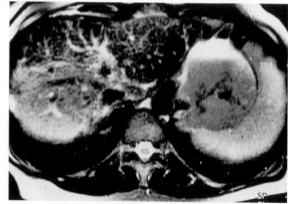

b

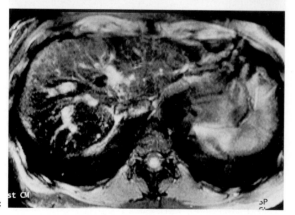

c

Fig. 6.21 a–c. Fifty-four year old female with an 18-year history of sclerosing cholangitis. a Unenhanced CT demonstrates pneumobilia and a large hypodensity of liver segment 8. Because of the history of primary sclerosing cholangitis, cholangiocarcinoma and cholangitis were the main differential diagnoses. b T2-weighted breath-hold FSE demonstrates a hyperintense mass lesion of segment 8, which was hypointense in T1-weighted sequences. The differential diagnosis did not change. c T2*-weighted gradient-echo sequence following administration of superparamagnetic ferrum oxide particles. Increased hypointensity in segment 8 rules out the possibility of cholangiocarcinoma and leads to the diagnosis of segmental cholangitis, due to a stenosis of the segment duct seen later at ERC

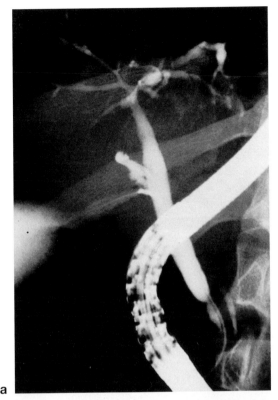

a

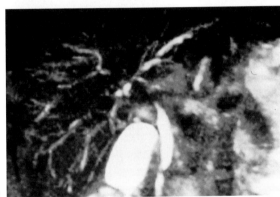

b

Fig. 6.22 a,b. Fifty-five year old male with a long-standing history of sclerosing cholangitis. **a** ERC shows the typical beading of intrahepatic ducts with dilated and narrowed duct segments. **b** Like ERC, MIP of HASTE images demonstrates the changing duct caliber

ingly role in the investigation of primary sclerosing cholangitis, because ERC places the patient at a higher risk of cholangitis and impairs liver function in these patients (BEUERS et al. 1992). Further studies combining T1-weighted fat-suppressed imaging and MRC techniques need to be conducted to determine the potential of MRI to replace ERC in the diagnosis and follow-up of sclerosing cholangitis.

6.8
Biliary Neoplasms

6.8.1
Gallbladder Carcinoma

Gallbladder cancer is a rare neoplasm occurring in patients older than 60 years of age with a female predominance. There is a strong association with cholecystolithiasis (75% of patients with gallbladder cancer). The most common histologic type is adenocarcinoma. The characteristic findings include a mass filling or replacing the gallbladder lumen or a thickening of the gallbladder wall protruding in the lumen or with diffuse infiltration of the liver, duodenum, and pancreas. If the gallbladder wall thickening exceeds 10mm, this finding is highly suggestive for gallbladder cancer.

The tumor presents with low signal intensity on T1-weighted images and is moderately hyperintense with T2-weighted sequences (Fig. 6.23). Therefore, extension of the tumor into the liver is best seen with T2-weighted sequences, while extension to the pancreas and duodenum is well shown with coronal fat-suppressed T1-weighted sequences after administration of gadolinium.

6.8.2
Cholangiocarcinoma

Cholangiocellular carcinoma is a primary malignancy of the bile ducts that is more commonly associated with ulcerative colitis, usually in patients with pre-existing sclerosing cholangitis. Other risk factors include aniline exposure, liver fluke infestation, and choledochal cysts. Patients are commonly older than 60 years and present with jaundice and weight loss in over 75% of cases. Histologically, these tumors are mucus-secreting adenocarcinomas. In 50% of cases, cholangiocellular carcinoma arises at the junction of the left and right hepatic ducts; these typical cholangiocellular carcinomas are called Klatskin tumors (Fig. 6.24). In terms of frequency, this tumor type is followed by the central cholangiocellular carcinomas (arising from the common hepatic or bile duct), while peripheral cholangiocellular carcinomas (arising from the intrahepatic branches) have a lower frequency. The peripheral cholangiocellular carcinomas do not cause early bile duct obstruction and cholestasis and are therefore mostly diagnosed at a later stage. If CT or MRI reveals high-grade biliary duct obstruction with ductal wall

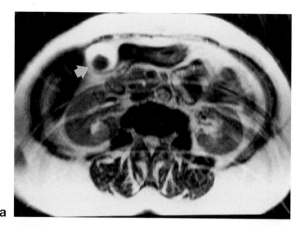

a

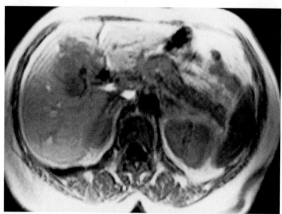

b

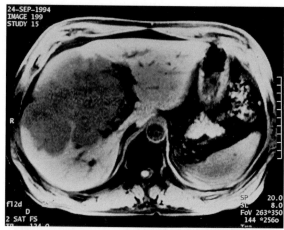

a

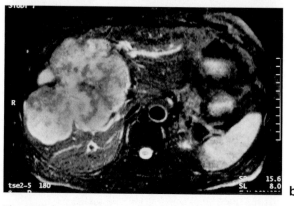

b

Fig. 6.23 a,b. Seventy-four year old female with a gallbladder carcinoma. **a** T2-weighted breath-hold FSE image shows a hypointense round stone inside the gallbladder lumen (*arrow*). This is a typical finding in gallbladder cancer, because almost 80% of these patients show cholecystolithiasis. There are some artifacts due to patient movement during acquisition resulting from subcutaneous fat. **b** T1-weighted GRE image 20 min after administration of 0.1 mmol Gd-DTPA. The solid tumor delineates as a hypovascular hypointense mass replacing the gallbladder and slightly dilated bile ducts of the left liver lobe. There was no uptake of Gd-EOB, because no hepatocytes are present in this tumor type

Fig. 6.24 a,b. Eighty-one year old male with painless jaundice revealing central cholangiocellular carcinoma. **a** T1-weighted fat-suppressed GRE image shows a 14 cm central cholangiocarcinoma with low signal intensity compared with normal liver tissue. **b** T2-weighted FSE image shows the hyperintense tumor with mild signs of biliary dilatation of both lobes. The gallbladder is located in an atypical position, lateral to the tumor

thickness exceeding 5 mm, this finding should be reported as highly suggestive for a cholangiocellular carcinoma.

Gadolinium-enhanced fat-suppressed sequences show medium-grade enhancement of the tumor compared with surrounding structures. Therefore, these sequences allow for superior delineation of the tumor extension compared with CT. Also cholangiocellular carcinomas in the intrapancreatic portion of the common bile duct present with better delineation (low signal intensity) in the pancreas (high signal intensity) on fat-suppressed T1-weighted scans (Fig. 6.25). Peripheral cholangiocellular carcinomas

often present as large intrahepatic masses with low signal intensity on T1- and moderate signal intensity on T2-weighted images. Peripheral cholangiocellular carcinomas more often show dilated bile ducts in the periphery of the tumor, but definitive differentiation from other tumor entities is not possible with MRI.

6.8.3
Periampullary Carcinoma

Periampullary carcinomas arise in the region of the ampulla. Risk factors for periampullary carcinoma include ulcerative colitis, *Ascaris* infection, and Gardner's syndrome. Tumor growth causes obstruction of both the common bile duct and the pancreatic

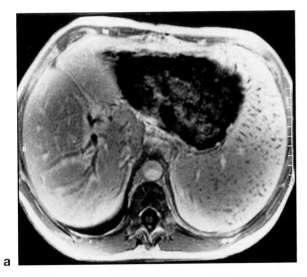

a

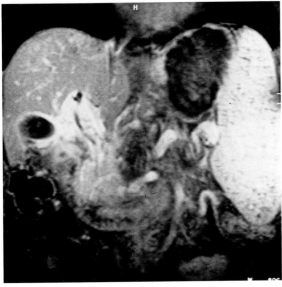

b

Fig. 6.25 a,b. Sixty-four year old female presenting with diffuse cholangiocarcinoma. **a** Axial T1-weighted fat-suppressed GRE after administration of Gd-DTPA shows solid tumor tissue adjacent to the central biliary ducts, inseparable from adjacent portal veins. **b** Coronal T1-weighted fat-suppressed GRE after administration of Gd-DTPA shows the diffuse tumor infiltration of the gallbladder and pancreatic head. Note also the hypointense presentation of splenosis.

duct. Therefore, the presenting symptoms are the same as those of adenocarcinoma of the pancreatic head. However, the 5-year survival rate (85%) is much better compared with pancreatic cancer, if a Whipple procedure is performed in patients with localized lesions.

On T1-weighted fat-suppressed images the tumor presents with low signal intensity in the ampullary region, surrounded by high signal intensity pancreas. Heterogeneous enhancement is seen on gadolinium-enhanced scans.

6.8.4
Cystadenoma and Cystadenocarcinoma

Biliary cystadenoma and cystadenocarcinoma show histologic similarities to cystadenomas and cystadenocarcinomas of the ovary and pancreas. They consist of mucin-secreting columnar epithelium and usually occur in middle-aged women, who present with diffuse abdominal pain and occasionally jaundice. US shows an intrahepatic hypoechoic mass, while CT demonstrates a hypodense uni- or multiloculated cystic mass. MRI features consist of hypointensity on T1- and hyperintensity on T2-weighted scans relative to the liver. In most cases, septations are better seen on T2-weighted scans. Mural nodules as solid parts of the lesion sometimes occur in cystadenoma and are common and larger in cystadenocarcinomas. They present with relative hypointensity on T1-weighted scans and moderate hyperintensity on T2-weighted scans. Small septal calcifications may be present in cystadenomas, while cystadenocarcinomas often have thick mural and septal calcifications which present with low intensity on both T1- and T2-weighted scans. The differential diagnosis should include hepatic cyst, hydatid cyst, choledochal cysts, hepatic abscess, and cystic metastases. An important feature for the differentiation is the hyperintensity of mucin on T1-weighted imaging, which allows for differentiation from other cystic lesions, if present.

6.9
Summary

Recent advances in MRI include the development of fast and ultrafast imaging sequences and better gradient systems and coil designs. For the imaging of the biliary system, the increased imaging speed allows both increased spatial resolution and faster image acquisition times. The combined use of fast gradient systems and array coils allows for fast breath-hold imaging with sufficient T1 and T2 weighting. Therefore, the known superior contrast resolution of MRI is now accompanied by higher spatial resolution. These developments necessitate a reevaluation of new MR techniques in comparison with spiral CT.

Unenhanced T2-weighted breath-hold MRI allows for superior delineation of the extension of solid lesions, such as cholangiocellular carcinoma and gallbladder carcinoma, into the liver, and not only because of its multiplanar capabilities. T1-weighted fat-suppressed imaging results in accurate delineation of the extension of tumors in the pancreatic and suprapancreatic portions of the common bile duct and seems to be a valuable tool for the imaging of the bile duct wall. Specific biliary contrast agents, currently under clinical investigation, may provide an adjunct or alternative to current scintigraphic functional tests.

Especially the development of fast T2-weighted techniques with high spatial resolution has broadened the indications for MRI for evaluation of the biliary system. MRC techniques for several field strength, FSE or GRE sequence derivatives have been published. Therefore, the implementation of MRC is possible on virtually every scanner. Excellent results regarding the diagnosis of biliary dilatation, stones, stenoses, and malignancies have been reported for FSE sequences using both breath-hold and non-breath-hold techniques. These studies, conducted with ERC correlation in smaller patient groups, have to be confirmed in larger studies. However, the replacement of purely diagnostic ERC seems possible and economically efficient in the absence of a high probability that endoscopic intervention will be necessary.

References

Barish MA, Yucel EK, Soto JA, Chuttani R, Ferrucci JT (1995) MR cholangiopancreatography: efficacy of three-dimensional turbo spin-echo technique. Am J Roentgenol 165:295–300

Baron RL (1987) Common bile duct stones: reassessment of criteria for CT diagnosis. Radiology 162:419–424

Beuers U, Spengler U, Sackmann M, Paumgartner G, Sauerbruch T (1992) Deterioration of cholestasis after endoscopic retrograde cholangiography in advanced primary sclerosing cholangitis. J Hepatol 15:140–143

Bilbao MK, Dotter CT, Lee TG, Katon RM (1976) Complications of endoscopic retrograde cholangiopanreatography (ERCP): a study of 10000 cases. Gastroenterology 70:314–320

Chezmar JL (1991) Magnetic resonance imaging of the liver. Technique. Radiol Clin North Am 29:1251–1258

Feinberg DA, Hale JD, Watts JC, Kaufman L, Mark A (1986) Halving MR imaging time by conjugation: demonstration at 3.5 kG. Radiology 161:527–531

Gauger J, Holzknecht N, Lackerbauer CA, Sittek H, Fiedler KE, Petsch R, Reiser M (1996) Breathhold imaging of the upper abdomen using a circular polarized-array coil: comparison with standard body coil imaging. MAGMA 4:93–104

Guibaud L, Bret PM, Reinhold C, Atri M, Barkun AN (1994) Diagnosis of choledocholithiasis: value of MR cholangiography. Am J Roentgenol 163:847–850

Guibaud L, Bret PM, Reinhold C, Atri M, Barkun AN (1995) Bile duct obstruction and choledocholithiasis: diagnosis with MR cholangiography. Radiology 197:109–115

Hall-Craggs MA, Allen CM, Owens CM, et al. (1993) MR cholangiography: clinical evaluation in 40 cases. Radiology 189:423–427

Hamm B, Vogl TJ, Branding G, Schnell B, Taupitz M, Wolf KJ, Lissner J (1992) Focal liver lesions: MR imaging with Mn-DPDP-initial clinical results in 40 patients (see comments). Radiology 182:167–174

Hamm B, Staks T, Muhler A, et al. (1995) Phase I clinical evaluation of Gd-EOB-DTPA as a hepatobiliary MR contrast agent: safety, pharmacokinetics, and MR imaging. Radiology 195:785–792

Hennig J, Nauerth A, Friedburg H (1986) A fast imaging method for clinical MR. Magn Reson Med 3:823–833

Ishizaki Y, Wakayama T, Okada Y, Kobayashi T (1993) Magnetic resonance cholangiography for evaluation of obstructive jaundice. Am J Gastroenterol 88:2072–2077

Laing FC, Jeffrey RB, Wing VW (1984) Improved visualization of choledocholithiasis by sonography. Am J Roentgenol 143:949–952

Laub G, Simonetti O, Nitz W (1995) Single-shot imaging of the heart with HASTE (abstract). In: Proceedings of the Society of Magnetic Resonance in Medicine and the European Society for Magnetic Resonance in Medicine and Biology. Society of Magnetic Resonance in Medicine, Berkeley, Calif, p 246

Laubenberger J, Buchert M, Schneider B, Blum U, Hennig J, Langer M (1995) Breath-hold projection magnetic resonance-cholangio-pancreaticography (MRCP): a new method for the examination of the bile and pancreatic ducts. Magn Reson Med 33:18–23

Low RN, Sigeti JS, Francis IR, Weinman D, Bower B, Shimakawa A, Foo TK (1994) Evaluation of malignant biliary obstruction: efficacy of fast multiplanar spoiled gradient-recalled MR imaging vs spin-echo MR imaging, CT, and cholangiography. Am J Roentgenol 162:315–323

Margosian PM (1986) Faster MR imaging: imaging with half the data. Health Care Instrum 1:195–197

Matsui O, Kadoya M, Takashima T (1989) Intrahepatic periportal abnormal intensity on MR images: an indication of various hepatobiliary diseases. Radiology 171:335–338

McCarthy S, Hricak H, Cohen M, Fisher MR, Winkler ML, Filly RA, Margulis AR (1986) Cholecystitis: detection with MR imaging. Radiology 158:333–336

Meiboom S, Gill D (1958) Modified spin-echo method for measuring nuclear relaxation times. Rev Sci Instrum 29:688–691

Miyazaki T, Yamashita Y, Tsuchigame T, Yamamoto H, Urata J, Takahashi M (1996) MR cholangiopancreatography using HASTE (half-Fourier acquisition single-shot turbo spin-echo) sequences. Am J Roentgenol 166:1297–1303

Morimoto K, Shimoi M, Shirakawa T, Aoki Y, Choi S, Miyata Y, Hara K (1992) Biliary obstruction: evaluation with three-dimensional MR cholangiography. Radiology 183:578–580

Panasen P, Partanen K, Pikkarainen P, Alhava E, Pirinen A, Janatuinen E (1992) Ultrasonography, CT and ERCP in the diagnosis of choledochal stones. Acta Radiol 33:53–56

Pavone P, Laghi A, Catalano C, et al. (1996) Lithiasis of the common bile duct: the role of cholangiography and magnetic resonance. Radiol Med (Torino) 91:420–423

Reinhold C, Guibaud L, Genin G, Bret PM (1995) MR cholangiopancreatography: comparison between two-dimensional fast spin-echo and three-dimensional gradient-echo pulse sequences. J Magn Reson Imaging 5:379–384

Reinhold C, Bret PM, Guibaud L, Barkun ANG (1996) MR cholangiopancreatography: potential clinical applications. Radiographics 16:309–320

Sananes JC, Bonnet M, Lecesne R, Raymond JM, Couzigou P, Laurent F, Drouillard J (1995) Magnetic resonance cholangiography using HASTE sequence (abstr). In: Proceedings of the Society of Magnetic Resonance in Medicine and the European Society for Magnetic Resonance in Medicine and Biology. Society of Magnetic Resonance in Medicine, Berkeley, CA, p 1453

Schulte SJ, Baron RL, Teefey SA, Rohrmann C Jr, Freeny PC, Shuman WP, Foster MA (1990) CT of the extrahepatic bile ducts: wall thickness and contrast enhancement in normal and abnormal ducts. Am J Roentgenol 154:79–85

Schumacher KA, Wallner B, Weidenmaier W, Friedrich JM (1991) Biliary obstruction: MR-cholangiography with a rapid gradient-echo sequence (2D CE-Fast). Fortschr Röntgenstr 155:332–336

Seifert E (1977) Endoscopic retrograde cholangiopancreatography. Am J Gastroenterol 68:542–549

Soto JA, Barish MA, Yucel EK, Ferrucci JT (1995) MR cholangiopancreatography: findings on 3D fast spin-echo imaging. Am J Roentgenol 165:1397–1401

Soto JA, Barish MA, Yucel EK, Siegenberg D, Ferrucci JT, Chuttani R (1996) Magnetic resonance cholangiography: comparison with endoscopic retrograde cholangiopancreatography. Gastroenterology 110:589–597

Takehara Y, Ichijo K, Tooyama N, et al. (1994) Breath-hold MR cholangiopancreatography with a long-echo-train fast spin-echo sequence and a surface coil in chronic pancreatitis. Radiology 192:73–78

Taourel P, Bret PM, Reinhold C, Barkun AN (1996) Anatomic variants of the biliary tree: diagnosis with MR cholangiopancreatography. Radiology 199:521–527

Teefey SA, Baron RL, Rohrmann CA, Shuman WP, Freeny PC (1988) Sclerosing cholangitis: CT findings. Radiology 169: 635–639

Vogl TJ, Pegios W, McMahon C, Balzer J, Waitzinger J, Pirovano G, Lissner J (1992) Gadobenate dimeglumine – a new contrast agent for MR imaging: preliminary evaluation in healthy volunteers. Am J Roentgenol 158:887–892

Wallner BK, Schumacher KA, Weidenmaier W, Friedrich JM (1991) Dilated biliary tract: evaluation with MR cholangiography with a T2-weighted contrast-enhanced fast sequence. Radiology 181:805–808

Weissleder R, Stark DD, Compton CC, Simeone JF, Ferrucci JT (1988) Cholecystitis: diagnosis by MR imaging. Magn Reson Imaging 6:345–348

Wielopolski PA, Zuo C, Clouse M, Buff B (1995) Breath-hold 3D cholangiography using RARE and segmented echo planar imaging readouts (abstract). In: Proceedings of the Society of Magnetic Resonance in Medicine and the European Society for Magnetic Resonance in Medicine and Biology. Society of Magnetic Resonance in Medicine, Berkeley, Calif., p 1448

Zimmon DS, Falkenstein DB, Riccobono C, Aaron B (1975) Complications of endoscopic retrograde cholangiopancreatography. Gastroenterology 69:303–309

7 Advanced MR Imaging Techniques for the Pancreas, with Emphasis on MR Pancreatography

T. Helmberger and S. Gryspeerdt

CONTENTS

7.1 Introduction

Due to advances in scanner and sequence technology, pancreatic magnetic resonance imaging (MRI) has improved considerably over the past ten years, providing a valuable alternative to computed tomography. First described as long ago as the mid 1980s, specifically fluid-sensitive sequences have undergone increasing improvement, allowing MR hydrography (MR urography, MR cholangiography) to be adopted as a more or less routine technique since the beginning of the 1990s (Hennig et al. 1986). However, visualization of the pancreatic duct by MRI is much more challenging than visualization of the bile ducts owing to the smaller structures.

Like MR cholangiography (MRC), MR pancreatography (MRP) is based on T2-weighted imaging. The principle is to display the fluid-filled pancreatic duct systems by using a heavily T2-weighted sequence and suppressing the background simultaneously.

The efficacy of MRP has to be proved by comparison with endoscopic retrograde pancreaticography (ERP). While ERP is still the gold standard for examination of the pancreatic duct and includes the option of interventional procedures, it does have a

T. Helmberger, MD, Department of Diagnostic Radiology, Klinikum Großhadern, Ludwig-Maximilians University, Marchioninistrasse 15, D-81377 Munich, Germany
S. Gryspeerdt, MD, Department of Radiology, University Hospitals K.U. Leuven, Herestraat 49, B-3000 Leuven, Belgium

number of drawbacks: (a) patient sedation is needed; (b) contrast material is needed; (c) an experienced operator is required; (d) successful intubation of the duct is possible only in 70%–91% of cases; (e) prestenotic or preocclusive opacification is circumscribed or impossible; (f) cannulation causes pancreatitis in 1%–2% of cases; (g) the mortality is 0.2% and the morbidity, 1%–7%; (h) in the case of failed ERCP/ERP, the transhepatic approach to the pancreatic duct is impossible (Bilbao et al. 1976; Ghazi and Washington 1989; Teplick et al. 1991).

Ultrasonography and computed tomography (CT) are inadequate for visualization of the pancreatic duct due to the frequency of intestinal artifacts (ultrasonography) or limited spatial and contrast resolution (CT).

As a result of the technical prerequisites, MRP is limited in terms of spatial resolution and the depiction of calculi, and is subject to artifacts due to patient motion. However, the benefits of MRP are convincing: (a) sedation is not required; (b) contrast material is not required; (c) there is less user/operator dependence; (d) visualization is not limited by stenosis or occlusion; (e) it can provide cross-sectional plus three-dimensional projection imaging.

7.2 Technique

In the following, MRI of the pancreatic parenchyma is discussed only briefly because technical details are presented in subsequent specific chapters (8–10). A comparison of different imaging techniques by Mitchell et al. (1995) showed that T1-weighted fat-suppressed images, by increasing the intrinsic contrast, had significant advantages for the depiction of the pancreatic borders and the pancreatic parenchyma. While T2-weighted fast spin-echo images were found to be superior to spin-echo T2-weighted images, motion artifacts remained the major limiting factor for the evaluation of the pancreatic duct in the axial plane (MITCHELL et al. 1995). A recent advantageous innovation in fast (turbo) spin-echo imaging has been the half-Fourier single-shot turbo spin-echo imaging (HASTE) technique. Using the HASTE technique, the pancreas can be evaluated in a subsecond image time, providing images free of motion artifacts. Although randomized studies in respect of the pancreas remain to be performed, encouraging initial results using the HASTE technique have already been reported (SEMELKA et al. 1996).

Optimal evaluation of inflammation requires optimization of the detection of structures with increased water content. This can be achieved by obtaining T2-weighted fat-suppressed images (MITCHELL et al. 1995). However, since T2-weighted fat-suppressed images result in a considerable reduction in the delineation of pancreatic parenchyma, they should be used in conjunction with other non-fat-suppressed T2-weighted images. Disadvantages of this technique are the need for an additional sequence, prolonging the investigation time, and the inability to obtain axial images that are identical to the no-fat saturation images. A new "double-echo" HASTE technique, recently presented by BOSMANS et al. (1996), seems a suitable means of overcoming these problems. In this technique an RF excitation pulse is followed by a long echo train of which the first part is used for an image with a short TE (60 ms) and the second part for an image with a later echo (TE 439 ms). Advantages of this technique are the fact that both images are obtained from the same anatomic position and the absence of any need for breath-holding.

For evaluation of the function of pancreatic parenchyma, gadolinium-DTPA-enhanced images are acquired. Fast low-angle shot (FLASH) images obtained immediately after the administration of gadolinium allow evaluation of the viability of pancreatic parenchyma in cases of acute pancreatitis, and of the degree of fibrosis in cases of chronic pancreatitis (SEMELKA and ASCHER 1993).

In addition to the advantages deriving from optimization of the sequences, the signal-to-noise and contrast-to-noise ratios in abdominal imaging have been improved by the use of phased-array surface coils instead of the body coil (CAMPEAU et al. 1995). However, the incomplete coverage of the abdomen by the surface coils is still a limitation.

In summary, a current pancreatic imaging protocol might include axial (fast) gradient-echo T1-weighted imaging with or without breath-hold and with and without fat suppression, axial (and coronal) fast spin-echo T2-weighted imaging with breath-hold, and the very promising technique of (double-echo) HASTE imaging with or without breath-hold (Fig. 7.1).

The range of heavily T2-weighted sequences includes variants of gradient-echo (e.g., PSIF, SSFP, CE-FAST, CE-GRASS), fast spin-echo (2D/3D fast SE), and multi-echo, "EPI-hybrid" sequences (RARE, HASTE) (DOOMS et al. 1986; HENNIG et al. 1986; WALLNER et al. 1991; MORIMOTO et al. 1992; TAKEHARA et al. 1994; BARISH et al. 1995; LAUBENBERGER et al. 1995; MACAULAY et al. 1995; MCDERMOTT and NELSON 1995; REINHOLD et al. 1995; SOTO et al. 1995). In addition, methods can be distinguished according to the acquisition time (breath-hold vs non-breath-hold) and the means of image acquisition (e.g., thick-slab, projection imaging vs multislice plus 3D reformation).

Non-breath-hold imaging usually takes the form of gradient-echo or fast spin-echo imaging with 3D reformation. Adjusted to the needs of a heavy T2 weighting, these sequences produce adequate representation of the pancreatic duct. However, despite acquisition averaging, motion can still compromise image quality. In addition, multi-spin-echo sequences (fast or turbo spin-echo) suffer from a distorted point spread function resulting in reduced resolution, and from J-coupling effects causing increased signal intensity of fat (WALLNER et al. 1991; CONSTABLE and GORE 1992; MORIMOTO et al. 1992; MCDERMOTT and NELSON 1995; REINHOLD et al. 1995; SOTO et al. 1995).

Due to "real" T2 weighting, EPI-hybrid sequences (RARE, i.e., rapid acquisition relaxation enhanced, and HASTE) show superior contrast to gradient-echo imaging (HENNIG et al. 1986). Furthermore, the originally low signal intensity of subminute fast spin-echo imaging can be compensated by using surface (phased-array) coils. Thus, a valuable gain in signal-to-noise and contrast-to-noise ratios can be achieved, combined with excellent spatial resolution (LAUBENBERGER et al. 1995).

Because of the excellent projection display of the pancreatic duct system and the high in-plane resolution on 2D imaging, a combined MRP protocol consisting of a RARE and a HASTE sequence may be preferred. Such studies are ideally performed on high-field scanners equipped with a surface coil (e.g., four-element body–phased-array surface coil).

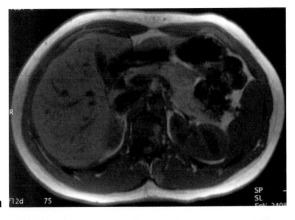
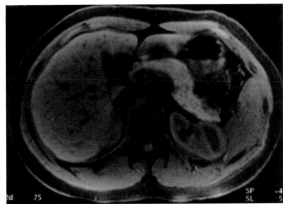
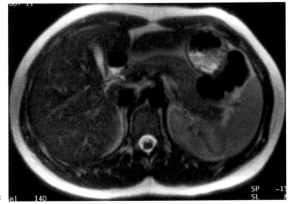

Fig. 7.1 a–c. MRI of the normal pancreas. **a** Artifact-free delineation of the pancreas on non-fat-suppressed gradient-echo breath-hold T1-weighted imaging (TR 140 ms, TE 4.1 ms, flip angle 75°, FOV 240 × 320, matrix 144 × 256, 18 × 5 mm, TA 20 s). Increased intrinsic parenchymal contrast can be provided by using frequency selective fat suppression (**b**; TR 155 ms, TE 4.8 ms, flip angle 75°, FOV 240 × 320 mm, matrix 132 × 256, 5 × 5 mm, TA 20 s). Breath-hold HASTE imaging (TR ~, TE_{eff} 60 ms, echo spacing 4.3 ms, ETL 72, FOV 240 × 320 mm, matrix 160 × 256, 18 × 8 mm, TA 19 s) offers excellent T2 contrast without the limitations of conventional spin-echo or fast spin-echo T2-weighted imaging (**c**)

The RARE sequence produces an ERCP-like projection image (LAUBENBERGER et al. 1995). In this single-shot sequence [TR 11.5 ms, TE_{eff} 1200 ms, matrix 256 × 256, field of view (FOV) 250–320 mm, slab 60–80 mm, TA 5.3 s] a train of progressively phase-encoded spin-echoes is generated by a series of 180° refocusing pulses (Fig. 7.2a). The effective echo time of 1200 ms is determined by the position of the zero point of phase encoding. Thus, a heavy T2 weighting can be provided.

Planned on an axial GRE T1-weighted localizer, a thick slab is angulated parallel to the pancreatic duct in the coronal plane. With a slab thickness of between 80 and 100 mm the pancreas can be covered in most cases. Sometimes multiple angulations are needed following the curved shape of the pancreas. With a slab thickness of maximally 100 mm and careful slab positioning, overlap from fluid-containing structures such as the spinal canal, stomach, and urinary system usually can be avoided.

RARE imaging is done during an inspiration breath-hold of about 5 s. This procedure is recommended because most patients feel more comfort-able than with expiration. Additionally, due to the short acquisition time this sequence is suitable even for severely ill patients. In our experience of about 400 patients who have undergone MR cholangio- and pancreatography, no patient has been unable to hold their breath for 5 s.

In principle, HASTE imaging is based on the RARE technique (SANANES et al. 1995). However, by using the half-Fourier technique the readout of the k-space can be reduced dramatically (Fig. 7.2b). Thus, data collection takes about 450 ms per slice. Using this technique [TR theoretically infinite, TE_{eff} 87 ms, echotrain length 140, matrix 256 × 256, FOV 240–300 mm, SL (slices) 17, slice thickness 3 mm, TA 23 s], stationary fluids present a bright signal due to the heavy T2 weighting while soft tissue and circulating fluids contribute no signal. Due to inadequate signal loss, a slice thickness of less than 3 mm is inappropriate. With an in-plane resolution of about 0.9 × 1.2 mm, the resulting anisotropy is still considerable.

The study can be performed in an axial or oblique coronal slice orientation parallel to the pancreas

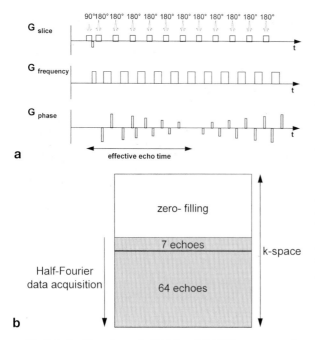

a

b

Fig. 7.2 a,b. Flow chart of a RARE and HASTE sequence. **a** In RARE imaging the remaining transversal magnetization after the first 180° pulse is used to provoke the next echoes with a progressive phase encoding. **b** HASTE imaging basically uses the RARE technique. However, by reading only half the k-space (half Fourier technique) the acquisition time for the single slice can be shortened enormously

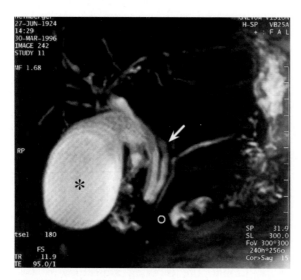

Fig. 7.3 a,b. Maximum intensity projection reconstruction of HASTE MRP. In addition to the nondilated pancreatic duct, the common bile duct and the distal inserting cystic duct (*arrow*) are demonstrated. Note the enlarged gallbladder (*)

(Fig. 7.3). Routinely, 3D reconstruction (maximum intensity projection) of the single slices is not necessary due to the 3D overview provided by RARE imaging. However, in cases where RARE imaging fails, a reformatted, ERCP-like presentation based on RARE imaging is helpful.

Using the different MRP techniques described above, the sensitivity for the detection of ductal dilatation and stenoses ranges between 75% and 100% and between 62% and 75%, respectively (MORIMOTO et al. 1992; BARISH et al. 1995; LAUBENBERGER et al. 1995; SANANES et al. 1995). In our own experience with breath-hold RARE and HASTE imaging the sensitivity/specificity for detecting dilatations and stenoses is 100%/91.6% and 64.7%/91.6%, respectively, using ERP as the reference investigation (49 patients; data presented at RSNA 1996).

7.3
Clinical Applications of MR Pancreatography

7.3.1
Normal Pancreatic Duct and Variants

The diameter of the normal pancreatic duct is less than 2 mm. The rate of successful visualization varies according to the MRP technique, from 23% with gradient-echo imaging (REINHOLD et al. 1995) to up to 91% with different fast spin-echo variants (BARISH et al. 1995; BRET et al. 1995; MACAULAY et al. 1995; REINHOLD et al. 1996). Furthermore, some authors consider nonvisualization of the duct as a sign of normality (BARISH et al. 1995). Studies in volunteers have demonstrated that RARE and HASTE imaging during breath-hold demonstrates the normal duct in 100% of cases (LAUBENBERGER et al. 1995; own data, submitted for publication). Comparison with ERCP indicates that with RARE and HASTE imaging side branches of the nondilated duct are not depicted routinely. In our experience, the ductal course within the papilla of Vater is seen only incidentally, the most likely reason being that in normal individuals the papillary sphincter is closed without stimulation.

While ERCP identifies an abnormality of the ductal system within the pancreatic head in cases of pancreas divisum, in many cases the duct of Santorini is not visualized due to technical problems in cannulating the minor papilla. In contrast, BRET et al. (1995) diagnosed pancreas divisum in up to 14% of 289 patients by MRP as an incidental finding, using a 2D fast spin-echo sequence and a phased-array coil with a high level of accuracy (Fig. 7.4).

7.3.2
Pathologic Conditions of the Pancreatic Duct

Magnetic resonance pancreatography routinely depicts the dilated and nondilated pancreatic duct, and in addition dilated ducts proximal to an occlusion that are not accessible with ERCP. However, MRP has limited ability to demonstrate the obstructive cause because only the fluid-containing duct is displayed. Calculi either cannot be seen or are confused with air bubbles post ERCP. In such cases, additional axial T1- and T2-weighted imaging is helpful.

There is only limited experience in the use of MRI for the imaging of acute pancreatitis, but MRP seems to be able to show the pancreatic duct, whether it is dilated or not, as well as the surrounding fluid (Fig. 7.5).

In chronic pancreatitis, MRP matches ERCP in the delineation of the dilated and irregularly formed pancreatic duct and dilated side branches (Fig. 7.6). Pancreatic pseudocysts are only demonstrated by ERCP in the presence of communication with the

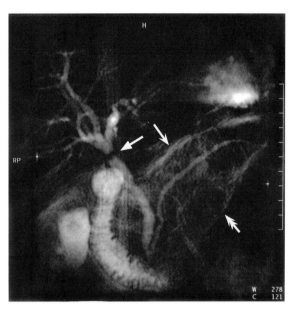

Fig. 7.5. In this patient with alcohol-induced acute pancreatitis, MRP using HASTE (oblique coronal orientation) reveals a nondilated pancreatic duct with thin side branches and a small rim of fluid surrounding the gland (*arrows*). Note the additional slight stricture of the common hepatic duct (*double arrow*) with a history of stone-induced biliary inflammation

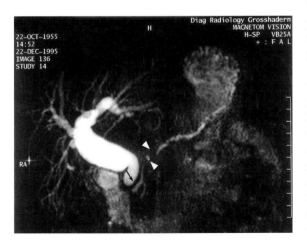

Fig. 7.4. In this 41-year-old female patient with alcohol-induced pancreatitis, RARE imaging reveals a persistent duct of Santorini (*arrow*) in addition to inflammatory irregularity and stenosis (*as heads*) of the pancreatic duct. Note the excellent demonstration of the biliary system dilated due to a swollen papilla. The intrapapillary biliary and pancreatic ducts are not depicted

duct. If there is no communication, the cyst will be missed by ERCP or a mass effect is merely appreciated indirectly. In contrast, MRP reveals communicating and noncommunicating cysts routinely (Fig. 7.7) and, when both T1- and T2-weighted MRI is performed, offers additional information about the content of the cyst and the relationship to other organs (Fig. 7.8).

In general, for the clinical workup of pancreatic tumors, cross-sectional imaging and ERCP are necessary. During recent years, technical advances have established MRI as a technique comparable to CT for the characterization of pancreatic tumors. On the other hand, ERCP is often limited in imaging the affected duct: (a) in pancreatic head tumors cannulation of the duct is often impossible; (b) in more distally located tumors, the proximal duct can be visualized, but not the duct distal to the neoplastic occlusion. These limitations can be overcome by MRP. MRP is able (a) to delineate pancreatic as well as biliary ducts in papillary or pancreatic head tumors, (b) to estimate the length of tumorous ductal occlusion, and (c) to depict the dilated duct distal to the occlusion or stenosis (Fig. 7.9).

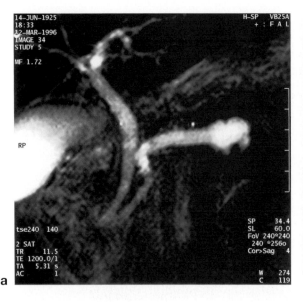

a

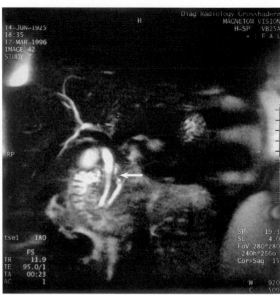

b

Fig. 7.6 a,b. In this 64-year-old female with a clinical history of chronic pancreatitis, ERCP failed in cannulating the pancreatic duct. RARE imaging (**a**) reveals a dilats proximal duct with a club-like swelling in the region of the pancreatic body. The signal loss in the very proximal part of the duct (*arrow*) on coronal HASTE imaging (**b**) was proved to be a calculus that could not be reliably seen on RARE imaging. Note that the biliary and the pancreatic duct can be followed into the papillary region on both RARE and HASTE imaging

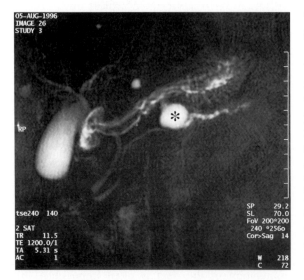

Fig. 7.7. In this 58-year-old female with known chronic pancreatitis, MRP depicts a noncommunicating pseudocyst (*), whereas ERCP revealed only signs of a mass effect. RARE imaging demonstrates the normal proximal duct as well as dilatation of the distal duct due to compression by the cyst

7.4
Conclusion

While the biliary system can be opacified by percutaneous transhepatic cholangiography and by ERCP, visualization of the pancreatic duct is routinely possible only by ERP. MRP offers a noninvasive, reproducible alternative without the limitations and disadvantages of ERP, such as the need for sedation and analgesia, the risk of induction of pancreatitis, the frequent failure of cannulation, the lack of visualization of the pancreatic duct distal to an occlusion, and the need for separate cannulation of the biliary system. However, the diagnostic value of MRP may be restricted by fluid-containing structures (e.g., duodenum, stomach, ascites) that may surround the pancreas and by signal loss due to hemorrhage, calculi, or proteinaceous excretion within the duct.

Discussion as to the "best" sequence for MRP continues, mainly on the basis of the hard- and software capabilities of the current MRI systems. Recent studies indicate that the most reliable results are provided by 3D fast spin-echo imaging in non-breath-hold and by EPI-hybrid imaging in breath-hold MRP. For every sequence used, there seems to be agreement on the advantage of using surface

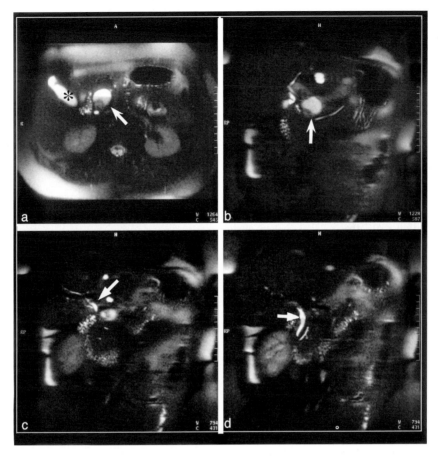

Fig. 7.8 a–d. ERCP showed a kink in the pancreatic duct that was interpreted as a congenital anomaly. No mass effect was seen. In the area of the kink, MRP (axial HASTE imaging at subsequent levels) delineates a cyst containing a soft tissue mass (**a, b,** *arrow*) that was surgically proven to be an adenocarcinoma of the pancreas. The proximal and distal pancreatic duct shows a normal caliber (**b, d**). The gallbladder (*) and parts of the common bile duct (*double arrow*) are also demonstrated (**a, c, d**)

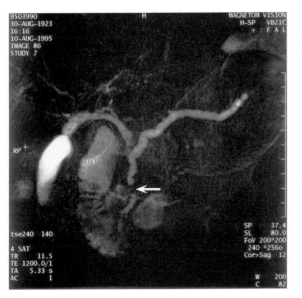

Figure 7.9. In this patient with adenocarcinoma of the pancreas, ERCP displayed the duct only within the pancreatic head, while MRP reveals the tumor-induced occlusion (*arrow*) together with the slightly dilated duct proximal to the occlusion

(body) coils due to the benefit in terms of signal intensity (GUIBAUD et al. 1994; OUTWATER and GORDON 1994; TAKEHARA et al. 1994; BARISH et al. 1995; GUIBAUD et al. 1995; LAUBENBERGER et al. 1995; MACAULAY et al. 1995; MCDERMOTT and NELSON 1995; REINHOLD et al. 1995; SANANES et al. 1995; SOTO et al. 1995; REINHOLD et al. 1996).

No matter which MRP technique gains acceptance, MRP is extending MRI and may prove the method of choice for noninvasive screening of the pancreatic duct to assess the need for further interventional procedures. In consequence, ERP will become an exclusively therapeutic instrument, and ultimately an impact on diagnostic and therapeutic cost-effectiveness can be anticipated.

References

Barish MA, Yucel EK, Soto JA, Chuttani R, Ferrucci JT (1995) MR choalangiopancreatography: efficacy of three-dimensional turbo spin-echo technique. AJR 165:295–300

Bilbao M, Dotter C, Lee T, Katon R (1976) Complication of retrograde cholangiopancreaticography (ERCP). A study of 10 000 cases. Gastroenterology 70:314–320

Bosmans H, Kiefer B, Gryseerdt S, Van Hoe L, Marchal GJ, Baert AI (1996) Single-shot half-Fourier double-echo MR imaging acquisition: promising clinical applications. 82nd scientific assembly and annual meeting, RSNA 12/1–12/6 1996 (Suppl). Radiology 201:529

Bret P, Reinhold C, Taourel P, Barkun A, Atri M (1995) Pancreas divisum: evaluation with MR imaging. Proceedings of the Societ of Magnetic Resonance. 3. Scientific meeting and exhibition, SMR/ESMRMB, Nice, France. Book of abstracts, vol 3:1452

Campeau NG, Johnson CD, Felmlee JP, Rydberg JN, Butts RK, Ehman RL, Riederer SJ (1995) MR imaging of the abdomen with a phased-array multicoil: prospective clinical evaluation. Radiology 195:769–776

Constable R, Gore J (1992) The loss of small objects in variable TE imaging: implications for FSE, RARE, and EPI. Magn Reson Med 28:9–24

Dooms G, Fisher M, Higgins C, Hricak H, Goldberg H, Margulis A (1986) MR imaging of the dilated biliary tract. Radiology 158:337–341

Ghazi A, Washington M (1989) Endoscopic retrograde cholangiopancreatography, endoscopic sphincterotomy and biliary drainage. Surg Clin North Am 69:1249–1274

Guibaud L, Bret P, Reinhold C, Atri M, Barkun A (1994) Diagnosis of choledocholithiasis: value of MR cholangiography. AJR 163:847–850

Guibaud L, Bret P, Reinhod C, Atri M, Barkun A (1995) Bile duct obstruction and choledocholithiasis: diagnosis with MR cholangiography. Radiology 197:109–115

Hennig J, Nauerth A, Friedburg H (1986) RARE imaging: a fast imaging method for clinical MR. Magn Reson Med 3:823–833

Laubenberger J, Büchert M, Schneider B, Blum U, Hennig J, Langer M (1995) Breath-hold projection Magnetic Resonance-cholangio-pancreaticography (MRCP): a new method for the examination of the bile and pancreatic ducts. Magn Reson Med 33:18–23

Macaulay S, Schulte S, Sekijima J, et al. (1995) Evaluation of a non-breath-hold MR cholangiography technique. Radiology 196:227–232

McDermott V, Nelson R (1995) MR cholangiopancreatography: efficacy of three-dimensional turbo spin-echo technique (letter). AJR 165:301–302

Mitchell DG, Winston CB, Outwater EK, Ehrlich SM (1995) Delineation of the pancreas with MR imaging: multiobserver comparison of five pulse sequences. J Magn Reson Imag 5:193–199

Morimoto K, Shimoi M, Shirakawa T, Aoki Y, Choi S, Miyata Y, Hara K (1992) Biliary obstruction: evaluation with three-dimensional MR cholangiography. Radiology 183:578–580

Outwater E, Gordon S (1994) Imaging the pancreatic and biliary ducts with MRI. Radiology 192:19–21

Reinhold C, Guibaud L, Genin G, Bret P (1995) MR cholangiopancreatography: comparison between two-dimensional fast spin-echo and three-dimensional gradient-echo pulse sequences. J Magn Reson Imaging 4:379–384

Reinhold C, Bret P, Guibaud L, Barkun ANG, Genin G, Atri M (1996) MR cholangiopancreatography: potential clinical application. Radiographics 16:309–320

Sananes J, Bonnet M, Lecesne R, Raymond J, Couzigou P, Laurent F, Drouillard J (1995) Magnetic resonance cholangiography using HASTE sequence. Optimization and clinical evaluation in extrahepatic cholestasis. Proceedings of the Society of Magnetic Resonance. 3. Scientific meeting and exhibition, SMR/ESMRMB, Nice, France. Book of abstracts, vol 3:1453

Semelka RC, Ascher SM (1993) MR imaging of the pancreas. Radiology 188:593–602

Semelka RC, Kelekis NL, Thomasson D, Brown MA, Laub GA (1996) HASTE MR imaging: description of technique and preliminary results in the abdomen. J Magn Reson Imaging 6:698–699

Soto J, Barish M, Yucel E, Siegenberg D, Chuttani R, Ferrucci J (1995) Pancreatic duct: MR cholangiopancreatography with a three-dimensional fast spin-echo technique. Radiology 196:459–464

Takehara Y, Ichijo K, Tooyama N, et al. (1994) Breath-hold MR cholangiopancreatography with a long-echo-train fast spin-echo sequence and a surface coil in chronic pancreatitis. Radiology 192:73–78

Teplick S, Flick P, Brandon J (1991) Transhepatic cholangiography in patients with suspected biliary disease and non-dilated intrahepatic bile ducts. Gastrointest Radiol 16:193–197

Wallner B, Schumacher K, Weidenmaier W, Friedrich J (1991) Dilated biliary tract: evaluation with MR cholangiography with a T2-weighted contrast-enhanced fast sequence. Radiology 181:805–808

8 Acute and Chronic Pancreatitis

S. Gryspeerdt, L. Van Hoe, and A.L. Baert

CONTENTS

8.1
Introduction

While computed tomography (CT) and ultrasound (US) have proven to be invaluable for the evaluation of the pancreatic parenchyma in patients with acute or chronic pancreatitis, assessment of the pancreatic duct and biliary tree by US or CT remains difficult. This is a serious shortcoming, since gallstone pancreatitis accounts for 62% of all cases of acute pancreatitis (Winslet et al. 1992), and the diagnosis of

chronic pancreatitis requires an accurate evaluation of subtle ductal changes. Until recently, endoscopic retrograde cholangiopancreatography (ERCP) and percutaneous transhepatic cholangiography (PTC) were the only techniques providing good visualization of the pancreaticobiliary tree. The invasive nature of both techniques, however, carries an inherent mortality and morbidity of, respectively, 1% and 7% (Lenriot et al. 1993). Pancreatitis is one of the most frequently encountered complications of ERCP (Sherman and Lehman 1991).

Magnetic resonance (MR) imaging combines the advantages of cross-sectional imaging techniques, such as US and CT, with the ability to visualize the pancreaticobiliary tree, as in ERCP and PTC. The use, advantages, and limitations of MR imaging for the evaluation of acute and chronic pancreatitis will be discussed.

8.2
Technique

Details of advanced MR imaging techniques for the pancreas have already been discussed in Chap. 7.

A current imaging protocol would preferably consist of axial breath-hold fast low-angle shot (FLASH) or non-breath-hold turbo FLASH sequences for T1-weighted images, and breath-bold half-Fourier single-shot turbo spin-echo (HASTE) (double-echo HASTE if available) for T2-weighted images. T2-weighted imaging is performed in the axial plane, as well as in the coronal plane. The latter is performed perpendicular to the pancreas as well as through the pancreatic tail. To reduce partial volume averaging, we use thin slices of 5 mm. In this way, detailed images are obtained that include invaluable information concerning the pancreatic duct as well as the pancreatic parenchyma. Especially images with a long TE are very reliable in demonstrating ductal changes as well as small pseudocysts (Fig. 8.1). The disadvantage of the thin-slice HASTE technique is the inability to obtain projectional images

S. Gryspeerdt, MD, Department of Radiology, University Hospitals K.U. Leuven, Herestraat 49, B-3000 Leuven, Belgium
L. Van Hoe, MD, Department of Radiology, University Hospitals K.U. Leuven, Herestraat 49, B-3000 Leuven, Belgium
A.L. Baert, MD, Professor, Department of Radiology, University Hospitals K.U. Leuven, Herestraat 49, B-3000 Leuven, Belgium

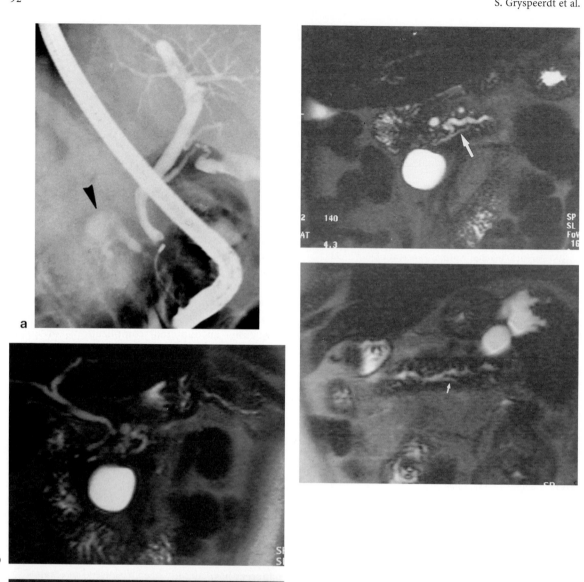

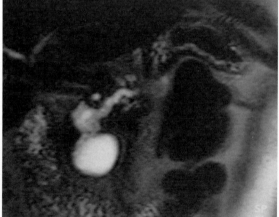

Fig. 8.1 a–e. Chronic pancreatitis in a 55-year-old, critically ill patient, who was unable to maintain a 5-s breath-hold: use of double-echo single-shot half-Fourier turbo spin-echo imaging in the detection of pseudocysts with splenic extension after incomplete ERCP. **a** ERCP shows the distal pancreatic duct and a single pseudocyst (*arrowhead*). There is no visualization of the proximal pancreatic duct. **b–d** Coronal T2-weighted images with TE 439 ms, obtained through the pancreatic head, show the pseudocyst, already known from ERCP, and additionally a second large as well as multiple small pseudocysts in the pancreatic head and a small ventral pancreatic duct (*arrow*). **e** A coronal T2-weighted image with TE 439 ms through the pancreatic tail shows pseudocysts extending from the pancreatic tail into the splenic hilum and upper pole. The irregular dilatation of the proximal pancreatic duct (not seen on ERCP) and its side branches (*arrow*) is clearly appreciated

without postprocessing. For the purpose of obtaining projectional images, comparable with cholangiopancreatography, we currently use the rapid acquisition by repeated echoes (RARE) technique. The RARE technique, however, requires a short 5-s breath-hold period. For critically ill patients, in whom breath-holding is impossible, images with a long TE (obtained with double-echo HASTE technique) are used instead (Fig. 8.1).

8.3
Evaluation of the Normal Pancreatic Parenchyma and Normal Pancreatic Duct

The normal pancreas exhibits a relatively high signal intensity on T1-weighted images. Immediately after the administration of contrast material, the pancreas shows a capillary blush, reflecting normal vasculature. On 10 min postcontrast FLASH images, the pancreas has a diminished signal intensity relative to fat (SEMELKA et al. 1991; BRAILSFORD et al. 1994).

On T2-weighted images, normal pancreas appears isointense to the liver parenchyma. Until recently, T2-weighted imaging of the pancreas was considerably impaired by motion artifacts. Recently, however, the use of HASTE and other turbo spin-echo sequences has proved reliable in delineating the pancreatic parenchyma.

Using magnetic resonance cholangiopancreatography (MRCP), the normal pancreatic duct may be visualized in up to 66% of cases in the pancreatic head, and in 31% of cases in the pancreatic body (MACAULEY et al. 1995). The rather low sensitivity for detecting a normal nondilated pancreatic duct is one of the weak points of MRCP (MACAULEY et al. 1995; OUTWATER and GORDON 1994; SOTO et al. 1995b; TAKEHARA et al. 1994).

8.4
Evaluation of Anatomic Variants That May Be Responsible for Recurrent Episodes of Pancreatitis

Anatomic variants that may be responsible for acute or chronic pancreatitis include pancreas divisum, annular pancreas, anomalous junction of the common bile duct and the pancreatic duct, and biliary cysts.

8.4.1
Pancreas Divisum

Pancreas divisum occurs in 5%–10% of patients undergoing ERCP and thus constitutes the most frequent congenital ductal anomaly of the pancreas (SUGAWA et al. 1987). Pancreas divisum originates in a failure of complete fusion of the dorsal and ventral pancreas: the common bile duct and ventral pancreatic duct drain into the duodenum through the major papilla, and the dorsal pancreatic duct drains through the minor papilla. Both chronic and acute pancreatitis have been reported to be associated with pancreas divisum (BERNARD et al. 1990; WARSHAW et al. 1983).

A recent study reported on the diagnosis of pancreas divisum with MRCP (BRET et al. 1996). Axial images were found to be most reliable for the detection of pancreas divisum in the majority of patients. MRCP typically shows an atrophic ventral duct posterior and to the left of the common bile duct on axial images (Fig. 8.2).

Compared with ERCP, MRCP suffers from inferior spatial resolution Although the diagnosis of pancreas divisum can be made with MRCP, the inferior resolution represents a limitation of the technique that has the following consequences:

1. The ventral duct is not appreciated in many cases [17 out of 25 patients in the study by BRET et al. (1996)]; consequently the diagnosis of pancreas divisum frequently relies upon the identification of a common bile duct terminating in the duodenum separately from the dorsal pancreatic duct. Associated findings typically seen on ERCP, such as a tapered pancreatic duct demonstrating early arborization, also remain undiagnosed on MRCP.

2. MRCP does not always allow differentiation between complete and incomplete pancreas divisum.

3. Direct diagnosis of stenosis of the accessory ampulla, responsible for recurrent episodes of acute pancreatitis, is impossible with MRCP. Stenosis, however, results in dilatation of pancreatic ducts that can be diagnosed on MRCP.

8.4.2
Annular Pancreas

In annular pancreas, the head of the pancreas completely encircles the duodenum, usually in its second portion. This results in duodenal obstruction in approximately 50% of patients during childhood. Annular pancreas causes chronic pancreatitis in ap-

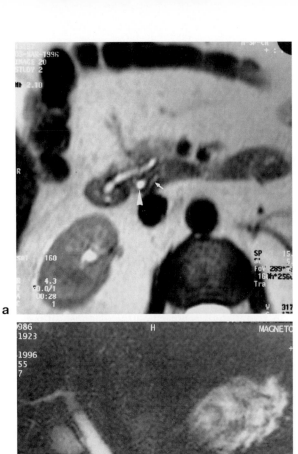

a

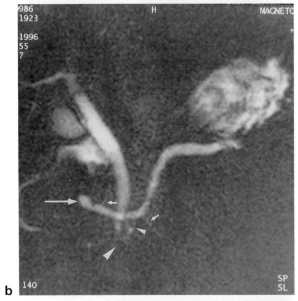

b

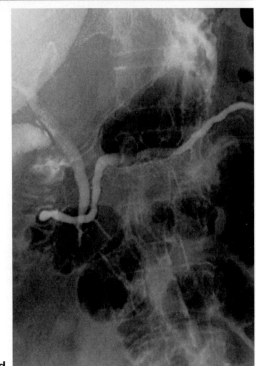

d

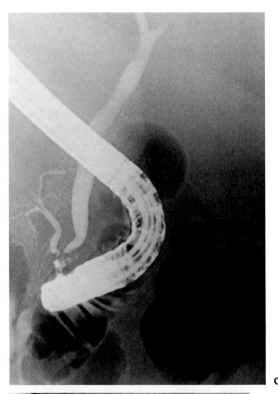

c

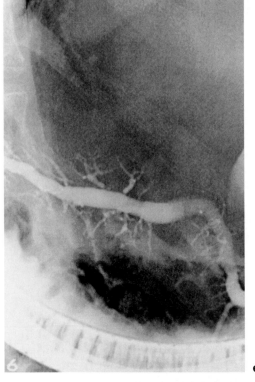

e

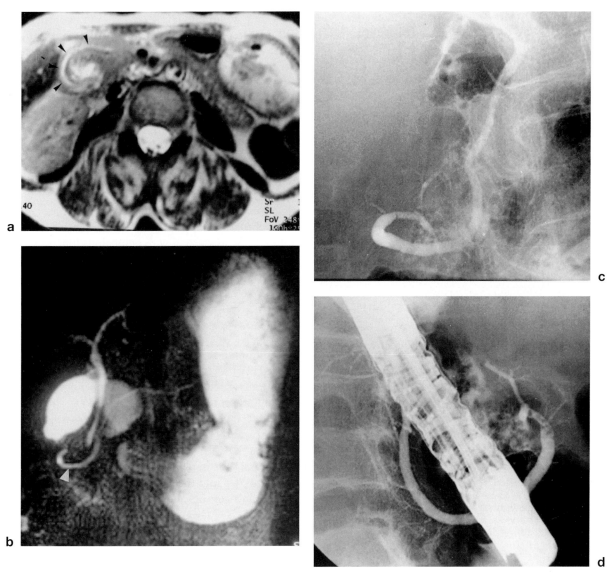

Fig. 8.3 a–d. Annular pancreas. **a** Axial T2-weighted image shows the main pancreatic duct (*arrowheads*) encircling the duodenum. **b** Single-shot MR pancreatogram using the RARE technique more clearly depicts the main pancreatic duct (*arrowhead*) that encircles the duodenum. **c,d** ERCP confirms the presence of annular pancreas. There is a slight dilatation of the main pancreatic duct as well as slight irregular dilatation of the side branches representing mild chronic pancreatitis. These minor changes are not noted on MRCP

◄

Fig. 8.2 a–e. Chronic pancreatitis in a patient with pancreas divisum and "Santorino-cele." **a** Axial T2-weighted images show a small ventral duct posterior (*arrow*) and medial of the common bile duct (*arrowhead*). The dorsal pancreatic duct drains into the duodenum through the papilla minor. There is a focal dilatation of the intramural portion of the dorsal pancreatic duct: Santorino-cele. **b** Single-shot MR pancreatogram using the RARE technique more clearly depicts the relationship between the papilla major (*arrowhead*) and minor (*arrow*). There is also visualization of the ventral pancreatic duct (*small arrowhead*), as well as some dilated side branches of the ventral (*small arrow*) and dorsal pancreatic duct (*small arrow*). **c–e** ERCP confirms the presence of pancreas divisum (**c**), Santorino-cele (**d**), and mild chronic pancreatitis (**d,e**). Both MRCP and ERCP demonstrate dilatation of side branches of the ventral and dorsal pancreatic duct in the pancreatic head (*small arrows* and *arrowheads* in **b**, **d** and **e**). ERCP additionally reveals mild dilatation of the side branches in the pancreatic tail (**e**), not appreciated on MRCP

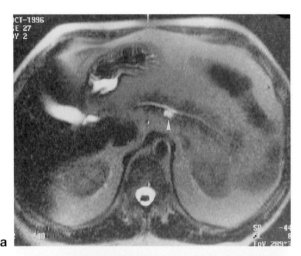

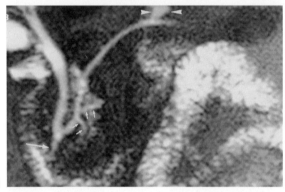

Fig. 8.4 a,b. Long common channel in a patient with chronic pancreatitis. **a** Axial T2-weighted image with long TE (439 ms) shows a small intrapancreatic pseudocyst (*arrowhead*). **b** Single-shot MR cholangiopancreatogram using the RARE technique demonstrates the presence of a long common channel (*arrow*) as the probable cause of chronic pancreatitis. The RARE image also shows the pancreatic pseudocyst (*arrowheads*) as well as mild dilatation of side branches in the pancreatic head (*small arrows*)

proximately 15%–20% of patients (Van der Horst 1961). MRCP diagnoses annular pancreas by demonstrating an encirclement of the duodenum by the pancreatic duct (Fig. 8.3).

8.4.3
Anomalous Junction of Common Bile Duct and Pancreatic Duct

Anomalous junction of the pancreaticobiliary ductal system is defined as a union of the common bile duct and pancreatic duct occurring outside the duodenum and beyond the influence of the sphincter of Boyden. Different types of anomalous junction are:

(a) a long common channel (>4–5 mm), (b) insertion of the common bile duct into the pancreatic duct, and (c) a more complex union of the ducts (Rizzo et al. 1995). Anomalous junction can be detected on MR pancreatography. Especially a long common channel can be appreciated on projectional images. However, no studies have investigated the exact anatomic correlation between the pancreatic duct and the common bile duct on ERCP and MRCP. It thus remains questionable whether MRCP can reliably distinguish between the different types of normal and abnormal union. The finding of an abnormal union may nevertheless be important since chronic relapsing pancreatitis has been reported to be associated with anomalous junction of the pancreaticobiliary ducts (Fig. 8.4).

8.4.4
Biliary Cysts

Five different types of biliary cyst have been described (Todani et al. 1977): type I, choledochocyst; type II, diverticulum; type III, choledochocele; type IV, multiple communicating intra- and extrahepatic duct cysts; type V, Caroli's disease. Of these five types of biliary cyst it is type III, choledochocele, that may cause pancreatitis. An analogous bulbous dilated intramural portion of the main pancreatic duct that herniates into the duodenum has also been described and can be called a Santorino-cele. Such a Santorino-cele may also cause recurrent pancreatitis (Fig. 8.2).

8.5
Acute Pancreatitis

8.5.1
Definition and Possible Role of Magnetic Resonance Imaging

The Cambridge symposium defined acute pancreatitis as an acute inflammatory disease of the pancreas, typically causing abdominal pain, and usually associated with raised pancreatic enzyme levels in blood or urine (Axon 1989; Sarner and Cotton 1984; Freeny 1989). The Marseille symposium proposed the same clinical definition and included pathomorphology (Freeny 1989). According to the severity, pancreatitis is classified as either mild (no multisystem failure and uncomplicated recovery) or severe (multisystem failure and/or development of a

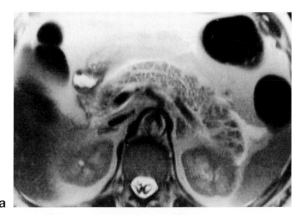

a

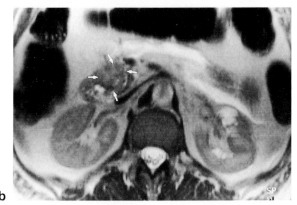

b

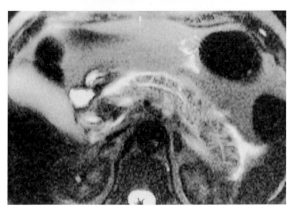

c

Fig. 8.5 a–c. Double-echo single-shot half-Fourier turbo spin-echo imaging in the detection of acute pancreatitis secondary to adenocarcinoma of the pancreatic head. **a,b** Images with TE 60 ms show the peripancreatic fluid collections (**a**) and a pancreatic adenocarcinoma, seen as a slightly hyperintense mass in the pancreatic head (*arrows*, **b**). **c** Pancreatic edema causes an increased signal intensity of the pancreatic parenchyma on T2-weighted images. This is more clearly depicted on images with a long TE (439 ms) than on those with a short TE (**a**)

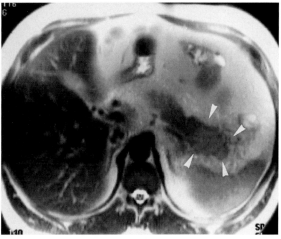

Fig. 8.6. Acute pancreatitis. Axial T2-weighted images show a focal enlargement and increased signal intensity of the pancreatic tail (*arrowheads*)

more severe form. Considering this clinical classification, it is clear that in the evaluation of the patient suffering from acute pancreatitis the radiologist has to answer two questions:

1. Is there necrosis of the pancreatic parenchyma?
2. How severe are the peripancreatic inflammatory changes?

A third obvious question to be answered is the presence of underlying abnormalities. In this respect, MR imaging is useful for the diagnosis of an underlying unsuspected pancreatic carcinoma. Pancreatitis due to carcinoma (Fig. 8.5) is, however, less frequent than pancreatitis due to alcohol abuse or biliary pancreatitis.

Two reports emphasized the utility of early ERCP and sphincterotomy in cases of biliary pancreatitis (e.g., pancreatitis caused by common bile duct stones) (NEOPTOLEMOS et al. 1988; FAN et al. 1993). Comparison of MRCP and ERCP reveals that MRCP is not suitable for the immediate treatment of pancreatitis. The complications that are related to ERCP, however, occur more frequently in patients with pancreatitis. A role for MRCP might thus lie in the primary investigation of patients referred with a suspected diagnosis of acute pancreatitis. If a common bile duct stone is detected as the cause of pancreatitis, ERCP can be performed subsequently; otherwise, the patient may be spared ERCP. However, a significant problem to be expected when evaluating the frequently physically ill patients suffering from acute pancreatitis is the inability to obtain images using a breath-hold technique; axial images obtained

complication, for example pseudocysts). In the mild form, peripancreatic fat necrosis and interstitial edema may be recognized but gland necrosis is absent. Gland necrosis is frequently present in the

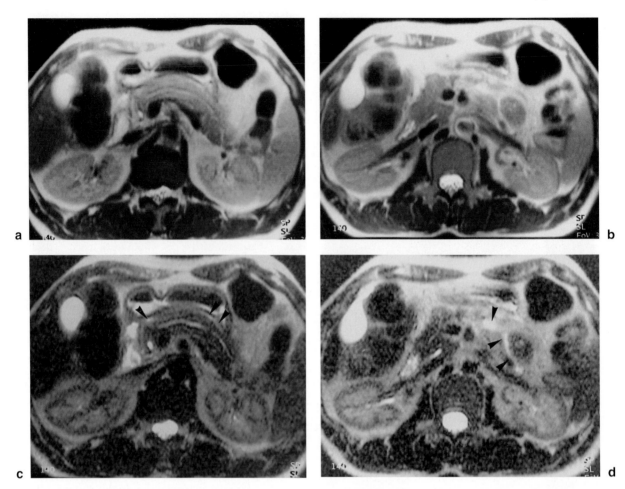

Fig. 8.7 a–d. Double-echo single-shot half-Fourier turbo spin-echo imaging in the detection of acute pancreatitis. Patient referred with clinical and laboratory signs of acute pancreatitis. **a,b** Images with TE 60 ms show no obvious abnormalities. **c,d** Corresponding images with TE 439 ms show a small amount of fluid around the pancreas (*arrowheads*, **c**) and in the small bowel mesentery (*arrowheads*, **d**), suggestive of acute pancreatitis

using the single-shot turbo spin-echo sequence (HASTE) resolve this problem (SEMELKA et al. 1996; BOSMANS et al. 1996).

8.5.2
Imaging Findings

The MR appearance of uncomplicated, acutely inflamed pancreatic parenchyma is a normal signal intensity of fat-suppressed images with normal enhancement on contrast-enhanced images. Typical morphologic changes may include focal enlargement, hyperintense strands in the peripancreatic fat tissue, and increased signal intensity of the pancreas on T2-weighted images (Figs. 8.5, 8.6). The latter imaging finding is attributed to the accumulation of fluid within the pancreas. In more advanced cases, fluid can accumulate in peripancreatic tissue and the lesser sac. The presence of fluid in peripancreatic tissue and the lesser sac is best shown on unenhanced T1-weighted FLASH images, on which the fluid appears as hypointense strands or fluid collections against a background of hyperintense fat. Other sequences that demonstrate the presence of fluid in the peripancreatic tissue are T2-weighted fat-suppressed images and double-echo T2-weighted images. The latter sequence is especially useful in demonstrating small fluid collections surrounding the pancreatic tissue (Fig. 8.7). Compared with images obtained with T2-weighted fat-suppressed sequences, heavily T2-weighted images do not suffer from blurring of the pancreas, which reduces the conspicuity of small fluid collections.

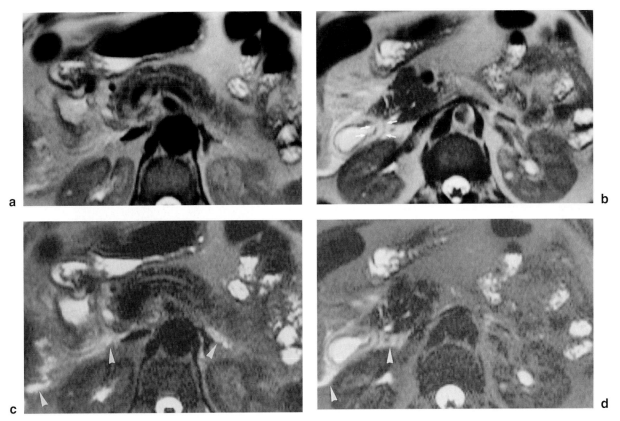

Fig. 8.8 a–d. Patient with acute pancreatitis, causing narrowing of the second duodenum. **a,b** Images with TE 60 ms show thickening of the duodenal wall (*allows*) due to acute pancreatitis of the pancreatic head. **c,d** Fluid collections (*arrowheads*) are more clearly depicted on images with TE

The percentage of pancreatic necrosis is an important prognostic indicator in patients suffering from more severe acute pancreatitis. Similar to contrast-enhanced CT (BALTHAZAR 1989), dynamic gadolinium-enhanced MR imaging may be useful for determination of this parameter, as necrosis is extremely sensitive to contrast enhancement (BROWN and SEMELKA 1995); a limitation, however, is that patients with florid pancreatitis may be unable to cooperate sufficiently to allow a standard MR examination. Besides the percentage of pancreatic necrosis, the presence of fluid accumulation correlates extremely well with mortality (BALTHAZAR et al. 1990). MR imaging is superior to CT in demonstrating the extent of fluid accumulation on coronal images (SAIFUDDIN et al. 1993). Moreover it has been shown that death does not occur when no extrapancreatic spread of fluid collection is found on CT performed within 48 h after admission (MEYER et al. 1992). Since MR imaging is superior in te characterization of the complex nature of associated fluid collections (LEE et al. 1992), it might play an invaluable role in the evaluation of patients with acute pancreatitis.

8.5.3
Complications

8.5.3.1
Gastrointestinal Complications

The stomach and especially the duodenal loop are affected in patients presenting with acute pancreatitis (SAFRIT and RICE 1989). Pathologic findings such as thickening of the gastric and duodenal folds may be observed on MR imaging. Duodenal narrowing or stenosis due to acute pancreatitis as well as gastric varices in cases of thrombosis of the splenic vein (see below) are other findings on MR imaging (Fig. 8.8). Anatomic relations result in a continuation between the body of the pancreas and the trans-

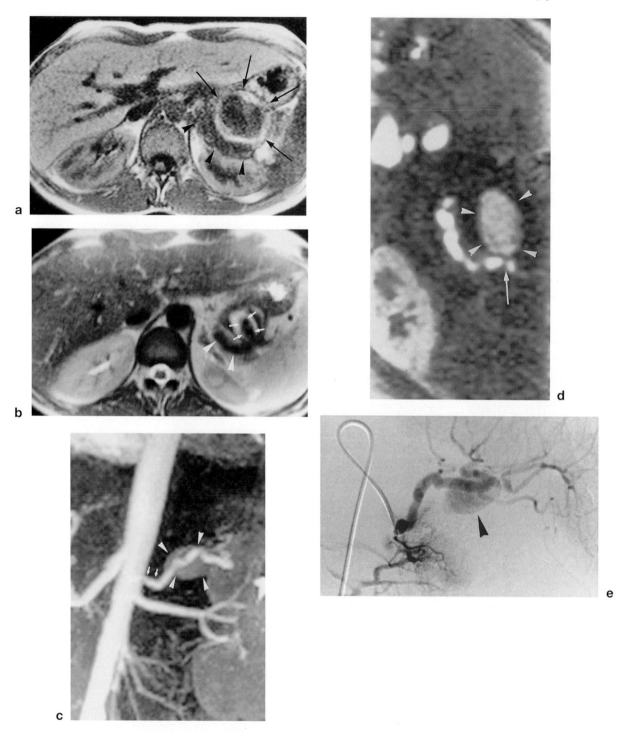

Fig. 8.9 a–e. Pancreatic pseudoaneurysm. The patient has a history of chronic pancreatitis and recurrent upper gastrointestinal bleeding. **a** Axial T1-weighted images show the pseudoaneurysm (*arrow*) ventral to the pancreatic tail (*arrowhead*). There is a hyperintense rim, representing clotted blood. **b** Axial T2-weighted images show a signal void in the pseudoaneurysm (*arrows*), allowing differentiation from pseudocyst. The hypointense foci in the pancreatic tail represent calcification (*arrowheads*). **c** Gadolinium-enhanced three-dimensional time-of-flight acquisition shows filling of the pseudoaneurysm (*arrowheads*), adjacent to the splenic artery (*arrows*) **d** Image obtained in the plane of the splenic artery shows erosion of the splenic artery (*arrow*) adjacent to the pseudoaneurysm (*arrowheads*). **e** Digital subtraction angiography confirms the filling of a pseudoaneurysm (*arrowhead*), adjacent to the splenic artery

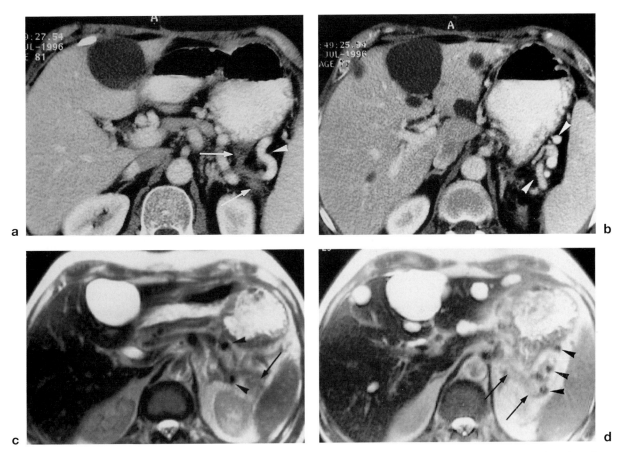

Fig. 8.10 a–d. Splenic vein thrombosis secondary to acute pancreatitis. **a,b** Axial CT images show the thrombosed splenic vein (*arrows*) and multiple collateral vessels (*arrowheads*). Note the presence of multiple biliary cysts. **c,d** On corresponding axial T2-weighted images, the thrombosed splenic vein appears as a slightly hyperintense strand (*arrows*). Collateral veins are seen as multiple tortuous structures with signal void (*arrowheads*)

verse mesocolon and small bowel mesentery, and between the tail of the pancreas and the splenic flexure of the colon. As emphasized by MEYER et al. (1992), exudation of pancreatic enzymes along these mesenteric pathways can produce pathologic findings involving the small bowel and colon.

8.5.3.2
Biliary Complications

Although transient cholestasis may occur because of compression of the common bile duct due to the edema and inflammatory swelling of acute pancreatitis, common bile duct stenosis usually is the result of periductal fibrosis from long-standing chronic pancreatitis (ROHRMANN and BARON 1989). Evaluation of the common bile duct in the setting of acute pancreatitis should include a search for common bile duct stones as a causative factor.

8.5.3.3
Vascular Complications

8.5.3.3.1
ARTERIAL COMPLICATIONS

The artery that is most commonly involved in acute pancreatitis is the splenic artery. Other vessels frequently involved in pancreatitis are the pancreaticoduodenal and gastroduodenal arteries (VUJIC 1989). Arteries that are less frequently involved are the gastrohepatic and small intrapancreatic arteries. Acute bleeding causing life-threatening complications may occur; these patients are generally not evaluated by MR imaging.

Beside acute bleeding, erosion of an artery may result in the formation of pseudoaneurysms (Fig. 8.9). The blood within a pseudoaneurysm is either hyperintense on T1-weighted images or gives rise to a signal void in the pseudoaneurysm, allowing it to be differentiated from pancreatic pseudocysts. Gadolinium-enhanced three-dimensional time of fight acquisition allows differentiation of the artery causing the pseudoaneurysm.

8.5.3.3.2
VENOUS COMPLICATIONS

Thrombosis of the portal and splenic veins is the most frequently encountered vascular complication of pancreatitis (Fig. 8.10). Splenic vein thrombosis causes formation of gastric varices. Gastric varices are seen as multiple tortuous structures with signal void on T2-weighted images, whereas the thrombosed splenic vein exhibits hyperintensity on T2-weighted images. Three different collateral pathways may be encountered:

1. Venous drainage via short gastric veins into the right and left gastric veins and then into the portal vein
2. Collateral circulation through the left and right gastroepiploic veins and superior mesenteric vein
3. Retroperitoneal venous collateral drainage via the left renal vein and inferior vena cava (VUJIC 1989)

8.5.3.4
Splenic Complications

Pancreatitis with splenic involvement may result in intrasplenic pseudocysts, splenic hemorrhage, hematoma, and rupture, inflammation of splenic vessels with pseudoaneurysms, and splenic infarction (FISHMAN et al. 1995). The relation of the splenic pseudocysts with the pancreatic tail is ideally evaluated on coronal T2-weighted images (Fig. 8.1e).

8.6
Chronic Pancreatitis

8.6.1
Definition and Possible Role of Magnetic Resonance Imaging

Chronic pancreatitis is defined as a continuing inflammatory process of the pancreas, characterized by morphologic changes and permanently impaired pancreatic function as revealed by pancreatic function tests (AXON 1989; SARNER and COTTON 1984; FREENY 1989). Patients with chronic pancreatitis may have acute exacerbations.

Two major anatomic forms have been described: chronic calcifying pancreatitis and chronic obstructive pancreatitis. The obstructive form is most frequently caused by carcinoma and stones, while alcoholism accounts for approximately 75% of all cases of chronic calcifying pancreatitis.

Microscopically, the main features include dilatation of ducts and acini, and perilobular and intralobular sclerosis.

Imaging strategies in patients with chronic pancreatitis are thus directed to evaluate fibrosis, calcifications and secondary ductal changes, as well as carcinoma or intraductal stones.

Ductal changes related to chronic pancreatitis can be detected with various imaging modalities. The most sensitive method for the detection of ductal abnormalities in patients with suspected chronic pancreatitis is ERCP. ERCP has the major advantage of unparalleled resolution and can detect subtle changes at an early stage. The main disadvantage of ERCP is the associated morbidity and mortality of 7% and 1% respectively, mainly related to the fact that ERCP requires direct injection of contrast material in the pancreatic ducts (PONETTE et al. 1994). Other limitations are the fact that the technique is operator dependent, with unsuccessful cannulation of the common bile duct or pancreatic duct occurring in 3%–9% of cases (LENRIOT et al. 1993; ASSOULINE et al. 1993). It is in this respect that MR cholangiography offers major possible advantages: there is no related morbidity and mortality, and the technique is operator independent. The challenge is, however, to achieve an accuracy comparable to that of ERCP.

Magnetic resonance cholangiopancreatography is particularly useful in the evaluation of the pancreatic duct in patients in whom ERCP is unsuccessful or incomplete (Fig. 8.1). In the study by SOTO et al. (1996), chronic pancreatitis was found to be a major cause of unsuccessful or incomplete ERCP: chronic pancreatitis was found in seven out of 20 patients in whom ERCP was unsuccessful, and in five out of seven patients in whom ERCP showed complete pancreatic duct obstruction. In this particular group of patients, a twofold role of MRCP can be postulated:

1. MRCP may help to determine whether antegrade or retrograde cannulation should be attempted.
2. By depicting the obstructed segment as well as the obstruction itself, MRCP might be helpful in differentiating tumoral from nontumoral (e.g., inflammatory) obstruction.

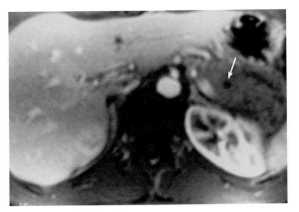

Fig. 8.11. Gadolinium-enhanced T1-weighted turbo FLASH image in a patient with chronic pancreatitis. The pancreas shows low signal intensity and diminished 1-s contrast enhancement. Note the small pseudocysts (*arrow*)

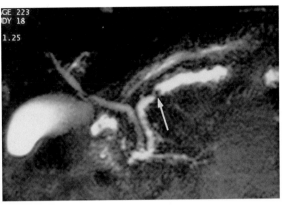

Fig. 8.12. Chronic pancreatitis with pancreatic duct stone. Single-shot MR pancreatogram using the RARE technique demonstrates an intraductal focus of low signal intensity representing a pancreatic duct stone (*arrow*). There is also irregular dilatation of the main and accessory pancreatic ducts

8.6.2
Imaging Findings

8.6.2.1
Detection of Fibrosis and Calcifications

Fibrosis, calcifications, and atrophy are the main histologic features in chronic pancreatitis. Although very small calcifications are usually not seen on MR images, larger calcifications are seen as small signal-void foci. Fibrosis results in: (a) diminished proteinaceous fluid content of the glandular elements and (b) diminished vascularity. This explains the diminished signal intensity of the pancreas on fat-suppressed images, and the diminished capillary blush immediately after contrast agent injection. Patients in whom the pancreas showed low signal intensity regions and diminished 1-s contrast enhancement on MR imaging were found to have calcifications on CT (SEMELKA et al. 1993). However, similar findings were also obtained in patients with clinically suspected chronic pancreatitis and no calcifications on CT examinations. This apparent discrepancy is explained by the presence of fibrosis. Since fibrosis is the precursor of calcifications, MR may detect changes associated with chronic pancreatitis earlier than CT (SEMELKA and ASCHER 1993) (Figure 8.11).

8.6.2.2
Detection of Ductal Changes

Comparison with the results of ERCP has shown that MRCP results in an underestimation of main pancreatic duct dilatation (SOTO et al. 1995a,b; MACAULEY

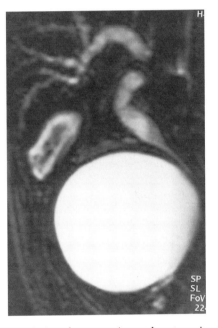

Fig. 8.13. Depiction of a pancreatic pseudocyst causing dilatation of the biliary system in a 50-year-old alcoholic patient. Single-shot MR cholangiopancreatogram using the RARE technique shows a gradual tapering obstruction and lateral deflection of the common bile duct due to an adjacent pseudocyst

et al. 1995; TAKEHARA et al. 1994). The principal reason for this is that during ERCP there is slight overdistention of the pancreatic ducts due to the direct injection of contrast material. A second reason is related to post-processing, such as the use of the maximum intensity projection, New imaging techniques might therefore improve evaluation of the pancreatic ducts in the future.

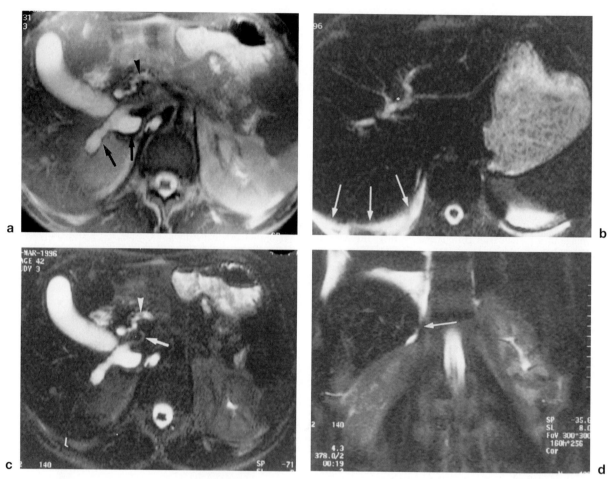

Fig. 8.14 a–d. Pancreatic pleural effusion in a patient with acute exacerbation of chronic pancreatitis. **a** Axial T2-weighted images with TE 60 ms show a retroperitoneal fluid collection between the pancreatic head and the upper pole of the right kidney (*arrows*). **b** Axial T2-weighted images with TE 439 ms show a right pleural effusion (*arrows*). **c,d** Axial and coronal T2-weighted images with TE 439 ms clearly show the rupture of the pancreatic duct (*arrow* in **c**) and a fistula between the retroperitoneal fluid collections and a pleural effusion (*arrow* in **d**). The rupture of the pancreatic duct (**c**) is clearly seen on images with TE 439 ms, but only retrospectively on the images with TE 60 ms (**a**). A small ductal stone is also more clearly seen on images with TE 439 ms (*arrowheads* in **a** and **c**)

Pancreatic duct strictures can be detected, but there is a major risk of false-positive findings due to the underestimation of the diameter of the pancreatic duct (Soto et al. 1995b; Macauley et al. 1995; Takehara et al. 1994). Evaluation of axial images might help to distinguish between real and pseudo-strictures. One should also be aware of pseudonarrowing in the absence of pancreatic duct dilatation (Soto et al. 1995b).

It has been shown that MRCP is an excellent modality for the evaluation of main pancreatic duct stones (Fig. 8.12), with reported sensitivities of 100% (Soto et al. 1995b; Macauley et al. 1995; Takehara et al. 1994).

Side branch dilatation can also be detected in patients with chronic pancreatitis. Subtle changes may, however, remain undetected (Fig. 8.2).

8.6.3
Complications

8.6.3.1
Biliary Complications

Cholestasis, cholangitis, fistulization affecting the hepatobiliary system, and secondary biliary cirrhosis constitute the spectrum of biliary complications that may be encountered in the setting of chronic pancreatitis (Rohrmann and Baron 1989). The most typical finding is a dilated common bile duct due to inflammatory stricture. The typical configuration of the common bile duct stricture in chronic pancreatitis is a gradual tapering (Fig. 8.13). Other possible configurations are the "hourglass" configuration of alternating stenosis and dilatation, or a

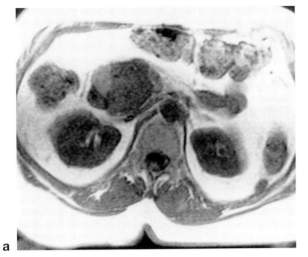

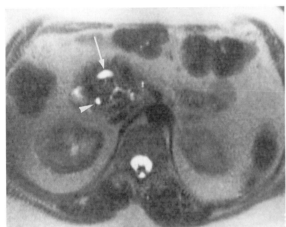

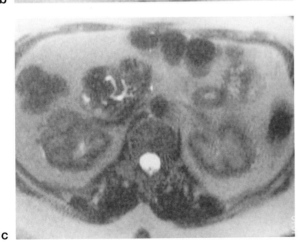

Fig. 8.15 a–c. Chronic pancreatitis causing pseudotumoral mass of the pancreatic head. **a** T1-weighted image shows an enlarged, hypointense pancreatic mass in the ventral pancreas, suggesting the diagnosis of pancreatic carcinoma. Note the normal signal intensity of the dorsal pancreas. **b,c** Axial T2-weighted images (TE 439 ms) show the Santorini duct (*arrow*), the common bile duct (*arrow head*), and some ventral pancreatic ducts. The latter are seen within the mass and show irregular dilatations. The presence of dilated pancreatic ducts within the mass suggests the diagnosis of chronic pancreatitis rather than pancreatic carcinoma

laterally deflected bile duct due to an adjacent pancreatic pseudocyst (ROHRMANN and BARON 1989). Especially the relation of tapered biliary stricture to an adjacent pancreatic pseudocyst is ideally evaluated on MRCP (Fig. 8.1). Choledocholithiasis can evolve secondary to the stenosis and is also evaluated on MRCP images.

8.6.3.2
Vascular Complications

Arterial bleeding, pseudoaneurysms, and venous thrombosis are seen in patients with acute as well as chronic pancreatitis. Imaging findings are discussed in Sect 8.5.3.3, on acute pancreatitis.

8.6.3.3
Pancreatic Pseudocysts

In cases of pseudocyst formation, ERCP may result in a false-negative diagnosis if the pancreatic pseudocyst does not communicate with the main pancreatic duct (Fig. 8.1a). In this respect, MRCP offers a major advantage in demonstrating pancreatic cysts, as well as their relation to the pancreatic duct (SOTO et al. 1996).

8.6.3.4
Pancreatic Pleural Effusion

A pancreatic pleural effusion is defined as a massive fluid accumulation in the thorax with a high amylase content resulting from a disrupted pancreatic duct (Fig. 8.14). It is reported that in adults the cause of most cases of pancreatic disruption is chronic relapsing pancreatitis. Acute alcoholic pancreatitis occurring in patients with chronic alcoholism is the most frequently encountered clinical setting (UCHIYAMA et al. 1992). Another cause of pancreatic pleural effusion is trauma. MR imaging using heavily T2-weighted images as well as coronal views nicely demonstrates the rupture of the pancreatic duct and also the connection of the peripancreatic fluid collection with pleural effusion.

8.6.4
Differentiating Chronic Pancreatitis from Pancreatic Carcinoma

Since pancreatic carcinoma may cause acute pancreatitis, or arise in patients with known chronic

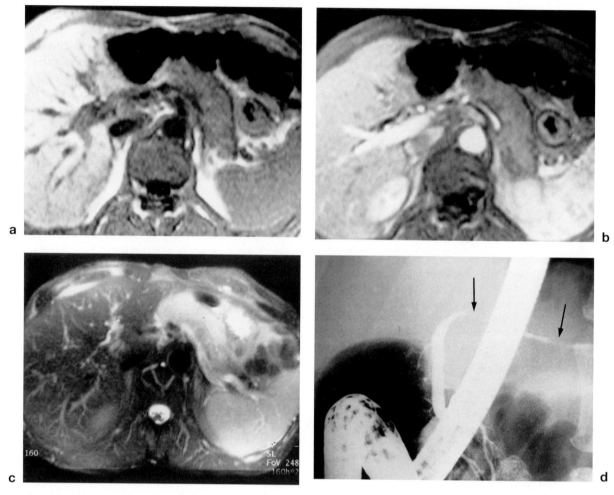

Fig. 8.16 a–d. Non alcoholic duct destructive chronic pancreatitis of the pancreatic tail, causing pseudotumoral mass. **a,b** T1-weighted images show an enlarged hypointense pancreatic tail (**a**), exhibiting absence of the normal blush on dynamic gadolinium-enhanced images (**b**). **c** T2-weighted fat-suppressed images show the pancreatic body and tail to be hyperintense. **d** ERCP shows narrowing of the pancreatic duct in the pancreatic body and tail (*arrows*) in the absence of irregular dilatation of the side branches, suggesting the presence of pancreatic carcinoma of the pancreatic body and tail. Pathologic examination revealed the presence of autoimmune pancreatitis affecting the pancreatic body and tail

pancreatitis, it is the main differential diagnosis to be taken into account when a focal mass is detected in a patient with acute or chronic pancreatitis. The following findings are in favor of pancreatitis:

1. Irregular dilatation of the pancreatic duct
2. The presence of dilated ducts and small pseudocysts within the mass (Fig. 8.15)
3. Intraductal or parenchymal calcifications
4. A less pronounced degree of atrophy of the pancreatic parenchyma
5. Gradual (not abrupt) narrowing of the dilated pancreatic gland or bile duct

More recently, the normal pancreatic parenchyma has been shown to enhance after the administration of MnDPDP. The pancreatic lesions did not enhance, and, therefore, a marked increase in contrast between the lesion and the pancreas occurred (GEHL et al. 1993). MnDPDP therefore may be helpful in differentiating chronic pancreatitis from pancreatic carcinoma.

8.7
Non Alcoholic Duct Destructive Chronic Pancreatitis

The pathogenetic mechanisms involved in non alcoholic duct destructive chronic pancreatitis allow distinction between the necrosis–fibrosis sequence (e.g., alcoholism), and the destruction of acinar parenchyma (e.g., obstruction). Some cases, however, do not fit this classification and are suggestive of an autoimmune-based process (ECTORS et al. 1995; MAILLET et al. 1995).

On pathologic examination the changes in pancreatic parenchyma are characterized by dense inflammatory infiltrates surrounding the medium interlobular ducts. The inflammatory process leads to periductal fibrosis and secondary lesions in the acinar parenchyma.

On radiologic examination, these changes may simulate diffuse tumoral pathology. ERCP may show narrowing of the main pancreatic duct. Due to inflammation and fibrosis, mainly affecting the small to medium interlobular ducts, no filling of the side branches is noted. The narrowing or even stenosis of the main pancreatic duct in the absence of irregular dilatation of the side branches is suggestive of tumoral rather than inflammatory pathology.

On MRI, fibrosis results in a hypointense aspect of the affected parenchyma on T1-weighted images, and in absence of normal blush on dynamic enhanced FLASH images. The periductal inflammatory changes result in a hyperintense aspect of the pancreatic parenchyma on T2-weighted (fat-suppressed) images (Fig. 8.16) (Van Hoe et al. 1998).

References

Assouline Y, Liguroy C, Ink O, et al. (1993) Resultats actuels de la sphincterotomie endoscopique pour lithiase de la voie biliare principale. Gastroenterol Clin Biol 17:251–258

Axon AT (1989) Endoscopic retrograde cholangiopancreatography in chronic pancreatitis: Cambridge classification. Radiol Clin North Am 27:39–50

Balthazar EJ (1989) CT diagnosis and staging of acute pancreatitis. Radiol Clin North Am 27:19–37

Balthazar EJ, Robinson DL, Megibow AJ, Ranson JH (1990) Acute pancreatitis: value of CT in establishing prognosis. Radiology 174:331–336

Barish MA, Yucel EK, Soto JA, Chuttani R, Ferrucci JT (1995) MR cholangiopancreatography: efficacy of three-dimensional turbo spin-echo technique. AJR 165:295–300

Bernard JP, Sahel J, Giovannini M, Sarles H (1990) Pancreas divisum is a probable cause of acute pancreatitis: a report of 137 cases. Pancreas 5:248–254

Bosmans H, Kiefer B, Gryspeerdt S, Van Hoe L, Marchal G, Baert AL (1996) Single-shot half-Fourier double-echo MR imaging acquisition: promising clinical applications. Radiology 201(P):529

Brailsford J, Ward J, Chalmers AG, Ridgway J, Robinson PJ (1994) Dynamic MRI of the pancreas – gadolinium enhancement in normal tissue. Clin Radiol 49:104–108

Bret PM, Reinhold C, Taourel P, Guibaud L, Atri M, Barkun AN (1996) Pancreas divisum: evaluation with MR cholangiopancreatography. Radiology 199:99–103

Brown ED, Semelka RC (1995) Magnetic resonance imaging of the spleen and pancreas. Top Magn Reson Imaging 7:82–89

Campeau NG, Johnson CD, Felmlee JP, Rydberg JN, Butts RK, Ehman RL, Riederer SJ (1995) MR imaging of the abdomen with a phased-array multicoil: prospective clinical evaluation. Radiology 195:769–776

Ectors N, Maillet B, Aerts R, Geboes K, Donner A, Borchard F, Klöppel F (1995) Morphological features of auto-immune disease in chronic duct-destructive pancreatitis (abstract). Gastroenterology 108:351

Fan ST, Lai EC, Mok FP, Lo CM, Zheng SS, Wong J (1993) Early treatment of acute biliary pancreatitis by endoscopic papillotomy. N Engl J Med 328:228–232

Fishman EK, Soyer P, Bliss DF, Bluemke DA, Devine N (1995) Splenic involvement in pancreatitis: spectrum of CT findings. AJR 164:631–635

Freeny PC (1989) Classification of pancreatitis. Radiol Clin North Am 27:1–3

Gehl HB, et al. (1993) Mn-DPDP in MR imaging of pancreatic adenocarcinoma: initial clinical experience. Radiology 186:795–798

Ichikawa T, Nitatori T, Hachiya J, Mizutani Y (1996) Breath-held MR cholangiopancreatography with half-averaged single shot hybrid rapid acquisition with relaxation enhancement sequence: comparison of fast GRE and SE sequences. J Comput Assist Tomogr 20:798–802

Laubenberger J, Buchert M, Schneider B, Blum U, Hennig J, Langer M (1995) Breath-hold projection magnetic resonance-cholangio-pancreaticography (MRCP): a new method for the examination of the bile and pancreatic ducts. Magn Reson Med 33:18–23

Lee MJ, Rattner DW, Legemate DA, et al. (1992) Acute complicated pancreatitis: redefining the role of interventional radiology. Radiology 183:171–174

Lenriot JP, Le-Neel JC, Hay JM, Jaeck D, Millat B, Fagniez PL (1993) Cholangiopancreatographie retrograde et sphincterotomie endoscopique pour lithiase biliare. Gastroenterol Clin Biol 17:244–250

Macauley SE, Schulte SJ, Sekijima HJ, et al. (1995) Evaluation of a non-breath-hold MR cholangiography technique. Radiology 196:227–232

Maillet B, Ectors N, Geboes K, Donner A, Borchard F, Stolte M, Klöppel F (1995) Pathology of chronic idiopathic duct destructive pancreatitis (abstract). Pathol Res Pract 191:248

Meyer P, Clavien PA, Robert J, Hauser H, Rohner A (1992) Roel of imaging technics in the classification of acute pancreatitis. Dig Dis 10:330–334

Mitchell DG, Winston CB, Outwater EK, Ehrlich SM (1995) Delineation of pancreas with MR imaging: multiobserver comparison of five pulse sequences. J Magn Reson Imaging 5:193–199

Miyazaki T, Yamashita Y, Tsuchigame T, Yamamoto H, Urata J, Takahashi M (1996) MR cholangiopancreatography using HASTE (half-Fourier acquisition single-shot turbo spin-echo) sequences. AJR 166:1297–1303

Neoptolemos JP, Carr-Locke DL, London NJ, Bailey IA, James D, Fossard DP (1988) Controlled trial of urgent endoscopic retrograde cholangiopancreatography and endoscopic sphincterotomy versus conservative treatment for acute pancreatitis due to gallstones. Lancet 2:979–983

Outwater EK, Gordon SJ (1994) Imaging the pancreatic and biliary ducts with MR. Radiology 192:19–21

Ponette E, Brys P, Van Steenbergen W (1994) Endoscopic retrograde cholangiopancreatography. In: Baert AL, Delorme G (eds) Radiology of the pancreas. Springer, Berlin Heidelberg New York, pp 106–119

Reinhold C, Bret PM (1996) Current status of MR cholangio-pancreatography. AJR 166:1285–1295

Reinhold C, Guibaud L, Genin G, Bret PM (1995) MR cholan-giopancreatography: comparison between two-dimen-sional fast spin-echo and three-dimensional gradient-echo pulse sequences. J Magn Reson Imaging 4:379–384

Reinhold C, Bret PM, Guibaud L, Barkun ANG, Genin G, Atri M (1996) MR cholangiopancreatography: potential clinical applications. Radiographics 16:309–320

Reuther G, Kiefer B, Tuchmann A (1996) Cholangiography before biliary surgery: single-shot MR cholangiography versus intravenous cholangiography. Radiology 198:561–566

Rizzo RJ, Szucs RA, Turner MA (1995) Congenital abnor-malities of the pancreas and biliary tree in adults. Radiographics 15:49–68

Rohrmann CA, Baron RL (1989) Biliary complications of pan-creatitis. Radiol Clin North Am 27:93–104

Safrit HD, Rice RP (1989) Gastrointestinal complications of pancreatitis. Radiol Clin North Am 27:73–79

Saifuddin A, Ward J, Ridgway J, Chalmers AG (1993) Compar-ison of MR and CT scanning in severe acute pancreatitis: initial experiences. Clin Radiol 48:111–116

Sarner M, Cotton PB (1984) Classification of pancreatitis. Gut 25:756–759

Semelka RC, Ascher SM (1993) MR imaging of the pancreas. Radiology 188:593–602

Semelka RC, Kroeker MA, Shoenut JP, Kroeker R, Yaffe CS, Micflikier AB (1991) Pancreatic disease: prospective com-parison of CT, ERCP, and 1.5T MR imaging with dynamic gadolinium enhancement and fat suppression. Radiology 181:785–791

Semelka RC, Shoenut JP, Kroeker MA, Micflikier AB (1993) Chronic pancreatitis: MR imaging features before and after administration of gadopentate dimeglumine. J Magn Reson Imaging 3:79–82

Semelka RC, Kelekis NL, Thomasson D, Brown MA, Laub GA (1996) HASTE MR imaging – description of technique and preliminary results in the abdomen. J Magn Reson Imaging 6:698–699

Sherman S, Lehman GA (1991) ERCP- and endoscopic sphinc-terotomy-induced pancreatitis. Pancreas 6:350–367

Soto JA, Barish MA, Yucel EK, Ferrucci JT (1995a) MR cholangiopancreatography: findings on 3D fast spin-echo imaging. AJR 165:1397–1401

Soto JA, Barish MA, Yucel EK, Clarke P, Siegenberg D, Chuttani R, Ferrucci JT (1995b) Pancreatic duct MR cholangiopancreatography with a three-dimensional fast spin-echo technique. Radiology 196:459–464

Soto JA, Yucel EK, Barish MA, Chuttani R, Ferrucci JT (1996) MR cholangiopancreatography after unsuccessful or in-complete ERCP. Radiology 199:91–98

Sugawa C, Walt AJ, Nunez DC, Masuyama H (1987) Pancreas divisum: is it a normal anatomical variant? Am J Surg 153:62–67

Takehara Y, Ichijo K, Tooyama N, et al. (1994) Breath-hold MR cholangiopancreatography with a long-echo-train fast spin-echo sequence and a surface coil in chronic pan-creatitis. Radiology 192:73–78

Todani T, Watanebe Y, Narusue M, Tabuchi K, Okajima K (1977) Congenital bile duct cysts: classification, operative procedures, and review of thirty-seven cases including cancer arising from choledochal cyst. Am J Surg 134:263–269

Uchiyama T, Suzuki T, Adachi A, Hiraki S, Iizuka N (1992) Pancreatic pleural effusion: case report and review of 113 cases in Japan. Am J Gastroenterol 87:387–391

Van der Horst LF (1961) Annular pancreas. Arch Surg 83:249–252

Van Hoe L, Gryspeerdt S, Ectors N, Baert AL, Marchal G. (1998) Non alcoholic duct destructive chronic pancreatitis. Imaging findings. AJR 171 (in press)

Vujic I (1989) Vascular complications of pancreatitis. Radiol Clin North Am 27:81–91

Wallner BK, Schumacher KA, Weidenmaier W, Friedrich JM (1991) Dilated biliary tract: evaluation with MR cholangio-graphy with a T2-weighted contrast-enhanced fast se-quence. Radiology 181:805–808

Warshaw AL, Richter JM, Schapiro RH (1983) The cause and treatment of pancreatitis associated with pancreas divisum. Ann Surg 198:443–452

Winslet M, Hall C, London NJ, Neoptolemos JP (1992) Rela-tion of diagnostic serum amylase levels to etiology and severity of acute pancreatitis. Gut 33:982–986

9 Endocrine Tumors of the Pancreas

L. Van Hoe, S. Gryspeerdt, and A.L. Baert

9.1
Classification and Clinical Aspects

9.1.1
Functioning Endocrine Tumors

Nearly 85% of the endocrine pancreatic tumors are functioning tumors (Roche et al. 1994). They are named according to the main hormone produced, for example insulinoma or gastrinoma, and usually present with the clinical effects of excessive hormone production. The diagnosis is almost always made biochemically. In the following sections, the frequency, symptoms, size, location, and biologic behaviour of the most important types of endocrine tumors are described.

9.1.1.1
Insulinoma

Approximately 60% of all endocrine tumors of the pancreas are insulinomas. Patients typically suffer from hypoglycemia. The diagnosis is based on demonstrating inappropriately high insulin levels, together with hypoglycemia. Insulinomas are usually very small: 90% are less than 2 cm in size and 50% less than 1.3 cm (King et al. 1994). There is a uniform distribution between the head, body, and tail of the pancreas. Patients with type 1 multiple endocrine neoplasia (MEN) syndrome usually have multiple small tumors. Ectopic localization of insulinomas is rare. Approximately 16% of insulinomas are malignant, and malignant insulinomas tend to be larger than benign ones.

9.1.1.2
Gastrinoma

Gastrinomas are the second most common functioning tumor of the pancreas, accounting for approximately 18% of all islet cell tumors. They give rise to the Zollinger-Ellison syndrome, which comprises increased gastric acid secretion, diarrhea, and upper gastrointestinal ulceration. Ulcers in atypical locations, particularly if multiple and resistant to therapy, should raise the suspicion of a gastrinoma. The diagnosis is established by the demonstration of a raised fasting serum gastrin level with simultaneous high basal gastric acid output. Like insulinomas, gastrinomas tend to be small: their size is usually between 1 and 3 cm (King et al. 1994). Up to 90% of gastrinomas occur in the "gastrinoma triangle," which is the area bounded by the junction of the cystic and common bile ducts superiorly, the second and third portions of the duodenum inferiorly, and the junction between the head and body of the pancreas medially (Stabile et al. 1984). Importantly, between 30% and 43% of gastrinomas are found in the duodenal wall. These tumors are usually very small (<1 cm). In patients with type 1 MEN syndrome, most gastrinomas are located in the duodenal wall. They may also occur in local lymph nodes. Approximately 60% of gastrinomas are malignant. Metastatic spread occurs primarily to the liver and local lymph nodes.

L. Van Hoe, MD, Department of Radiology, University Hospitals K.U. Leuven, Herestraat 49, B-3000 Leuven, Belgium
S. Gryspeerdt, MD, Department of Radiology, University Hospitals K.U. Leuven, Herestraat 49, B-3000 Leuven, Belgium
A.L. Baert, MD, Professor, Department of Radiology, University Hospitals K.U. Leuven, Herestraat 49, B-3000 Leuven, Belgium

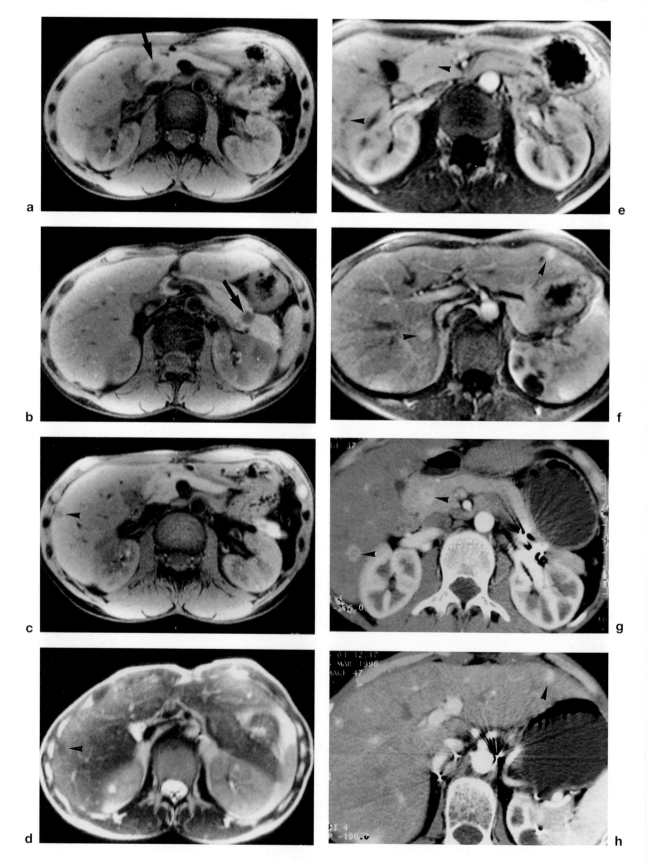

9.1.1.3
Glucagonoma

Approximately 2.3% of endocrine pancreatic tumors are glucagonomas. They produce a syndrome of glucose intolerance, anemia, weight loss, and rash. Unlike insulinomas and gastrinomas, glucagonomas are usually large (>2 cm). They are usually solitary, and the majority of glucagonomas are malignant (ROCHE et al. 1994).

9.1.1.4
Other Types of Functioning Endocrine Tumors

Vipomas (tumors secreting vasoactive intestinal peptides) account for approximately 1.8% of endocrine pancreatic tumors. They cause a syndrome of watery diarrhea and hypocalcemia (Verner-Morrison syndrome). Vipomas are usually large and are malignant in up to 60% of cases. Among the other types of functioning endocrine tumors (all with a relative frequency below 1%) are somatostatinoma, somatocrinoma, and carcinoid tumor. All of these rare tumors are usually large and thus easily detected.

9.1.2
Nonfunctioning Endocrine Tumors

Nonfunctioning endocrine tumors account for 15% of all endocrine pancreatic tumors. They do not usually present with symptoms until the tumor is large, and 30% are larger than 10 cm at the time of initial diagnosis (KING et al. 1994). Ninety-two percent of nonfunctioning tumors are malignant. In comparison with pancreatic adenocarcinomas, nonfunctioning endocrine tumors are relatively slow growing

and have a relatively high survival rate (60% at 3 years).

9.2
Role of Imaging

Diagnosis of functioning endocrine tumors is usually based on clinical symptoms and biochemical tests. The role of imaging studies is to guide the type of surgery performed. Therefore, accurate determination of the number of lesions and the exact localization of each lesion is mandatory. Ideally, imaging techniques should be able to detect all intra- and extrapancreatic tumors. This is a difficult task, particularly in the case of insulinomas and gastrinomas, because these tumors tend to be very small. In patients with multiple lesions, detection of only one lesion with preoperative imaging studies may lead to inappropriate surgery and to the persistence of clinical symptoms. Therefore, imaging studies should be optimized in order to allow the detection of very small lesions, and investigators should carefully scrutinize the entire pancreas.

In patients with nonfunctioning endocrine tumors the role of imaging is quite different. In these patients, the tumor is usually easily detected because of its large size. Characterization, on the other hand, is relatively more important. It is, for instance, mandatory to be able to differentiate these tumors from serous cystadenomas and adenocarcinomas.

9.3
Magnetic Resonance Imaging

9.3.1
Technique

Accurate detection of endocrine pancreatic tumors requires an optimized magnetic resonance (MR) technique. Crucial requirements are high-resolution imaging and fast imaging. High-resolution imaging can be obtained by use of body phased array coils. While it was initially believed that fast MR imaging would be impossible, several solutions were proposed in the mid-1980s. Two major independent approaches to reduce acquisition times in MRI are:

1. Replacement of the classic 90° excitation pulses by lower flip angles (gradient-echo MR imaging) (HAASE et al. 1986)

Fig. 9.1 a–h. Insulinoma with hepatic metastases. **a–c** Fat-saturated T1-weighted images show two pancreatic lesions (*arrows*, **a**, **b**) and a hepatic metastasis (*arrowhead*, **c**). All lesions are hypointense. **d** T2-weighted HASTE image shows hepatic metastasis as a hypointense nodule. The lesion in the pancreatic head was hypointense, too. The lesion in the pancreatic tail was isointense. **e,f** Dynamic contrast-enhanced images. The pancreatic head lesion is nearly isointense (*arrowhead*, **e**). The hepatic metastases show either ring enhancement (**e**) or homogeneous enhancement (**f**) (*arrowheads*). **g,h** Corresponding arterial-phase CT images show the lesions as enhancing nodules (*arrowheads*)

2. Generation of multiple echoes after a single excitation pulse [rapid acquisition by repeated echoes
(RARE), fast spin echo] (HENNIG et al. 1986)

Currently, high-resolution T1-weighted images
can be obtained within a very short time interval by
using a multislice breath-hold spoiled gradient-echo
sequence [e.g., fast low-angle shot (FLASH), magnetization-prepared gradient echo (MPGR)] (HAASE
1990). With currently available equipment, individual non-fat-suppressed T1-weighted images can
be obtained in less than 1 s ("single-shot" MR imaging). The major advantage of this technique is that
artifacts caused by patient motion or respiration are
completely avoided. Thus, high-quality images can
be obtained in every patient, irrespective of the
patient's condition. On the other hand, it has been
demonstrated that the conspicuity of pancreatic
tumors and the delineation of the pancreas from
surrounding fat is best on fat-suppressed images
(SEMELKA et al. 1993; MITCHELL et al. 1995). Fat
suppression on T1-weighted images renders the normal pancreas high in signal intensity due to the
presence of aqueous protein in the acini of the
pancreas. Currently, high-resolution fat-suppressed
T1-weighted images can be obtained during short
periods of breath-holding.

Since the introduction of new MR systems
equipped with stronger gradients and faster gradient
switching capability, it has become possible to fully
exploit the intrinsic advantages of the RARE sequence and to obtain T2-weighted images during
breath-holding. This technique is called breath-hold
fast spin echo (FSE) or turbo spin echo (TSE)
(REINIG 1995). A recently introduced evolution of
RARE is called HASTE (half-Fourier acquisition
single-shot turbo spin echo) (KIEFER et al. 1994). In
this technique, single-shot T2-weighted images can
be obtained in less than 1 s (±0.4 s). As in single-shot
gradient echo, artifacts caused by respiration or
patient motion are eliminated.

In summary, artifact-free T1-and T2-weighted
MR images can currently be obtained in less than a
second, which will most likely improve the detection

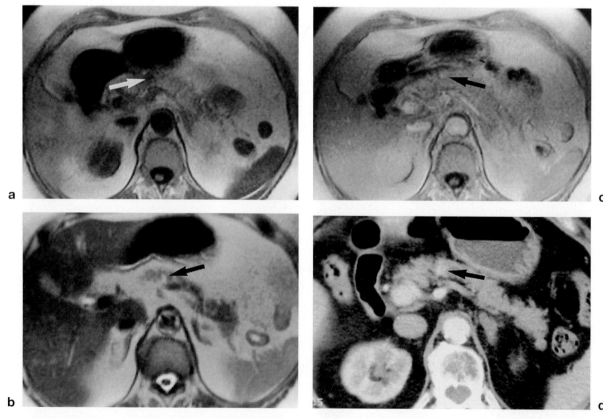

Fig. 9.2 a–d. Gastrinoma best seen on non-contrast-enhanced
scans. The lesion is hypointense on T1- (**a**) and partially
hyperintense on T2-weighted images (**b**) (*arrows*). It is only
slightly hyperintense on the dynamic contrast-enhanced
T1-weighted image (*arrow*, **c**). Corresponding CT image
(**d**) shows the tumor as an enhancing nodule (*arrow*)

of small pancreatic tumors. On the other hand, it has been shown that dynamic contrast-enhanced MR imaging may facilitate the detection of endocrine pancreatic tumors and hepatic metastases (SEMELKA et al. 1993). Dynamic gadolinium-enhanced imaging is usually performed using a multislice spoiled gradient-echo sequence. The normal pancreas enhances on the immediate postgadolinium images. Most endocrine tumors are richly vascularized and enhance even more than the pancreatic parenchyma.

9.3.2
Imaging Findings

Most islet cell tumors are well visualized on T1-weighted MR images due to (a) high inherent contrast between hypointense tumors and hyperintense pancreas on T1-weighted images (particularly fat-suppressed images), and (b) the frequently hypervascular nature of these tumors, which permits good conspicuity between intensively enhancing tumors

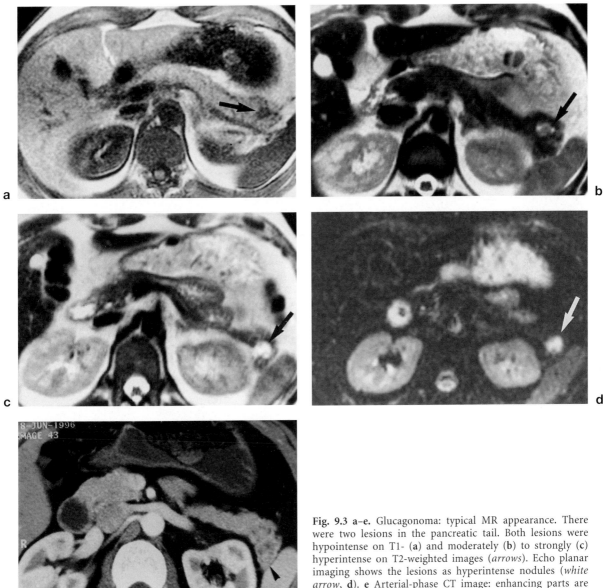

Fig. 9.3 a–e. Glucagonoma: typical MR appearance. There were two lesions in the pancreatic tail. Both lesions were hypointense on T1- (**a**) and moderately (**b**) to strongly (**c**) hyperintense on T2-weighted images (*arrows*). Echo planar imaging shows the lesions as hyperintense nodules (*white arrow*, **d**). **e** Arterial-phase CT image: enhancing parts are nearly isodense to the pancreas; conspicuity is related to the presence of cystic/necrotic areas (*arrowhead*)

relative to more moderate enhancement of normal pancreatic parenchyma on dynamic contrast-enhanced images. Furthermore, many endocrine pancreatic tumors are seen as hyperintense masses on T2-weighted images. SEMELKA et al. (1993) have shown that this holds true in particular for pancreatic gastrinomas.

Typically, endocrine pancreatic tumors display a hypointense aspect on T1-weighted MR images, a hyperintense aspect on T2-weighted images, and a hyperintense aspect on dynamic contrast-enhanced images (SEMELKA et al. 1993; KRAUS and Ros 1994; MITCHELL et al. 1992; PAVONE et al. 1993). However, the MR imaging appearance of the different types of endocrine tumors may be variable (Figs. 9.1–9.5). Some tumors may, for instance, be isointense or even hypointense on T2-weighted images (Figs. 9.1, 9.4). Moreover, endocrine tumors may be invisible on contrast-enhanced images, because both the tumor and the surrounding tissue enhance significantly (Fig. 9.1). Therefore, a combination of different types of images (T1-weighted, T2-weighted, and dynamic gadolinium-enhanced) is mandatory to detect as many lesions as possible. The same holds true for the detection and characterization of hepatic metastases. Gastrinoma metastases usually have very high signal intensity on T2-weighted images and may mimic hemangiomas. It has been demonstrated that the addition of delayed contrast-enhanced T1-weighted images is mandatory to differentiate metastases of gastrinomas from liver hemangiomas (BERGER et al. 1996).

On dynamic contrast-enhanced images, endocrine tumors may appear as homogeneously enhancing masses or may show ring-like enhancement. The latter pattern of enhancement is most commonly seen in insulinomas (SEMELKA and ASCHER 1993).

Gastrinomas and insulinomas tend to be small. Occasionally, they contain cystic components. Functioning tumors other than insulinomas and gastrinomas are usually relatively large and heterogeneous.

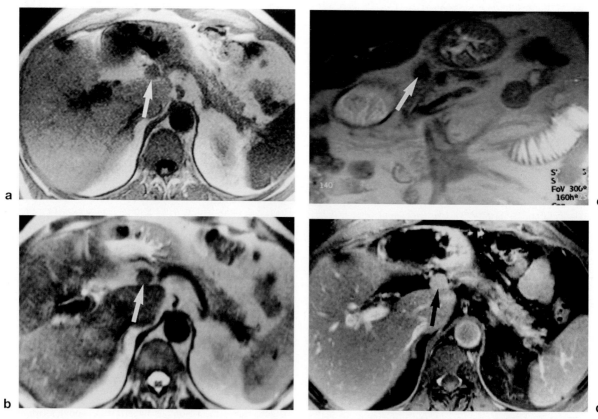

Fig. 9.4 a–d. Insulinoma in pancreatic neck with atypical signal intensity on T2-weighted images. The lesion is hypointense on T1- (**a**) and T2-weighted images (**b, c**) (*white arrows*) and is partially located outside the pancreas. It is slightly hyperintense on the dynamic contrast-enhanced image (*arrow*, **d**)

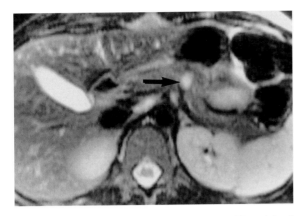

Fig. 9.5. Insulinoma: typical MR appearance. T2-weighted image shows insulinoma as a hyperintense nodule (*arrow*)

Nonfunctioning endocrine tumors are usually large and commonly contain zones of intratumoral hemorrhage and/or necrosis. Unlike adenocarcinomas, they are not typically associated with ductal ectasia. Mucinous cystic neoplasms, solid and papillary cystic tumors, and hypervascular pancreatic metastases should be considered in the differential diagnosis.

9.3.3
Comparison with Other Techniques

Controversy exists about the optimal diagnostic strategy in patients with clinical signs and laboratory findings suggestive of functioning endocrine tumors (KING et al. 1994). Many different techniques, including transabdominal and endoscopic ultrasonography, computed tomography, MR imaging, arteriography, transvenous sampling, and octreotide scanning have been proposed by different authors (KING et al. 1994; ROCHE et al. 1994; ROSCH et al. 1992; ROSSI et al. 1989). Because of the many recent technical advances in the different methods, no large studies have get compared different state-of-the-art techniques. Therefore, determination of the optimal diagnostic strategy warrants further study.

A particularly interesting comparison is that between spiral CT and ultrafast MR imaging. Currently, no studies have compared these two state-of-the-art techniques. Recently, good results have been obtained with dual-phase contrast-enhanced spiral CT. In a recent study, all endocrine tumors large than 0.5 cm could be detected with this technique (VAN HOE et al. 1995). Arterial-phase CT

with water as an oral contrast medium has also been shown to be valuable in the detection of extra-pancreatic gastrinoma localizations (WINTER et al. 1996). In our preliminary experience, dual-phase spiral CT and ultrafast MRI have comparable sensitivity for the detection of endocrine pancreatic tumors.

It should be kept in mind that all morphologic studies (ultrasonography, CT, MRI) tend to miss very small lesions. While glucagonomas, vipomas, and nonsecreting endocrine tumors are usually rather large, the mean size of insulinomas and gastrinomas is below 2 cm. Therefore, accurate detection of such tumors with morphologic studies is certainly a difficult task, and it will probably remain beyond the scope of both spiral CT and ultrafast MRI to detect all pancreatic insulinomas and gastrinomas. This is a crucial problem, particularly in patients with MEN syndrome, because these patients often have multicentric and small tumors or more diffuse areas of hypersecretion. There is no doubt that, in these patients, techniques based on the detection of hypersecretion (e.g., transvenous sampling) may provide important additional information.

Finally, several studies have suggested that preoperative palpation and/or peroperative ultrasonography may be more sensitive than any other technique (GALIBER et al. 1988; GORMAN et al. 1986; GRANT et al. 1988; ROCHE et al. 1994). Thus, in some patients, all preoperative imaging techniques currently available may fail to provide sufficient information to decide on the optimal surgical approach.

References

Berger JF, Laissy JP, Limot O, Henry-Feugeas MC, Cadiot G, Mignon M, Schouman-Claeys E (1996) Differentiation between multiple liver hemangiomas and liver metastases of gastrinomas: value of enhanced MRI. J Comput Assist Tomogr 20:349–355

Galiber AK, Reading CC, Charboneau JW, et al. (1988) Localisation of pancreatic insulinoma: comparison of pre- and intraoperative US with CT and angiography. Radiology 166:405–408

Gorman B, Charboneau JW, James EM, et al. (1986) Benign pancreatic insulinoma: preoperative and intraoperative sonographic localization. AJR 147:929–934

Grant CS, van Heerden J, Charboneau JW, James EM, Reading CC (1988) Insulinoma: the value of intraoperative sonography. Arch Surg 123:843–848

Haase A (1990) Snapshot FLASH MRI. Applications to T1, T2, and chemical-shift imaging. Magn Reson Med 13:77–89

Haase A, Frahm J, Matthaei KD (1986) FLASH imaging: rapid NMR imaging using low flip angles. J Magn Reson 67:258–266

Hennig J, Nauerth A, Friedburg H (1986) RARE imaging: a fast imaging method for clinical MR. Magn Reson Med 3:823–833

Kiefer B, Grässner J, Hausman R (1994) Image acquisition in a second with half-Fourier acquisition single-shot turbo spin echo. Magn Reson Imaging 4 (Suppl):86–87

King CMP, Reznek RH, Dacie JE, Wass JAH (1994) Imaging islet cell tumors. Clin Radiol 49:295–303

Kraus BB, Ros PR (1994) Insulinoma: diagnosis with fat-suppressed MR imaging. AJR 162:69–70

Mitchell DG, Cruvella M, Eschelman DJ, Miettinen MM, Vernick JJ (1992) MRI of pancreatic gastrinomas. J Comput Assist Tomogr 16:583–585

Mitchell DG, Winston CB, Outwater EK, Ehrlich SM (1995) Delineation of pancreas with MR imaging: multiobserver comparison of five pulse sequences. J Magn Reson Imaging 5:193–199

Pavone P, Mitchell DG, Leonetti F, et al. (1993) Pancreatic beta-cell tumors: MRI. J Comput Assist Tomogr 17:403–407

Reinig JW (1995) Breath-hold fast spin-echo MR imaging of the liver: a technique for high-quality T2-weighted images. Radiology 194:303–304

Roche A, Baert AL, Therasse E, Rigauts H, Marchal G (1994) Endocrine tumors of the pancreas. In: Baert AL (ed) Radiology of the pancreas. Springer, Berlin Heidelberg New York, pp 197–234

Rosch T, Lightdale CJ, Botet JF, et al. (1992) Localization of pancreatic endocrine tumors by endoscopic ultrasonography. N Engl J Med 326:1721–1726

Rossi P, Allison DJ, Bezzi M, et al. (1989) Endocrine tumors of the pancreas. Radiol Clin North Am 27:129–161

Semelka RC, Ascher SM (1993) MR imaging of the pancreas. Radiology 188:593–602

Semelka RC, Cumming MJ, Shoenut JP, Magro CM, Yaffe CS, Kroeker MA, Greenberg HM (1993) Islet cell tumors: comparison of dynamic contrast-enhanced CT and MRI with dynamic gadolinium enhancement and fat suppression. Radiology 186:799–802

Stabile BE, Morrow DJ, Passaro E Jr (1984) The gastrinoma triangle: operative implications. Am J Surg 147:25–31

Van Hoe L, Gryspeerdt S, Marchal G, Baert AL, Mertens L (1995) Helical CT for the preoperative localization of islet cell tumors of the pancreas: value of arterial and parenchymal phase images AJR 165:1437–1439

Winter TC, Freeny PC, Nghiem HV (1996) Extrapancreatic gastrinoma localization: value of arterial-phase helical CT with water as an oral contrast agent. AJR 166:51–52

10 Nonendocrine Tumors of the Pancreas

R.C. Semelka and H.B. Marcos

10.1
Magnetic Resonance Imaging Techniques

Current magnetic resonance (MR) techniques have been shown to be effective at imaging the pancreas and evaluating pancreatic diseases. These techniques include: (a) breath-hold spoiled gradient echo, which avoids phase artifact caused by respiration and peristalsis, (b) T1-weighted fat-suppressed spoiled gradient echo or spin echo, which removes chemical shift artifact and improves the dynamic range of the intra-abdominal tissue signal intensities, (c) immediate postgadolinium spoiled gradient echo, which maximizes contrast between tumor and pancreas, and (d) single shot T2-weighted echo train spin echo [e.g., half-Fourier acquisition single-shot turbo spin echo (HASTE)], which evaluates the caliber of the common bile and pancreatic ducts and assesses the complexity of pseudocyst fluid composition. These techniques are generally most reliable at ≥1.0 T. T2-weighted fat-suppressed spin-echo imaging is useful to improve the conspicuity of high signal intensity masses such as islet cell tumors, or for detection of associated liver metastases (Semelka and Ascher

R.C. Semelka, MD, Director of MR Services and Associate Professor of Radiology, Department of Radiology, University of North Carolina, Chapel Hill, NC 27599-7510, USA
H.B. Marcos, MD, Clinical Research Fellow in MR Services, Department of Radiology, University of North Carolina, Chapel Hill, NC 27599-7510, USA

1993; Semelka et al. 1990, 1991b, 1993; Chezmar et al. 1991).

Magnetic resonance cholangiography (MRCP) is a recently introduced noninvasive method. MRCP images can generate 3D data display that demonstrates the appearance of the biliary and pancreatic ducts to assess for ductal obstruction, dilatation, stricture, stones, or abnormal duct pathways. MRCP may be performed as motion-averaged long TR/TE echo train sequences or as breath-hold or breathing-independent sequences such as HASTE (Soto et al. 1995).

Our standard MR protocol includes: T1-weighted fat-suppressed imaging (spoiled gradient-echo or spin-echo imaging), nonsuppressed spoiled gradient-echo imaging, and postgadolinium spoiled gradient-echo imaging in the capillary phase and interstitial phase (1–5 min post contrast) (Semelka et al. 1991b).

The normal pancreas is isointense relative to the liver on T1-weighted images and hyperintense relative to the liver on T1-weighted fat-suppressed images (Fig. 10.1) (Semelka et al. 1991a). The higher signal intensity on the fat-suppressed images reflects the presence of aqueous protein in the glandular elements of the pancreas (Mitchell et al. 1991; Semelka et al. 1990). On immediate postgadolinium images the pancreas shows a uniform capillary blush which renders it higher in signal intensity than liver and adjacent fat. On delayed postgadolinium images (5–10 min), the pancreas has a diminished signal intensity relative to fat (Chezmar et al. 1991; Semelka et al. 1991b).

10.2
Mass Lesions

10.2.1
Adenocarcinoma

Pancreatic ductal adenocarcinoma accounts for 95% of the malignant tumors of the pancreas and is the

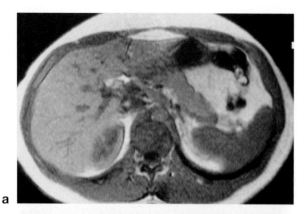

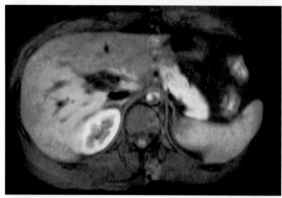

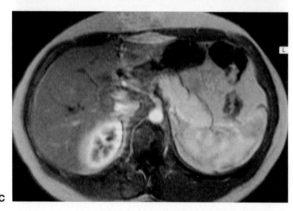

Fig. 10.1a–c. Normal pancreas. T1-weighted spoiled gradient-echo (**a**), T1-weighted fat-suppressed spin-echo (**b**), and immediate postgadolinium spoiled gradient-echo (**c**) images. Normal pancreas is lower in signal intensity than background fat on the precontrast spoiled gradient-echo image (**a**), and moderately high in signal intensity on the precontrast T1-weighted fat-suppressed image (**b**). On the immediate postgadolinium image (**c**), a uniform capillary blush is apparent

fourth most common cause of cancer death in the United States (BORING et al. 1991). Pancreatic cancers are more common in males and blacks (WARSHAW and FERNANDEZ-DEL CASTILLO 1992). The age range for tumor occurrence is the 4th

through the 8th decade, with tumor incidence peaking in the 8th decade (MOOSSA 1982).

Pancreatic cancers have a poor prognosis, with a 5-year survival of 5%. Approximately 60% of pancreatic adenocarcinomas occur in the head, 15% in the body, and 5% in the tail; 20% have diffuse involvement (CLARK et al. 1985).

Histologically, pancreatic cancer has a dense cellularity and sparse vascularity, which accounts for the low signal intensity of the tumor on T1-weighted images (both nonsuppressed and fat-suppressed sequences) and the diminished enhancement on immediate postgadolinium spoiled gradient-echo images.

Pancreatic cancer manifests late. At initial presentation, 65% of patients have advanced local disease or distant metastases, 21% have localized disease with spread to regional lymph nodes, and only 14% have tumor confined to the pancreas. This reflects the lack of a distinct capsule around the gland and the rich lymphatic supply, which allows rapid infiltration of the tumor into peripancreatic tissues and regional lymph nodes. The most common sites of metastases are liver, regional lymph nodes that include peripancreatic, periaortic, pericaval, periportal, and celiac lymph nodes, peritoneum, and lungs (CUBILLA and FITZGERALD 1979).

Ductal adenocarcinoma appears as a focal hypointense solid mass on T1-weighted fat-suppressed images and dynamic contrast-enhanced images (Figs. 10.2, 10.3). This tumor is usually relatively isointense with pancreas on T2-weighted images (SEMELKA et al. 1996a). Pancreatic cancer may cause changes of chronic pancreatitis distal to the mass lesion because of obstruction of the main pancreatic duct. This causes low signal intensity of the background pancreatic tissue on noncontrast T1-weighted image, which results in poor contrast with the low signal intensity tumors. Even in the presence of chronic pancreatitis, tumors are demarcated as low signal intensity masses in a background of higher signal intensity pancreas on immediate postgadolium spoiled gradient-echo images.

The majority of tumors (60%) occur in the head of the pancreas, where they tend to present earlier than tumors in the body or tail, as they cause obstruction of the common bile duct and jaundice. Painless jaundice is the classical presenting feature of pancreatic cancer. Pancreatic cancer arising in the head of the pancreas causes abrupt obstruction of the common bile duct and the pancreatic duct. This appearance is termed the double duct sign (BARON et al. 1983) and can be observed on MRCP studies

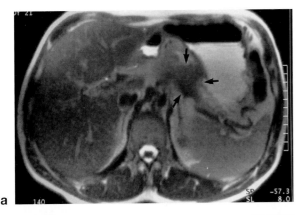

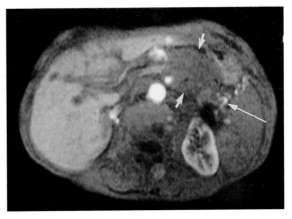

Fig. 10.3. Pancreatic cancer. Immediate postgadolinium spoiled gradient-echo image. A large pancreatic mass (*arrows*) is present arising from the body and tail of the pancreas. The mass enhances minimally on the immediate postgadolinium spoiled gradient-echo image. Varices are present along the greater curvature of the stomach (*arrow*) due to thrombosis of the splenic vein

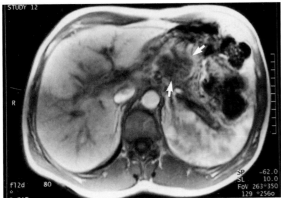

Fig. 10.2a,b. Ductal adenocarcinoma. HASTE (a) and immediate postgadolinium spoiled gradient-echo (b) images. A large mass is present arising from the body of the pancreas (*arrows*). Oral administration of water achieved gastric distention and improved demonstration of stomach wall invasion on the HASTE image. Heterogeneous minimal enhancement of the tumor mass is noted on the immediate postgadolinium spoiled gradient-echo image (b)

(SOTO et al. 1995). Enlargement of the head of the pancreas with dilatation of the common bile and pancreatic ducts and atrophy of the body and tail of the pancreas are commonly seen with advanced cancer of the pancreatic head.

The secondary features which assist in the diagnosis of pancreatic cancer include the presence of lymphadenopathy, encasement of the celiac axis or superior mesenteric artery, and liver metastases (Fig. 10.4). The only secondary feature that is absolutely diagnostic for pancreatic cancer is liver metastases as the other features may also be rarely observed in chronic pancreatitis (WITTENBERG et al. 1982).

A recent study evaluated the ability of MR imaging using T1-weighted fat-suppressed imaging and dynamic gadolinium chelate-enhanced spoiled gradient-echo imaging to detect the presence of pancreatic tumor in patients in whom spiral CT findings

were inconclusive (SEMELKA et al. 1996a). The study was performed in 16 patients with findings indeterminate for pancreatic cancer on spiral CT. Immediate postgadolinium spoiled gradient-echo imaging was found to be the most sensitive approach to detect pancreatic cancer, particularly in the head of the pancreas. Both immediate postgadolinium spoiled gradient-echo and T1-weighted fat-suppressed imaging performed well at excluding pancreatic cancer and both were significantly superior to spiral CT.

Chronic pancreatitis may uncommonly cause focal enlargement of the head of the pancreas with obstruction of the common bile duct and pancreatic duct (LAMMER et al. 1985). In these cases it may be difficult to distinguish focal chronic pancreatitis from adenocarcinoma of the head of the pancreas. In this setting, immediate postgadolinium spoiled gradient-echo images are the most useful for establishing the correct diagnosis, with definition of a focal lesion being consistent with tumor, while lack of de-monstration of a mass lesion is consistent with chronic pancreatitis. Large pancreatic tumors tend to remain of low signal intensity on early and late post-contrast images whereas smaller tumors may range from hypointense to hyperintense on delayed images.

Local extension of pancreatic cancer is well shown on noncontrast T1-weighted images (VELLET et al. 1992) and on interstitial phase gadolinium-enhanced fat-suppressed spoiled gradient-echo images. Peritoneal involvement with pancreatic cancer is best shown on interstitial phase gadolinium-enhanced

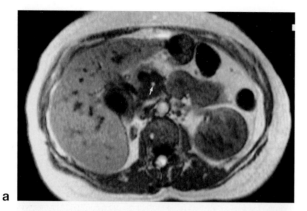

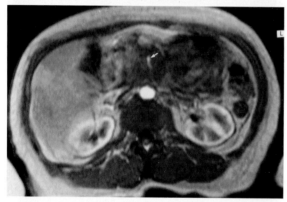

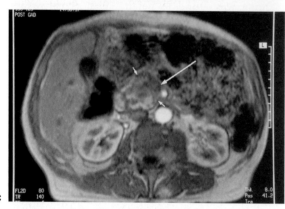

Fig. 10.4a–c. Pancreatic cancer with local extension and vascular encasement. T1-weighted spoiled gradient-echo (**a**), postgadolinium spoiled gradient-echo (**b**), and immediate postgadolinium spoiled gradient-echo (**c**) images in three different patients with ductal adenocarcinoma arising from the head of the pancreas. In the first patient low signal intensity tumor encases the hepatic artery (*arrow*, **a**). High signal intensity in the artery is due to time-of-flight effects. In the second patient a large pancreatic head cancer is noted to encase the superior mesenteric artery (*arrow*, **b**). In the third patient a pancreatic head cancer is identified (*arrows*, **c**). The superior mesenteric vein (*long arrow*, **c**), is thrombosed. The superior mesenteric artery is patent although tumor is closely apposed to the vessel

fat-suppressed spoiled gradient-echo images. Nodal disease is well shown using a combination of non-suppressed T1-weighted images, fat-suppressed T2-weighted images, and interstitial phase gadolinium-enhanced spoiled gradient-echo images (GABATA et al. 1994; PAVONE et al. 1991).

Liver metastases from pancreatic cancer typically appear as focal, irregular lesions which are moderately low in signal intensity on T1-weighted images, minimally high in signal intensity on T2-weighted images, and possess indistinct peripheral ring enhancement on immediate postcontrast spoiled gradient-echo images. Transient ill-defined increased perilesional hepatic parenchymal enhancement may also be observed on immediate postgadolinium images. The hypovascular nature of hepatic metastases permits the distinction between these lesions and cysts and hemangiomas even when lesions are 1 cm in diameter.

Magnetic resonance imaging is useful in the investigation of pancreatic cancer. MR imaging is particularly indicated in the examination of patients with diminished renal function or iodine contrast allergy, detection of small non-organ-deforming cancers, determination of tumor location for imaging-guided biopsy, evaluation of vascular involvement, and detection of associated liver lesions. Since surgery remains the main treatment of patients with pancreatic cancer, earlier detection of potentially curable disease may result in improved patient survival (WARSHAW and FERNANDEZ-DEL CASTILLO 1992).

10.2.2
Periampullary and Ampullary Tumors

Tumors arising in the vicinity of the ampulla of Vater are termed periampullary tumors. Ampullary tumors arise from the ampulla of Vater itself. These include both benign and malignant tumors. The majority are adenocarcinoma of the head of the pancreas (85%), with the following histologic types occurring less commonly: cholangiocarcinoma of the common bile duct (6%), duodenal adenocarcinoma (5%), and adenocarcinoma of the ampulla of Vater (4%) (BUCK and ELSAYED 1993). Patients with adenomas and adenocarcinomas of other sites of the gastrointestinal tract, particularly the colon, are also at higher risk of ampullary tumors (e.g., familial adenomatous polyposis syndromes).

Magnetic resonance imaging demonstrates a similar appearance to that of pancreatic adenocarcinoma. Periampullary and ampullary tumors have low signal intensity on T1- and T2-weighted images and diminished enhancement on immediate postgadolinium images (SEMELKA et al. 1997). Due to the common occurrence of chronic pancreatitis from obstruction of the pancreatic duct, immediate postgadolinium spoiled gradient-echo images are the most reliable at detecting tumors (Fig. 10.5).

10.2.3
Microcystic Adenoma

Microcystic adenoma is a benign neoplasm characterized by multiple tiny cysts. The tumor occurs in elderly patients and has an increased association with von Hippel-Lindau disease (MINAMI et al. 1989). Tumors range in size from 1 to 12 cm and have a mean diameter of 5 cm at presentation. A central scar may be present.

On MR images, the tumors are well defined and do not show invasion of fat or adjacent organs. On T2-weighted images, small cysts with intervening septations are demonstrated as a cluster of small grape-like structures. This appearance is more clearly seen on breath-hold images as the thin septations blur during a longer non-breath-hold sequence (Fig. 10.6).

Cystic pancreatic masses that contain cysts less than 1 cm in diameter most likely represent microcystic adenomas while masses that contain cysts greater than 2 cm mostly represent macrocystic adenoma or adenocarcinoma. Cysts that measure between 1 and 2 cm in diameter may be found in micro- or macrocystic adenoma (LEWANDROWSKI et al. 1992).

10.2.4
Macrocystic Adenoma or Adenocarcinoma

Macrocystic adenomas or adenocarcinomas are mucin-secreting tumors which are malignant or have malignant potential. They occur more frequently in females (6:1) and approximately one-half occur in people aged 40–60 years (COMPAGNO and OERTEL 1978). These tumors are frequently large (mean diameter 10 cm), multiloculated, and encapsulated. The most frequent location is in the body or tail of the pancreas. There is a great propensity for invasion of adjacent organs and tissues.

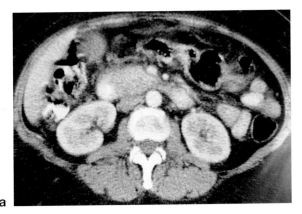

a

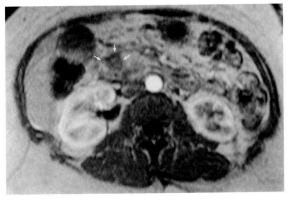

b

Fig. 10.5a,b. Ampullary carcinoma. Spiral CT scan image (a) and immediate postgadolinium spoiled gradient-echo image (b). Diffuse enlargment of the pancreatic head is demonstrated on the CT image with no definite mass apparent. A mass at the level of the ampulla is well shown on the immediate postgadolinium image, which demonstrates minimal heterogeneous enhancement (*arrows*, b)

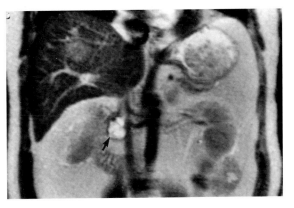

Fig. 10.6. Microcystic adenoma. Coronal T2-weighted HASTE image. A cystic lesion (*arrow*) is present in the head of pancreas, which contains microcysts measuring less than 1 cm in diameter and fine intervening septations. The fine septations are clearly defined on the breathing-independent HASTE image

Liver metastases are frequently identified at the time of initial diagnosis.

On gadolinium-enhanced T1-weighted fat-suppressed images, large irregular cystic spaces separated by thick septa are shown. Macrocystic adenomas are well-defined masses with septations of regular thickness and have no evidence of invasion of adjacent tissues or metastases. Low-grade malignant tumors may be very large.

Macrocystic adenocarcinomas may be very locally aggressive malignancies with extensive invasion of adjacent tissues and organs. Breathing-independent single-shot T2-weighted sequences (e.g., HASTE) demonstrate sharp definition of the internal architecture of cysts, which helps distinguish benign from malignant masses (Fig. 10.7).

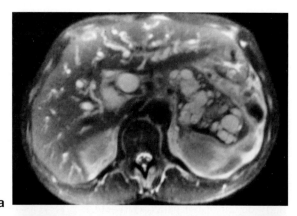

a

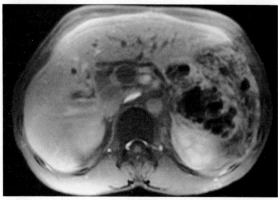

b

Fig. 10.7a,b. Macrocystic adenocarcinoma. T2-weighted fat-suppressed HASTE (a) and interstitial-phase gadolinium-enhanced T1-weighted fat-suppressed spoiled gradient-echo (b) images. A well-defined cystic mass arises from the body and tail of the pancreas. On the HASTE image (a) multiple high signal intensity cysts are appreciated that measure >2 cm in diameter. Intervening septations are thick and irregular. The cystic lesion is low in signal intensity on the T1-weighted fat-suppressed image (b), and enhancement of the septations is appreciated

These tumors may occasionally be of high signal intensity on T1-weighted images due to the presence of mucin. Liver metastases are generally hypervascular, commonly cystic, and may contain mucin. This presence of mucin in varying concentrations results in mixed low and high signal intensity on T1-weighted images and T2-weighted images. On immediate postgadolinium images, liver metastases have intense ring enhancement.

10.2.5
Solid and Papillary Epithelial Neoplasms

Solid and papillary epithelial neoplasms are rare tumors that have low-grade malignant potential and occur most frequently in females between 20 and 30 years of age (BALTHAZAR et al. 1984; OHTOMO et al. 1992). Solid and papillary epithelial neoplasms are commonly well-demarcated lesions containing high signal intensity on T1-weighted images consistent with hemorrhagic necrosis. Smaller tumors may not be hemorrhagic.

10.2.6
Lymphoma

Non-Hodgkin's lymphoma may involve peripancreatic lymph nodes or may directly invade the pancreas (ZEMAN et al. 1985). Intermediate signal intensity peripancreatic lymph nodes are well distinguished from normal high signal intensity pancreatic tissue on T1-weighted fat-suppressed images. Invasion of the pancreas is shown by loss of the normal high signal intensity of the pancreas on noncontrast T1-weighted fat-suppressed images.

10.2.7
Metastases

Metastases may involve peripancreatic lymph nodes or may invade the pancreas. Primary malignancies include neoplasms of the gastrointestinal tract, kidney, breast, lungs, prostate, and melanoma. MR imaging may be of value in the evaluation of pancreatic metastases in the context of a hypervascular primary malignancy.

A recent report described the MR appearance of renal cancer metastases to the pancreas. Metastases were low in signal intensity on T1-weighted images and high in signal intensity on T2-weighted

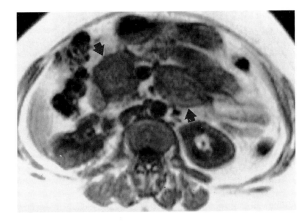

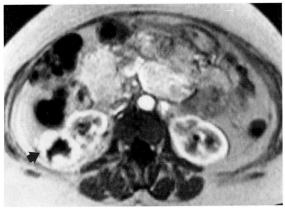

Fig 10.8. Pancreatic metastases from renal cancer. T1-weighted spoiled gradient-echo (**a**) and immediate postgadolinium spoiled gradient-echo (**b**) images. Metastases (*arrows*, **a**) are present diffusely involving the entire pancreas. The metastases are low in signal intensity on the precontrast image (**a**) and demonstrate intense enhancement on the immediate postcontrast image (**b**). A right renal cancer is also shown, which has intense peripheral enhancement on the immediate postgadolinium image (*arrow*, **b**)

images (Fig. 10.8). Small metastases measuring less than 1 cm in diameter usually enhance uniformly on immediate postgadolinium images while larger metastases have ring enhancement. Renal cancer metastases resemble the appearance of islet cell tumors (SEMELKA et al. 1996b).

Melanoma metastases may be of high signal intensity on T1-weighted images due to the paramagnetic properties of melanin.

10.3
Conclusions

Current MR techniques are very effective at evaluating the pancreas. The best clinical roles for MRI include: detection of pancreatic tumors, detection

of small non-organ-deforming ductal adenocarcinomas, characterization of cystic pancreatic masses, and differentiation of chronic pancreatitis from cancer.

References

Balthazar EJ, Subramanyam BR, Lefleur RS, Barone CM (1984) Solid and papillary neoplasm of the pancreas: radiographic CT, sonographic features. Radiology 150:39–40

Baron RL, Stanley RJ, Lee JKT, Koehler RE, Levitt RG (1983) Computed tomographic features of biliary obstruction. AJR 140:1173–1178

Boring CC, Squires TS, Tong T (1991) Cancer statistics, 1991. CA Cancer J Clin 41:19–51

Buck JL, Elsayed AM (1993) Ampullary tumors: radiologic-pathologic correlation. Radiographics 13:193–212

Chezmar JL, Nelson RC, Small WCA, Bernardino ME (1991) Magnetic resonance imaging of the pancreas with gadolinium-DPTA. Gastrointest Radiol 16:139–142

Clark LR, Jaffe MH, Choyke PL, Grant EG, Zeman RK (1985) Pancreatic imaging. Radiol Clin North Am 23:489–501

Compagno J, Oertel JE (1978) Mucinous cystic neoplasms of the pancreas with overt and latent malignancy (cystadenocarcinoma and cystadenoma): a clinicopathologic study of 41 cases. Am J Clin Pathol 69:573–580

Cubilla AL, Fitzgerald PJ (1979) Cancer of the pancreas (nonendocrine): a suggested morphologic clarification. Semin Oncol 6:285–297

Friedman AC, Liechtenstein JE, Dachman AH (1983) Cystic neoplasms of the pancreas: radiological-pathological correlation. Radiology 149:45–50

Gabata T, Matsui O, Kadoya M, et al. (1994) Small pancreatic adenocarcinomas: efficacy of MR imaging with fat suppression and gadolinium enhancement. Radiology 193: 683–688

Lammer J, Herlinger H, Zalaudek G, Hofler H (1985) Pseudotumorous pancreatitis. Gastrointest Radiol 10:59–67

Larson RE, Semelka RC, Bagley AS, Molina PL, Brown ED, Lee JK (1994) Hypervascular malignant liver lesions: comparison of various MR imaging pulse sequences and dynamic CT. Radiology 192:393–399

Lewandrowski K, Warshaw A, Compton C (1992) Macrocystic serous cystadenoma of the pancreas: a morphologic variant differing from microcystic adenoma. Hum Pathol 23:871–875

Lowenfels AB, Maisonneuve P, Cavallini G, et al. (1993) Pancreatitis and the risk of pancreatic cancer. N Engl J Med 328:1433–1437

Minami M, Itai Y, Ohtomo K, Yoshida H, Yoshikawa K, Iio M (1989) Cystic neoplasms of the pancreas: comparison of MR imaging with CT. Radiology 171:53–56

Mitchell DG, Vinitski S, Saponaro S, Tasciyan T, Burk DL Jr, Rifkin MD (1991) Liver and pancreas: improved spin-echo T1-weighted images contrast by shorter echo time and fat suppression at 1.5 T. Radiology 178:67–71

Mitchell DG, Winston CB, Outwater EK, Ehrlich SM (1995) Delineation of pancreas with MR imaging: multiobserver comparison of five pulse sequences. J Magn Reson Imaging 5:193–199

Moossa AR (1982) Pancreatic cancer: approach to diagnosis, selection for surgery and choice of operation. Cancer 50:2689–2698

Ohtomo K, Furui S, Onoue M, Okada Y, Kusano S, Uchiyama G (1992) Solid and papillary epithelial neoplasm of the pancreas: MR imaging and pathologic correlation (abstr). Radiology 185(p):284

Pavone P, Occhiato R, Michelini O, et al. (1991) Magnetic resonance imaging of pancreatic carcinoma. Eur Radiol 1:124–130

Ros PR, Hamrick-Turner JE, Chiechi MV, Ross LH, Gallego P, Burton SS (1992) Cystic masses of the pancreas. Radiographics 12:673–686

Semelka RC, Ascher SM (1993) MRI of the pancreas – state of the art. Radiology 188:593–602

Semelka RC, Chew W, Hricak H, Tomei E, Higgins CB (1990) Fat-saturation MR imaging of the upper abdomen. AJR 155:1111–1116.

Semelka RC, Simm FC, Recht M, Lenz G, Laub GA (1991a) MRI of the pancreas at high field strength – a comparison of six sequences. J Comput Assist Tomogr 15:966–971

Semelka RC, Krocker MA, Shoenut JP, Krocker R, Yaffe CS, Micflikier AB (1991b) Pancreatic disease: prospective comparison of CT, ERCP, and 1.5-T MR imaging dynamic gadolinium enhancement and fat suppression. Radiology 181:785–791

Semelka RC, Shoenut JP, Kroeker MA, Micflikier AB (1993) Pancreas. In: Semelka RC, Shoenut JP (eds) Magnetic resonance imaging of the abdomen with CT correlation. Raven Press, New York, pp 84–98

Semelka RC, Kelekis NL, Molina PL, Sharp T, Calvo B (1996a) Pancreatic masses with indeterminate findings on spiral CT. Is there a role for MRI?. J Magn Reson Imaging 6:585–588

Semelka RC, Kelekis NL, Siegelman ES (1996b) MRI of pancreatic metastases from renal cancer. J Comput Assist Tomogr 20:249–253

Semelka RC, Kelekis NL, John G, Asher SM, Burdeny DA, Siegelman ES (1997) Ampullary carcinoma: demonstration by current MR techniques. J Magn Reson Imaging 7:153–156

Soto JA, Barish MA, Yucel EK, et al. (1995) Pancreatic duct: MR cholangiopancreatography with a three-dimensional fast spin-echo technique. Radiology 196:459–464

Vellet AD, Romano W, Bach DB, Passi RB, Taves DH, Munk PL (1992) Adenocarcinoma of the pancreatic ducts: comparative evaluation with CT and MR imaging at 1.5T. Radiology 183:87–95

Warshaw AL, Fernandez-del Castillo C (1992) Pancreatic carcinoma. N Engl J Med 326:455–465

Wittenberg J, Simeone JF, Ferrucci JT, Mueller PR, Van Sonnenberg E, Neff CC (1982) Non-focal enlargement in pancreatic carcinoma. Radiology 144:131–135

Zeman RK, Schiebler M, Clark LR, et al. (1985) The clinical and spectrum of pancreaticoduodenal lymph node enlargement. AJR 144:1223–1227

11 Adrenal Glands

T.H.M. Falke, A.P. van Gils, M.P. Sandler, T. Doesburg, and M.A. Cuesta

CONTENTS

11.1
Introduction

Adrenal evaluation with magnetic resonance imaging (MRI) has been performed ever since abdominal imaging with MR became feasible (Moon et al.

T.H.M. Falke, MD, Professor of Radiology, Department of Radiology, Free University Hospital Amsterdam, de Boelenlaan, P.O. Box 7057, 1007 MB Amsterdam, The Netherlands

A.P. van Gils, MD, Assistant Professor, Department of Radiology, Central Military Hospital, Heidelberglaan 100, 3584 CX Utrecht, The Netherlands

M.P. Sandler, MD, Professor of Radiology and Radiological Sciences, Assistant Professor of Medicine, Director of Nuclear Medicine, Vice-Chairman, Department of Radiology and Radiological Sciences, Vanderbilt University School of Medicine, 1161 21st Avenue South, Nashville, Tenn., USA

T. Doesburg, MD, Research Fellow, Free University Hospital Amsterdam, de Boelenlaan, P.O. Box 7057, 1007 MB, Amsterdam, The Netherlands

M.A. Cuesta, MD, Associate Professor of Endocrine Surgery, Director of Abdominal Surgery, Free University Hospital Amsterdam, de Boelenlaan, P.O. Box 7057, 1007 MB Amsterdam, The Netherlands

1983). Immediately differences in signal intensities between masses on T2-weighted images were noted simultaneously by various investigators (Reinig et al. 1986; Falke et al. 1986a; Glazer et al. 1986). These initial results were followed by other reports that investigated various pulse sequences (Gruss and Newhouse 1996), field strengths (Kier and McCarthy 1989), and different parameters in an attempt to reduce the scatter and overlap of data from adenomas and malignancies by using contrast-enhanced MRI (Krestin et al. 1989) and chemical shift ratios (Mitchell et al. 1992). The quest for the ultimate approach to differentiate lesions continues, often neglecting the basic fact that there is an intrinsic histologic limitation to the reduction of overlap between benign and malignant disorders of the adrenal gland (Reinig 1992; Falke and Sandler 1994).

Despite its great potential, MRI's advantages over computed tomography (CT) have been offset by image corruption due to a large number of artifacts. However, over the last several years, developments have steadily decreased many types of artifacts. By reducing other causes of image degradation, this progress has resulted in an increase in the relative importance of motion effects in abdominal MRI (Ehman et al. 1986). Among the many effects of motion, unsharpness has been the most important limiting factor in the widespread application of MRI to the adrenal glands. With the introduction of fast and ultrafast imaging techniques in conjunction with phased array coils, anatomic resolution has improved dramatically through the reduction of basic blurring. At present MRI provides a great deal of morphologic detail of the adrenal glands with greater specificity than CT or ultrasonography (US) (Falke et al. 1987). The major remaining limitation of endocrine imaging with MR is that it does not provide information on the functional status of an adrenal lesion. However, initial experiments have demonstrated the feasibility of designing contrast agents for MRI of the adrenal glands (Weissleder et al. 1993). Other classes of contrast agents, now under development, are designed to define the physiology of various tissue layers, for example, paramagnetic cholesterol derivates for adrenal function (MUEHLER et al. 1995).

Adrenal scintigraphy, although not providing anatomic detail as with MRI or functional information as in venous sampling, does provide unique metabolic information, in the form of the specific uptake of a radiopharmaceutical mimicking either an adrenal substrate (i.e., cholesterol) or hormone reuptake and storage (i.e., norepinephrine), not afforded by other anatomic means of localization (GROSS et al. 1992).

Abnormal adrenal cortical or medullary function results in distinct patterns of signs and symptoms of unregulated amounts of hormone. Careful biochemical evaluation allows these abnormalities to be distinguished and is important in a tailored approach to the diagnostic localization of the lesion(s) responsible.

A carefully planned approach to adrenal disorders, which considers all of the available technologies, can in virtually every instance identify and efficiently localize possible sources of abnormal adrenal function. Its findings may even antedate the overt clinical onset of manifestations of disease, providing optimal and cost-effective management of imaging resources (TELENIUS-BERG et al. 1987). Accurate localization and identification of mass lesions is important because it determines whether the patient can be cured by surgery through the posterior approach or endoscopic adrenalectomy. These techniques have been reported to be associated with less postoperative pain than open adrenalectomy, resulting in early postoperative mobilization and decreased hospital stay (CUESTA et al. 1996). Increasing experience with image protocols and interpretation has led MRI to become the modality of first choice in the majority of patients with endocrine disorders of the adrenal glands.

11.2
Adrenal Anatomy

The adrenal glands are paired structures which are located in the region of the upper poles of the kidneys (Fig. 11.1). The outer portion of the adrenal, the adrenal cortex, accounts for the bulk (80%) of the normal gland weight in the adult (SYMINGTON 1969). The right gland occupies a slightly more cephalad and lateral position in relation to the kidney than the left gland. The adrenals have a rich vascular supply

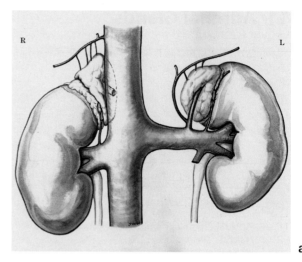

a

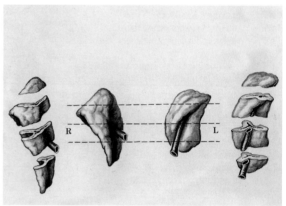

b

Fig. 11.1 a,b. Normal anatomy of the adrenal glands. a The main venous drainage is via the central vein. On the left side, this vein lies in the longitudinal axis of the gland. The left suprarenal vein joins the inferior phrenic vein before entering the left renal vein. The right central vein is very short and drains directly into the vena cava. b Cross-sectional adrenal anatomy. The shape of the adrenals on transverse sections shows considerable variation depending on the level of sectioning. (Artist's drawing after cryosectioned specimen.) (From GROSS et al. 1992)

with direct aortic, renal, phrenic, and lumbar arterial blood supply (MADSEN 1980). Venous drainage generally occurs via a single cortical vein into the inferior vena cava on the right, although anomalous drainage can occur via the hepatic vein (Fig. 11.1a). On the left, drainage generally is through the renal vein. The cortex is derived from mesodermal tissues, while the medulla is a neuroectodermal structure. Many sites in the abdomen and pelvis may harbor ectopic adrenocortical tissues, although true accessory adrenal glands consisting of both cortex and medulla are unusual. Accessory, separate cortical or medullary tissues may be found in the spleen, the retroperitoneum along the aorta, or the region of the pelvis. Extra-adrenal chromaffin cells may also be found in the intravagal, branchomeric visceral autonomic paraganglia or in the aortic sympathetic regions (Langman 1969; van Gils et al. 1990; Wilms et al. 1979).

On axial sections the right adrenal gland is situated above the upper pole of the right kidney and posterior to the inferior vena cava. Cranially and laterally the gland is in close relation with the posterior segment of the right lobe of the liver. The anterior–posterior (AP) axis of the gland courses parallel to the crus of the diaphragm in an oblique plane angulated 45° with respect to the sagittal plane. The tail of the right adrenal gland is visualized on the most cephalad slices and lies slightly lateral to the oblique plane through the AP axis of the head. On oblique/sagittal cuts the longitudinal axis is almost completely imaged in a single slice. Adrenal pseudomasses may be simulated on an imaging modality by the close anatomic relationship of normal or diseased surrounding structures, such as the inferior vena cava, the upper pole of the right kidney, or the gallbladder.

The left adrenal gland is situated posterior to the splenic vessels and is most often visualized at the level of the pancreatic tail. The head of the left gland is situated anteromedial to the left kidney just above the renal vein, and is visualized at a slightly lower level than the head of the right adrenal gland. The course of the left adrenal gland is usually not parallel to the diaphragm. The fundus of the stomach lies anterior and cranial to the tail of the left adrenal gland. The close relationship of the adrenal gland to surrounding structures may lead to the misinterpretation of a pancreatic mass as an adrenal pseudomass or may be confused with aneurysms of the splenic artery, an accessory spleen, retroperitoneal spleen, gastric diverticulum, retroperitoneal pulmonary sequestration, a normal or abnormal upper pole of the left kidney, tortuous splenic vessels, and varices (Berliner et al. 1982; Silverman 1986; Baker et al. 1982; Brady et al. 1985).

The right adrenal is triangular and has a smooth anterior surface. The left gland is elongated and crescent shaped, with a groove on the anterior surface from which the main suprarenal vein emerges. The shape of the normal adult adrenal gland is affected by the kidney (Kenney et al. 1985). If the kidney is present in the normal location in the renal fossa during fetal life, it exerts a mass effect on the large globular fetal adrenal, which results in a posteroinferior indentation. The adult human adrenal has a tripartite structure consisting of head, body, and tail, and

portions of the gland extend laterally to form the alae. The head of the adrenal glands is the most caudate part.

The shape of the adrenals shows considerable variation on cross-section, depending on the slice orientation and level of sectioning (Fig. 11.1b) (Gross et al. 1992; Wilms et al. 1979). On transverse and coronal sections, the shapes on the right are usually depicted as linear, inverted V and K configurations and the configurations on the left as linear, inverted V, triangular, and, most characteristically, star-shaped configurations, sometimes referred to as the "seagull sign." Shortening of one of the limbs may produce variations in these basic configurations. Linear configurations of the adrenal are due to the tail of the adrenal being sectioned out of the true perpendicular plane. In the sagittal plane, both adrenal glands show a dorsal curvature or bow-like configuration.

11.3
Adrenal Physiology and Pathophysiology

The adrenal cortex is functionally and anatomically subdivided into three histologic zones. Within each zone a principal adrenal steroid hormone is synthesized and secreted. Adrenal cortical dysfunction can be attributed to abnormalities of biosynthesis or hormone secretion in each zone (Neville and O'Hara 1985; Nelson 1980). Specific hormone abnormalities can be verified with appropriate biochemical testing. The principal mineralocorticoid hormone secreted within the outer portion of the cortex is aldosterone. Aldosterone secretion is augmented in response to a decrement of either body sodium or plasma volume. Serum potassium levels are also important in the control of aldosterone secretion.

The second principal division of the adrenal cortex is the zona fasciculata. This zone produces the principal glucocorticoid hormone, cortisol. The effects of cortisol are widespread and generally affect metabolism by a permissive action on numerous enzyme systems. Control of cortisol secretion is a result of a complex negative feedback loop which includes the hypothalamus, the anterior pituitary, and the adrenal cortex. Corticotropin-releasing factor (CRF) is secreted by the hypothalamus either in response to a decrement of circulating cortisol or as a result of other stimuli such as stress. ACTH secretion is stimulated by CRF and results in a direct increase in cortisol biosynthesis and subsequent secretion. The activity of the intra-adrenal enzymes responsible for the biosynthesis of glucocorticoids is also augmented by ACTH. The negative feedback of cortisol upon the anterior pituitary and hypothalamus and the subsequent effects on CRF and ACTH release serve as the basis for one of the oldest pharmacologic tests of adrenocortical function (GROSS et al. 1992). Administration of exogenous steroids provides a rapid method to test the integrity of the hypothalamic-pituitary-adrenal axis.

Adrenal androgens are secreted from the innermost zone of the adrenal cortex, the zone reticularis, and are androstenedione and dehydroepiandrosterone. These hormones are important for the maintenance of secondary sex characteristics in women and work in concert with gonadal steroids in this regard. Adrenal androgen secretion appears to be at least partially under the control of ACTH and hypothalamically derived CRF. But a putative androgen-secreting hormone, possibly luteinizing hormone (LH), and other factors have also been implicated in the control of androgen secretion from the inner adrenal cortex.

The principal catecholamine hormone secreted by the adrenal medulla is epinephrine, which is synthesized from the amino acid tyrosine (GROSS et al. 1992). Other catecholamine-secreting tissues in the body, e.g., sympathetic ganglia, lack the enzyme ethanolamine in methyltranferase, necessary for the conversion of norepinephrine (NE), a neurotransmitter, to the hormone epinephrine. The catechol-o-methyltransferase (COMT) enzyme appears to require high levels of glucocorticoids, i.e., cortisol, which are only present in the adrenal medulla as a result of its close approximation to the adrenal cortex and the venous drainage from the cortex to the medulla. Central nervous system control of adrenal medulla function is via the splanchnic nerves and the neurotransmitter acetylcholine. As a result the adrenal medulla functions similarly to a presynaptic neuron, but with epinephrine released as a hormone directly into the circulation. Stimulation of the adrenal medulla may occur in response to hypovolemia, hypoglycemia, hypotension, hypoxia, hypercapnea, acidosis, anxiety, and pain.

11.4
Imaging Techniques

Patients are best examined with T1- and T2-weighted breath-hold sequences using a phased array body coil for initial screening. The most useful orientation for imaging the adrenal area is the transverse plane. Additional T1-weighted spin-echo (SE) sequences *without* gradient moment nulling and with spatial presaturation should incorporate the shortest possible TE time and a TR ranging typically from 300 to 700 ms at mid and high field strengths. Breath-hold T2-weighted fast SE sequences often depict metastatic lesions and primary malignancies of the adrenal gland with lower signal relative to the liver than do conventional T2-weighted SE sequences, while depicting cysts and pheochromocytomas with a higher relative signal intensity. Breath-hold opposed-phase gradient-echo (GRE) imaging can be used to demonstrate loss in signal intensity compared with in-phase images to prove the presence of lipid-rich, steroid-accumulating cells of adrenocortical origin in adenomas (MITCHELL et al. 1996; BILBEY et al. 1995; TSUSHIMA et al. 1993; OUTWATER and MITCHELL 1994; SCHWARTZ et al. 1995; MAYO-SMITH et al. 1995). SE or GRE sequences can be repeated in combination with spectral fat suppression and/or an inversion prepulse to reduce ghosting artifacts from subcutaneous fat, especially if breath-hold sequences are not possible for any reason. An example of a basic fast imaging protocol used at our institution is given in Table 11.1.

In MRI, distinct visualization of the gastrointestinal tract is possible with orally administered paramagnetic agents. As in CT imaging, oral contrast agents in MRI will facilitate identification of normal adrenals and adrenal tumors by distinguishing them from normal intestinal structures. Preliminary results have demonstrated that contrast agents producing a low signal on T2-weighted images are often essential to distinguish fluid-filled bowel loops from neuroendocrine tumors, which usually have high signal intensities on T2-weighted images. Also the low signal intensity of oral contrast agents contributes to the reduction of artifacts from fluid-filled bowel loops (JACOBSEN et al. 1996).

The indications for intravenous administration of contrast agents during sectional imaging in patients suspected of having adrenal disease are the improvement of anatomic definition, differentiation of normal or anomalous vascular structures, identification of the upper pole of the kidneys, and characterization of the relative vascularity of the mass (FALKE et al. 1988; DE ROOS et al. 1988; SEMELKA et al. 1993; MITCHELL et al. 1995; KRESTIN et al. 1991; KOROBKIN et al. 1995, 1996b). Intravenous contrast agents such as Gd-DTPA enhance tissue specificity based on relative organ perfusion. As in CT, early, late, and delayed enhancement after 1 h may contrib-

Table 11.1. Basic protocol for MRI imaging of the adrenal glands at 1.5 T

TR (ms)	TE (ms)	FL	Acq.	TA (s)	ETL	SLT (mm)
T2-weighted multiple slice: fast spin echo (acronyms: TSE, RARE)						
3000	138	90°	1	10–20	15–33	5
T2-weighted single slice: half Fourier single shot TSE (acronym: HASTE)						
8000	87	90°	1	1–2	128	10
T1-weighted: fast gradient echo in-phase (acronyms: FLASH, FFE, SPGR)						
110–150	5	75°	1	16–20		5
T1-weighted: fast gradient echo out-of-phase (acronyms: FLASH, FFE, SPGR)						
110–150	7	75°	1	16–20		5

TR, repetition time; TE, echo time; FL, flip angle; Acq., number of acquisitions; TA, acquisition time; ETL, echo train length; SLT, slice thickness.

ute to the differentiation of benign from malignant adrenal masses (KOROBKIN et al. 1996b). However, MITCHELL et al. (1996) have recently demonstrated that contrast agents such as gadolinium increase the signal of water within fatty tissue, causing a paradoxical reduction in signal on opposed images. Because of the natural contrast between vascular structures and surrounding tissues in MRI, opacification of vessels with i.v. contrast agents as in CT is usually not necessary for delineation.

11.5
Adrenocortical Disorders with Overactivity

11.5.1
Primary Aldosteronism

Primary hyperaldosteronism (Conn's syndrome) is a clinical syndrome that is characterized by excessive production of aldosterone and low plasma renin levels. It is the cause of hypertension in 0.1%–0.5% of all cases of hypertension. Etiologies include single aldosterone-producing adenoma (±70%) and bilateral adrenocortical hyperplasia (15%–30%) (GROSS et al. 1992). However, the reported predominance of adrenal adenomas over hyperplasia and the supposed predilection of adenomas for the left adrenal gland are most likely the result of selection biases. In rare cases, primary aldosteronism is caused by macronodular hyperplasia, multiple aldosterone-producing adenomas, extra-adrenal adenoma, or unilateral hyperplasia (GROTH et al. 1985). Adrenal carcinoma producing primary hyperaldosteronism has been reported, but is also extremely rare. Adrenal adenoma in primary aldosteronism is often accompanied by non-hyperfunctioning secondary nodules of the adjacent gland, probably as a result of long-standing hypertension, and this may result in an equivocal histologic interpretation.

The diagnosis of primary hyperaldosteronism is usually suspected when hypertension and hypokalemia are present. Patient symptoms are related to the elevated blood pressure as well as episodic weakness, paresthesias, transient paralysis, and tetany due to hypokalemia (MELBY 1985). The biochemical profiles of these patients and saline suppression tests suggest the diagnosis. Postural plasma aldosterone and 18-OH-corticosterone tests provide an indication as to whether the patient has idiopathic hyperplasia or adrenal adenoma. However, a mismatch between response to physiologic maneuvers and morphologic findings on cross-sectional imaging does occur in a minority of cases. Such findings have led to a classification of primary hyperaldosteronism into subtypes including (a) primary hyperplasia (hyperplastic glands which mimic the response of aldosteronomas to physiologic maneuvers and unilateral adrenalectomy) and (b) the aldosterone-producing renin-responsive adenoma (morphologically an aldosteronoma that responds similarly to hyperplasia) (ROBERTS et al. 1985).

Magnetic resonance imaging is successfully applied in the visualization of the adrenal gland in primary aldosteronism. In contrast, venous sampling adds true information on hyperfunction not available from the other modalities (ROBERTS et al. 1985; DUNNICK et al. 1982). Because of the availability of less invasive localization techniques, venous sampling should be reserved for equivocal cases. The relative roles of CT, MRI, and venous sampling for localization are still under debate. Such widely ranging considerations as clinical circumstances, logistical availability, cost, and time factors all play a role.

Adrenal MRI is effective for the localization of adrenal aldosteronomas through the demonstration of a well-marginated, focal enlargement of the adrenal gland. The average size of aldosteronomas is approximately 1.5 cm, which is well within the spatial resolution of modern MRI scanners. About 15%–20% of the aldosteronomas are micronodules (≤1 cm) which may be missed when isointense to and buried deep within the gland parenchyma (GROTH et al. 1985). However, most small adenomas between 0.5 and 10 mm can be detected when a meticulous examination technique is applied.

In addition to the propensity for the smallest aldosteronomas to escape detection by MRI, the major limitation of MRI is that it provides anatomic but not histologic and functional information. MRI cannot differentiate between aldosteronoma, macronodules in nodular hyperplasia, and nonhyperfunctioning adenomas, especially when the lesion is solitary and isointense to the adjacent gland. Statistically, however, when a solitary adrenal mass in a normal sized gland is visualized by MRI and has the appropriate clinical and biochemical setting, it is extremely unlikely that it will be anything other than an aldosteronoma. In cases of multinodular hyperplasia the multiplicity of the nodules can usually be visualized with a more meticulous examination technique. In addition, in the event of equivocal MRI findings, postural plasma aldosterone and 18-OH-corticosterone tests provide an indication as to whether the patient has idiopathic hyperplasia or adrenal adenoma (DUNNICK et al. 1982). The accuracy of these tests in differentiating an aldosteronoma from adrenal hyperplasia is approximately 90%.

11.5.2
Cushing's Syndrome

The diagnosis of Cushing's syndrome is predominantly clinical and biochemical (GROSS et al. 1992; NELSON 1980). Clinical symptoms result from continued exposure to elevated plasma cortisol levels and include Cushing habitus, hirsutism, hypertension, diabetes mellitus, and osteoporosis. The diagnosis is confirmed by elevated serum cortisol levels throughout the day and sustained cortisol values following low-dose dexamethasone suppression. The syndrome may be produced by adrenal cortical hyperplasia in response to increased ACTH plasma levels or primary adrenal lesions, either adenoma, carcinoma, pigmented adrenocortical dysplasia, or marcronodular hyperplasia. ACTH-dependent Cushing's syndrome is usually pituitary driven and in a minority of cases is caused by paraendocrine production from cancer ("ectopic hormone syndrome"). Paraendocrine production of ACTH may result from various tumors, including oat cell carcinoma of the lung, pancreatic islet cell tumor, carcinoid, medullary carcinoma of the thyroid, pheochromocytoma, and thymoma (HOWLETT et al. 1986). Differentiation between the various causes of Cushing's syndrome is important because it determines whether the patient can be cured by surgery and also determines the surgical approach. Autonomous cortisol-producing tumors of the adrenal glands are generally treated with adrenalectomy whereas pituitary-driven Cushing's syndrome is treated with transsphenoidal resection of the pituitary adenoma. Treatment of ectopic ACTH-dependent Cushing's syndrome depends on the location and histology of the primary tumor.

Biochemical studies, including determination of plasma ACTH levels and response to high-dose dexamethasone, can be used to separate pituitary-driven Cushing's syndrome and ectopic ACTH-producing tumors from cortisol-producing adrenal neoplasias. Difficulties in the biochemical confirmation of hypercortisolism and differentiation between the forms of Cushing's syndrome may be encountered. In some patients with Cushing's syndrome the symptoms are suppressed after 1 mg of dexamethasone, for instance in situations where clearance of dexamethasone is delayed, during periodic hormonogenesis, when the creatinine clearance is poor, and where technical errors occur. Patients without Cushing's syndrome may have elevated levels of urinary free cortisol and failure to suppress plasma cortisol levels normally on 1 mg of dexamethasone due to mental depression, alcoholism, and stress-related events. An incidental non-hyperfunctioning adrenal tumor in such patients may be erroneously diagnosed as a hyperfunctioning adenoma or carcinoma. However, the greatest difficulty encountered in establishing a diagnosis based on biochemical analysis is the differentiation of pituitary Cushing's disease from paraendocrine ACTH secretion by tumors elsewhere (HOWLETT et al. 1986).

Inferior petrosal catheterization has been advocated as the initial study for the differentiation between pituitary and ectopic ACTH production in all patients, through the demonstration of a clear gradient (MILLER et al. 1990). However, venous sampling is not universally accepted as the initial technique to prove or disprove the presence of a pituitary microadenoma. Also controversy exists with regard to the accuracy of this technique for determination of the exact location of the adenoma once the pituitary gland has been established as the primary source of abnormal ACTH production.

11.5.2.1
Primary Adrenal Disorders

The main role of MRI of the adrenal gland in Cushing's syndrome is the localization or exclusion of a (unilateral) adrenal mass. The majority of cortisol-producing adrenal masses are larger than 2 cm in diameter and, therefore, well within the range of the spatial resolution of sectional imaging techniques (Figs. 11.2, 11.3). The absence of a mass on an imaging technique almost automatically indicates ACTH-dependent Cushing's syndrome. How-

ever, the presence of a mass may indicate a number of possibilities other than a cortisol-producing tumor. Differential diagnosis may include an incidental silent adrenal mass, an ACTH-producing pheochromocytoma, and a metastasis from an ACTH-producing occult lung carcinoma. Also in about 20%–23% of cases of pituitary-driven Cushing's syndrome, bilateral nodular hyperplasia is present, which denotes the presence of one or more prominent nodules visible to the naked eye on gross morphology. The incidence of such findings productive of Cushing's disease may vary between coun-

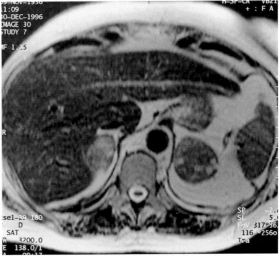

a

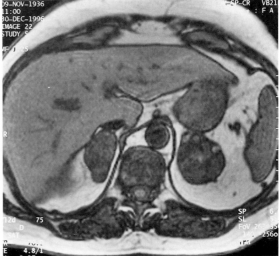

b

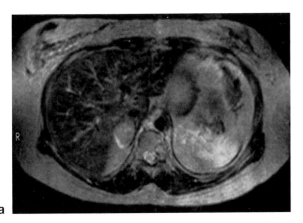

a

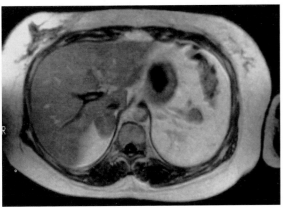

b

Fig. 11.2 a,b. Patient with a lipid-depleted right adrenal adenoma productive of Cushing's disease. **a** On T2-weighted sequences using SE there is an increased intensity relative to the liver. **b** The lesion enhances after intravenous injection of Gd-DTPA. (From GROSS et al. 1992)

Fig. 11.3 a,b. Patient with bilateral adrenal adenomas productive of Cushing's disease. **a** MRI demonstrates a bilateral mass of isointense signal relative to the spleen and an increased intensity relative to the liver on T2-weighted TSE. **b** On a FLASH 2D sequence with opposed phase there is a decrease in signal relative to the spleen, indicating the presence of fat

tries. Macronodular hyperplasia presents a possible pitfall because it may simulate a focal adenoma on an imaging technique if diffuse enlargement of the remaining gland is absent. In a small number of cases these patients may demonstrate impaired dexamethasone suppressibility in the presence of normal ACTH levels, making a clear-cut diagnosis of pituitary-dependent Cushing's syndrome difficult.

The occurrence of the cases described above, although exceptional, emphasizes the need to correlate imaging findings with biochemical evaluation.

On MRI adenomas have a low signal intensity relative to the liver on T2-weighted SE and fast low-angle shot (FLASH) images with opposed phase (Fig. 11.3). More commonly in Cushing's disease adenomas are lipid depleted and demonstrate isointensity or increased intensity relative to the liver on T2-weighted SE or opposed-phase GRE imgages (Fig. 11.2).

11.5.2.2
ACTH-Dependent Cushing's Syndrome

In the case of ACTH-dependent Cushing's syndrome, adrenal imaging can be helpful in excluding an adrenal tumor and in demonstrating adrenal hyperplasia. Gross enlargement without nodules is suggestive of paraendocrine ACTH production, whereas macronodular hyperplasia is more often found in long-standing pituitary-driven Cushing's syndrome. In addition, an imaging technique may demonstrate a pituitary adenoma or an occult ACTH-secreting tumor in the thorax or abdomen (DOPPMANN et al. 1989). Neuroendocrine tumors productive of ACTH are visualized on T2-weighted MRI by their high signal intensity. In the case of an occult tumor, identification of ACTH production can be obtained through immunostaining for ACTH or measurement of ACTH levels in an aspirated specimen (DOPPMANN et al. 1987), although false-negative results are quite common.

11.5.3
Androgen-Producing Disorders

Clinical symptoms in virilizing states are related to the age at onset of the disease, genetic sex, and severity of the hormonal disturbance (GROSS et al. 1992; NELSON 1980). In children, the clinical picture may include (intrauterine) virilization in females and pseudo pubertas praecox in males. Etiologies

include congenital adrenocortical hyperplasia, adrenal adenoma, adrenocortical carcinoma, and extra-adrenal pathologies such as idiopathic polycystic ovary syndrome and gonadal tumors. Congenital adrenocortical hyperplasia is the most common cause of virilizing states in childhood. This condition is usually the result of an inborn enzyme deficiency causing a partial block in adrenocortical steroid synthesis. When cortisol synthesis is affected, the pituitary gland correspondingly increases its release of ACTH in an attempt to normalize cortisol plasma levels. This compensatory mechanism leads to an increased release of steroids proximal to the impeded biochemical step.

The source of increased production of androgens in adults may also be adrenal, gonadal, or both. Nonclassic, adult onset or acquired 21-hydroxylase deficiency occurs far more commonly than the classic congenital hyperplasias. Androgen-secreting tumors of the adrenals and gonads are rare.

Traditional biochemical studies that employ hormonal suppression and stimulation tests are of limited value in tumor localization and helpful only in patients with steroidogenic enzyme deficiencies (TAYLOR et al. 1986). Many reports support a combined adrenal–ovarian source for the increased serum levels of androgens, with the ovary as major contributor in most instances. As a result of the flaws in the biochemical analysis of patients with hirsutism, in a number of patients imaging of both the adrenal and the gonadal area is necessary for the localization of the source of androgen excess.

Adrenal adenomas and carcinomas productive of androgens or precursor excess are usually larger than 2 cm and easily depicted by sectional imaging techniques. The morphologic appearances are similar to those of lipid-depleted adenomas and carcinomas described in other sections of this chapter.

Chronic adrenal cortical stimulation by excessive ACTH in congenital adrenal hyperplasia results in zona fasciculata-reticularis hyperplasia and gross enlargement of the adrenals which is easily depicted on MRI. Long-term overstimulation by ACTH may lead to transformation of adrenocortical hyperplasia into a macronodule or adenoma and possibly an adrenocortical carcinoma. These changes are unlikely to occur in childhood, but rather in older patients who, for a variety of reasons, have never received treatment. It is important not to confuse this entity with a primary virilizing adrenal tumor which requires surgical treatment. A specific diagnosis based on MRI is not possible without knowledge of the clinical and biochemical setting (FALKE et al. 1986b).

In childhood, the differentiation between primary adrenal tumor and hyperplasia does not provide a problem. US and MRI might be preferable in this group of patients because of the absence of ionizing radiation.

The possibility that MRI provides to screen adrenal glands and gonads with optimal plane selection and outstanding contrast is an advantage over CT and particularly suitable to differentiate an adrenal tumor from polycystic ovary syndrome (PCO) (MITCHELL 1992). This is especially true in patients with insufficient suppression on dexamethasone and normal androgen and LH levels. On MRI, the ovaries in PCO are enlarged (>4 cm) and demonstrate a characteristic peripheral zone of small cysts on the T2-weighted images. However, recent studies have demonstrated that some women presenting with characteristic clinical features of PCO have normal sized ovaries, depending on the clinical definition of PCO.

11.6
Adrenomedullary Disorders Associated with Overactivity

11.6.1
Functioning Paragangliomas

Functioning paragangliomas are catecholamine-secreting tumors originating from the autonomic nervous system. They may be situated anywhere from the neck to the bladder and, although rare in the general population (estimated incidence: 0.001%–0.002%), carry a considerable risk to those affected (SCHWARTZ et al. 1995). Given adequate localization, surgical cure is possible in the majority of cases. Because noninvasive localizing techniques are so accurate, considerable latitude in the surgical approach to a pheochromocytoma is allowable (TELENIUS-BERG et al. 1987; WILMS et al. 1979).

Paraganglion cells are derived from the neural crest and migrate in close association with the autonomic ganglion cells. The common feature of these cells is the presence of neurosecretory granules containing catecholamines and chromogranins in their cytoplasm. The tumors to which they give rise may be either catecholamine secreting or nonfunctional.

The original concept of a class of tumors known as paragangliomas has been extensively described. The WHO classification comprises the following categories (VAN GILS et al. 1990):

1. Pheochromocytomas, i.e., tumors arising from the adrenal medulla
2. Sympathetic paragangliomas arising from neuroendocrine cells associated with the sympathetic chain
3. Parasympathetic paragangliomas which are generally nonchromaffin and include the brachiomeric, vagal, and visceral autonomic paragangliomas
4. Paragangliomas not further specified

Pheochromocytomas are hormonally active in more than 90% of cases, whereas sympathetic paragangliomas are active in about 50% and parasympathetic paragangliomas in about 1%. In sporadic cases paragangliomas may secrete parathyroid hormone, calcitonin, gastrin, serotonin, and ACTH together with or instead of catecholamines. ACTH production may result in Cushing's syndrome and adrenal hyperplasia (GROSS et al. 1992; NELSON 1980).

There is an increased incidence of pheochromocytomas in patients with neuroectodermal disorders such as neurofibromatosis, tuberous sclerosis, Carney syndrome (ROY et al. 1994), and von Hippel-Lindau disease. From 5% to 10% of patients have family history of paraganglioma. These familial tumors show an increased tendency for multiplicity. Multiplicity, including bilateral pheochromocytomas, occurs in approximately 10% (FALKE et al. 1990; OUDKERK and FALKE 1981). Among children the prevalence of bilateral and multiple tumors is higher. Patients with sporadic or familial paragangliomas may have other associated tumors, e.g., multiple endocrine neoplasia (MEN) syndromes II and III, islet cell tumors, pituitary tumors, carcinoid, aldosteronomas, renal cell carcinomas, and the above-mentioned neuroectodermal tumors (FALKE et al. 1990). In contrast to sporadic pheochromocytoma, the pheochromocytomas in MEN II are asymptomatic in about half the patients and are only diagnosed because a raised suspicion exists (TELENIUS-BERG et al. 1987). An early diagnosis of adrenal medullary involvement in MEN syndromes may be suggested by abnormalities of epinephrine or its metabolites in plasma or urine. Diagnosis and localization of these clinically silent tumors is of the utmost importance, because these patients may develop fatal paroxysms during surgery for associated tumors or stenosis of the renal artery.

About 10% of functioning paragangliomas are malignant. Malignancy cannot be determined by microscopic appearance or local invasiveness but is defined by the presence of metastases located outside the region where normally paragangliomas are known to occur. However, malignancy probably occurs more often in tumors larger than 6 cm in diameter, in cases of local invasion, in extra-adrenal paragangliomas, and in dopamine-producing paragangliomas (Cuesta et al. 1996; van Gils et al. 1990).

A long-recognized feature of pheochromocytomas is the production of epinephrine, norepinephrine, and sometimes dopamine. However, the other types of paragangliomas can on occasion secrete the same substances, with the exception of epinephrine, as discussed previously. Co-production of chromogranin is usually present and be used to predict tumor size. Classically the secretion of pressor amines by the tumor produces paroxysmal hypertension associated with vasomotor crises, headache, pallor, and perspiration. The paroxysms may be spontaneous or can be elicited by exercise, bending over, pressure on the abdomen, induction of anesthesia, palpation of the tumor, intravenous injection of various drugs, and urination in the case of bladder localizations.

Clinical and surgical series tend to emphasize the correlation between the paroxysmal symptoms and the discovery of the tumor. Autopsy series, however, stress the relative frequency with which paragangliomas may remain undetected, despite the occurrence of hypertension in such cases (St John Sutton et al. 1981). Clinically silent tumors are not infrequent, so many potentially curable cases are not diagnosed during life. It can be expected that with the combined use of biochemical methods and MRI more clinically silent paragangliomas will be detected (Telenius-Berg et al. 1987).

Morphologic findings of pheochromocytoma on MRI include large variation in size, consistency, and margination of the tumors and significant enhancement in most cases after i.v. injection of contrast material (Table 11.2). On MRI the tumors have a low intensity on T1-weighted images and a very high intensity on T2-weighted SE and GRE images (Fig. 11.4) (Falke et al. 1986a; van Gils et al. 1990, 1991). In cases of extensive hemorrhage the intensity on T1-weighted images increases, and tumor intensity may exceed the intensity of the liver. Extra-adrenal paragangliomas have morphologic findings similar to pheochromocytomas, with the exception of many chemodectomas that demonstrate a decreased signal intensity due to increased stroma and the presence of flow void in multiple medium-sized vessels (Fig. 11.5) (van Gils et al. 1994).

Early changes of the adrenal medulla in MEN II or III syndrome may escape detection by MRI when the adrenergic shape and normal size are retained. Subtle changes in such cases could not be depicted on the basis of a change in signal intensity in normal or slightly enlarged glands.

It has been demonstrated that CT, MRI, and iodine-131 metaiodobenzylguanidine (^{131}I-MIBG) scintigraphy are comparable in their ability to localize pheochromocytomas. We found that this also applies for ^{123}I-MIBG scintigraphy (van Gils et al. 1991). The overall sensitivity of CT for the detection of functioning paragangliomas exceeds 90%. CT is limited in the localization of extra-adrenal sources of functioning paragangliomas, mainly because it is impractical to perform whole-body CT in each individual patient. It has been demonstrated that when CT is performed after localization of an extra-adrenal paraganglioma with other means, accuracy approximates 100%. The overall results of MRI are reported to be well above 95% because, as in MIBG scintigraphy, whole-body imaging can be performed

Table 11.2. Morphologic findings of adrenal tumors on MRI

A. Pheochromocytoma
Large variation in size, consistency, and margin
Can be cystic
Very high signal intensity on T2-weighted MRI
Usually significant enhancement

B. Non-hyperfunctioning adenoma
Small (<3 cm in diameter)
Smoothly marginated
Homogeneous
No perceptible wall
Isointense to the liver on T2-weighted MRI
Decreased signal on chemical shift images
No or almost no enhancement
Often multiple, uni- or bilateral (~50%)
No size increase during follow-up (>1 year)

C. Adrenocortical carcinomas
Usually larger than 6 cm in diameter
Irregular margin
Inhomogeneous
Intermediate increase in intensity on T2-weighted MRI
Substantial enhancement
Unilateral
Local invasion
Ancillary findings

D. metastases
Large variation in size
Inhomogeneous
Irregular margins
(Intermediate) increase in intensity on T2-weighted MRI
Substantial enhancement
Often bilateral
Ancillary findings

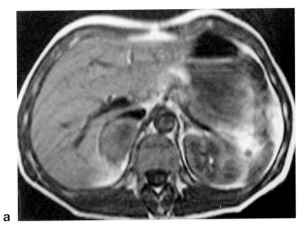

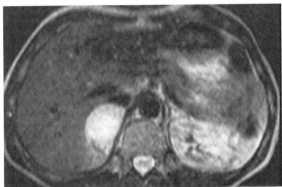

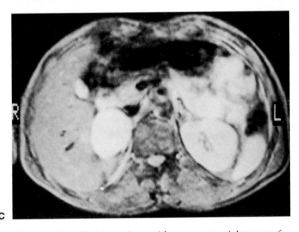

Fig. 11.4. Psychiatric patient with recurrent nightmares for 2 years demonstrates right pheochromocytoma on T1- (**a**) and T2-weighted (**b**) MRI. **c** GRE imaging of another patient shows a right adrenal pheochromocytoma of homogeneously increased signal intensity. (**c** from GROSS et al. 1992)

(VAN GILS et al. 1991). The overall sensitivity of ^{131}I-MIBG scintigraphy for localization of pheochromocytomas varies between 77% and 96% when imaging is performed in the appropriate clinical setting. The sensitivity of ^{131}I-MIBG scintigraphy for the detection of extra-adrenal paragangliomas can be as low as 67%. Comparison between ^{131}I-MIBG

and recently also ^{123}I-MIBG scintigraphy and MRI have demonstrated that MRI is at least equally effective in localizing functioning paragangliomas (VAN GILS et al. 1990, 1991).

11.6.2
Neuroblastoma and Ganglioneuroblastoma

Neuroblastoma is a sarcoma of the autonomic nervous system which occurs in children less than 5 years old (85%). Prognosis depends on the age of onset of the disease, but is usually poor after the neonatal period. Cytodifferentiation to a more benign ganglioneuroma may occur. All intermediate levels of differentiation between the neuroblastoma and ganglioneuroma are referred to as ganglioneuroblastoma (JAFFE 1976).

The tumors arise from primordial neural crest cells, and are found in a variety of locations. The adrenal medulla or adjacent retroperitoneum account for 50%–80% of the tumors. Clinical symptoms vary and are related to the rapid growth of the neoplasm and its secretory products (norepinephrine, dopa, or dopamine) which results in increased urinary levels of their metabolites (vanillylmandelic acid and 3-methoxyl-4-hydroxyphenolglycol).

Sectional imaging techniques have proven to be indispensable tools for diagnosing and following these tumors, and for demonstrating primary and metastatic disease as an aid in predicting tumor resectability. Particularly the dumbbell extension into, or primary location in, the epidural space of the spinal canal and the relation to major vessels are important preoperative and prognostic findings.

Of particular interest is the group of children with neuroblastoma with a good prognosis, namely children with neuroblastoma found incidentally during examination for another complaint. In children in whom the slightest possibility of a neuroblastoma is considered, a specific image modality without radiation hazard may be of use to exclude or detect neuroblastomas at an early stage and consequently improve prognosis.

Magnetic resonance imaging has many advantages in the assessment of neuroblastoma, similar to the advantages described in the previous section in respect of functioning paragangliomas (BERDON et al. 1992). Previous results have shown that MRI cannot differentiate functioning parangliomas from other sympathomedullary tumors, such as ganglioneuroblastomas and neuroblastomas, by signal intensity alone. The excellent contrast between

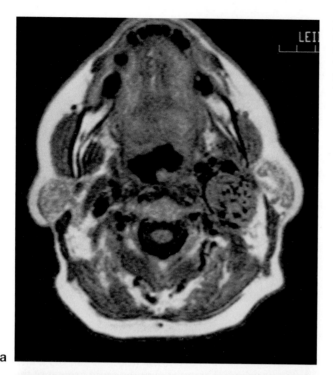

a

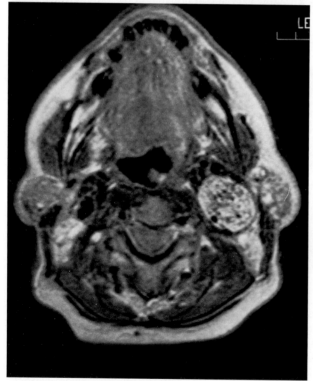

b

Fig. 11.5. Patient with a chemodectoma of the left carotid body. MRI demonstrates intermediate signal on T1-weighted images and increased signal on T2-weighted SE images. Note the "salt and pepper" appearance on the T1-weighted images due to abundant vessels. (From VAN GILS et al. 1990)

the high intensity of neuroblastoma locations and surrounding structures, including vessels, in combination with the multiplanar capability of MRI, greatly facilitate accurate detection and deter-

mination of the local extent of disease. In addition, dumbbell extension into the epidural space and compression of the spinal cord can be clearly identified with MRI, unlike with CT, and this has rendered myelograms obsolete. The facility of multiplanar imaging with MRI and the outstanding image contrast are advantages over CT and US with regard to screening of the whole body for the presence of multiple sites of involvement, including bone marrow metastases of the axial skeleton (NAJEAU et al. 1992; ALGRA et al. 1991).

The absence of a radiation hazard with MRI is of particular interest in pediatric patients and MRI should be applied as an initial screening technique before whole-body CT or isotope-tagged MIBG scintigraphy, which have unfavorable dosimetric properties.

11.7
Disorders Associated with a Normal Hormonal Activity

Establishing the nature of incidentally discovered adrenal masses has been a major concern in the imaging literature for more than a decade. Interest arises from the fact that the adrenal glands are frequently involved by metastatic disease (ABRAMS et al. 1950). Benign adrenal masses are also common and are usually detected as an incidental finding on an imaging procedure performed for an unrelated diagnostic problem. The number of such masses has increased substantially because of serendipitous detection of much smaller lesions by the new generation CT systems.

Silent adrenal masses are problematic because, once they have been discovered, their nature must be defined in order to exclude a metastatic lesion and, to a lesser degree, a pheochromocytoma or a primary adrenal carcinoma. Differentiation of silent adrenal masses in the imaging literature is focused on the positive identification of benign adrenocortical adenomas, which represent the most frequent incidental finding in the adrenal gland above the age of 50.

Adrenal masses are characterized by various morphologic criteria (Table 11.2). The size of an adrenal mass has been suggested as a cost-effective prognostic criterion to distinguish benign from malignant disease but fails as a single discriminator in individual patients if long-term follow-up studies are not performed (LEE et al. 1994). More recent criteria used with CT and MRI to distinguish adenomas from other masses include density or intensity indexes of adrenal masses on FLASH chemical shift MR images (MITCHELL et al. 1992; REINIG 1992; FALKE and SANDLER 1994; BILBEY et al. 1995; TSUSHIMA et al.

1993; OUTWATER and MITCHELL 1994; SCHWARTZ et al. 1995; MAYO-SMITH et al. 1995; LEE et al. 1991, 1994; VAN ERKEL et al. 1994; LEROY-WILLIG et al. 1987).

11.7.1
Adrenal Adenomas and Metastases

Discriminating parameters on CT and MRI for adrenal adenomas exploit the functional ability of the adrenal cortex to accumulate cholesterol esters (FALKE and SANDLER 1994; KOROBKIN et al. 1996a). In the normal adrenal cortex cholesterol is esterified and forms a pool of cholesterol ester substrate from which adrenal steroid hormones are synthesized in acute situations through ACTH-mediated de-esterification. Adrenal adenomas are thought to represent nontumorous overgrowth of adrenocortical cells usually from the zona fasciculata. They consist of cholesterol ester-laden clear cells, usually from the zona fasciculata, and are often seen at autopsy when the adjacent nonnodular cortex has become lipid-depleted as a result of the stress of dying. The lipid droplets, which no longer form a "stand-by" pool of cholesterol, probably consist of cholesterol esters in a quasi-crystalline phase, similar to cholesterol in atherosclerotic plaques.

Because of the high fat content, adrenal adenomas have a characteristic low density on CT and are easily identifiable on the basis of this criterion alone. On MRI, the short T2 relaxation time of the quasi-crystalline phase of cholesterol esters makes these lipids generally invisible on T2-weighted SE sequences with long echo times. As a result, adenomas are isointense to liver on T2-weighted SE images and demonstrate a high fat content on chemical shift imaging with a short echo time (Fig. 11.6), in contrast to metastases (Fig. 11.7). When an adenoma has low attenuation on CT, it will have a low intensity on T2-weighted SE and opposed-phase GRE sequences (OUTWATER et al. 1996), provided that the fat has not changes its liquid crystal phase from a semicrystalline to a liquid phase (FALKE and SANDLER 1994). Chemical shift MRI can demonstrate lipid within adrenocortical masses and thereby circumvents the theoretical problem of overlap in attenuation between adenomas with minimal fat and edematous or necrotic tumors on CT. However, in a practical sense, MRI does not add greatly to the CT findings in this category of adrenal masses. An exception may be the rare occurrence of collision tumors. It has been proposed that MRI can demonstrate and permit

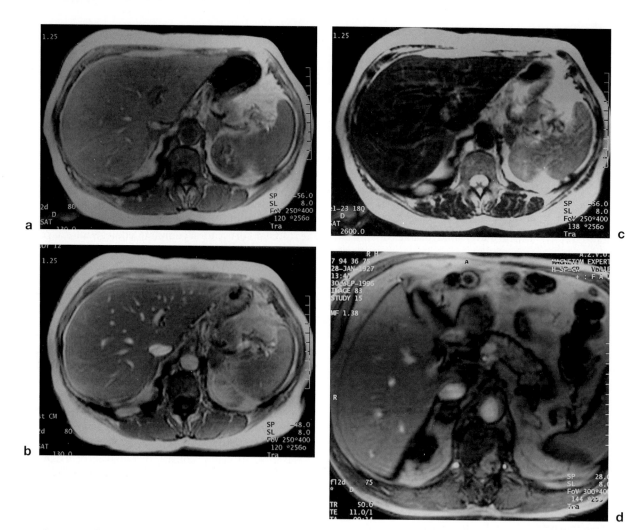

Fig. 11.6 a–d. Elderly patient with bilateral non-hyperfunctioning adenomas. T1-weighted FLASH 2D imaging (**a**) before and (**b**) after intravenous injection of Gd-DTPA demonstrates a nonenhancing lesion on the left side. **c** On the breath-hold TSE images there are bilateral small lesions of low signal intensity relative to the liver. **d** On breath-hold FLASH 2D images with opposed phase there is a significant decrease in signal intensity of the lesion on the right side, relative to the liver

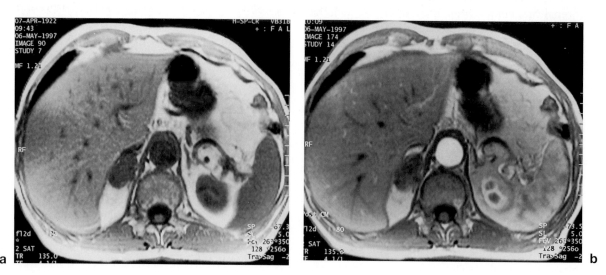

Fig. 11.7 a–h

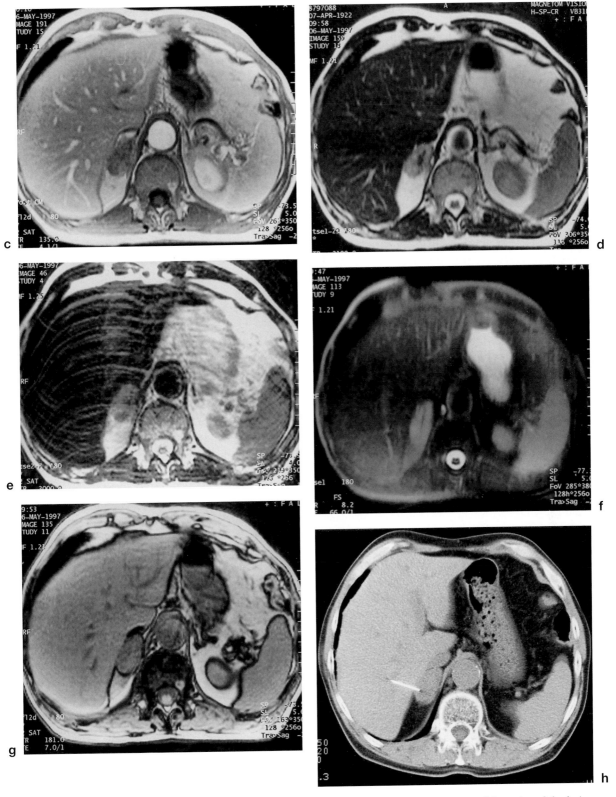

Fig. 11.7 a–h. Patient with lung cancer, who was a possible candidate for curative surgery, with a possible right adrenal metastasis on CT. **a** the mass has a decreased intensity on T1-weighted breath-hold GE images. There is no early enhancement of the lesion immediately following i.v. contrast material injection (**b**) but there is on late GE images (**c**). **d, e** Breath-hold and non-breath-hold T2-weighted images; breath-hold images demonstrate the difference in artifact reduction from respiratory motion and an increased intensity of the lesion relative to the liver. **f** Increased signal intensity relative to the liver is also seen on T2-weighted images with a HASTE sequence and spectral fat suppression. **g** On breath-hold opposed-phase GE imaging there is no loss in signal intensity, excluding the presence of lipid-rich cells. **h** CT-guided fine-needle biopsy proved the presence of metastatic disease

characterization of the separate components of collision tumors within the adrenal gland. Such findings can be crucial in planning and guiding subsequent percutaneous needle biopsy and patient care (SCHWARTZ et al. 1996).

Similar to the tissue of the fasciculata zone of the normal adrenal cortex, adrenal adenomas are poorly vascularized and demonstrate only mild enhancement and quick washout of intravenously injected contrast medium on dynamic CT or MRI studies (Fig. 11.6), in contrast to metastases (Fig. 11.7). This parameter has been used to improve classification of adrenal masses on contrast-enhanced CT and fast, dynamic contrast-enhanced MRI. Theoretically, enhancement parameters on dynamic studies can be expected to correlate with the attenuation and intensity measurements on CT and MRI, but this has not yet been examined in the literature.

Adenomas contain lipid-depleted cells from the zona reticularis that may predominate in 10%–30% of lesions. Such lesions have near isodensity to liver on CT and are hyperintense when compared with liver on T2-weighted MRI (Fig. 11.2). Under such circumstances CT and MRI attenuation intensity and enhancement parameters are likely to be indeterminate. It is this category that ends up in the cohort of silent adrenal masses that need further clarification by MRI or biopsy, if other morphologic parameters are inconclusive.

Benign, nonhypersecretroy, nonautonomous adrenal adenomas are but one manifestation of a whole spectrum of morphologic changes in the nodular adrenal cortex. The morphologic spectrum of adrenal nodules includes macronodules ("incidentaloma"), micronodules, and segmental hyperplasias in an otherwise normal adrenal gland. If the anatomic resolution of the images is sufficiently high, more of the morphologic spectrum can be visualized simultaneously in the same patient, permitting a specific diagnosis when considered in conjunction with the other discriminating parameters. The value of assessing the full spectrum of morphologic changes in nodular adrenals to clarify silent adrenal masses (instead of concentrating on the incidentaloma) has not been accorded much attention in the literature.

The role of MRI in respect of clinically silent adrenal masses detected with CT is presently under debate. Such widely ranging considerations as clinical circumstances, logistic availability, and cost and time factors all play their role in the evaluation. In practice, the majority of adenomas can be classified with a very high specificity on the basis of CT criteria. In these patients, it is not cost-effective to verity the

diagnosis with additional studies. MRI is useful in the remaining group of silent adrenal lesions because it can detect smaller quantities of fat (Fig. 11.3).

In our opinion, fine-needle aspiration biopsy of silent adrenal lesions that cannot be classified as adenomas on CT or MRI is, in general, essential and remains the most practical thing to do if a definite diagnosis (of metastatic disease) is crucial to patient managment (SILVERMAN et al. 1993).

11.7.2
Miscellaneous Lesions

11.7.2.1
Adrenocortical Carcinomas

Presenting signs and symptoms of malignant adrenocortical tumors depend on the nature of steroid overproduction, the size of the tumor, and the presence of metastases as well as the sex and age of the patient. Among the "functioning" carcinomas the following syndromes can be recognized: Cushing's syndrome (36%), Cushing's syndrome with virilization (20%), virilization (24%), feminization (6%), and mineralocorticoid excess (less than 1%; rarely without overproduction of other steroids) (OUTWATER et al. 1996; LUTON et al. 1990). The remaining tumors are clinically silent and are often referred to as "nonfunctioning carcinomas" (13%). Generally, corticosteroid production is low in malignant cortical tissue and for this reason tumors are usually quite large by the time they are diagnosed. When biosynthetic potency is even lower, as in non-hyperfunctioning carcinomas, patients present with abdominal pain, palpable mass, metastases, malaise, weight loss, and fever but without endocrine manifestations.

The most important biochemical criteria for the diagnosis of adrenocortical carcinoma are (relatively) increased production of precursor steroids using an extensive steroid profile and resistance to high-dose dexamethasone suppression. By these standards, true nonfunctioning carcinomas are extremely rare.

The role of imaging techniques lies in the determination of the adrenal origin of the tumor and the evaluation of the tumor extent in relation to surrounding structures. In addition, distant metastases in the liver, lung, and bone have to be localized. A small percentage of primary carcinomas of the adrenal cortex may be complicated by extension into the inferior vena cava, usually through invasion of the

Adrenal Glands

adrenal vein (Fig. 11.8) (FALKE et al. 1988). The presence of these findings still warrants surgical resection, since complete removal of the thrombus is often feasible. In the event of wall invasion and extension into surrounding tissues, debulking prior to chemotherapy might also be considered. Accurate demonstration of the presence and extension of tumor thrombus in the inferior vena cava prior to surgery is a prerequisite for successful surgical planning.

In patients with a small asymptomatic adrenal tumor incidentally discovered on an imaging modality there is always the issue of how to differentiate a silent adenoma from a small adrenocortical carcinoma. The incidence of occult adrenocortical carcinoma in such situations is estimated to be extremely low and can hardly be considered a realistic clinical problem.

The majority of the carcinomas are large enough (>6 cm in diameter) to be visualized by conventional radiographic methods such as plain abdominal films or intravenous urography, CT, or MRI (Figs. 11.8, 11.9). Although CT is usually applied, MRI is more appropriate for the staging and detection of recurrences (Fig. 11.8). Imaging modalities such as MRI

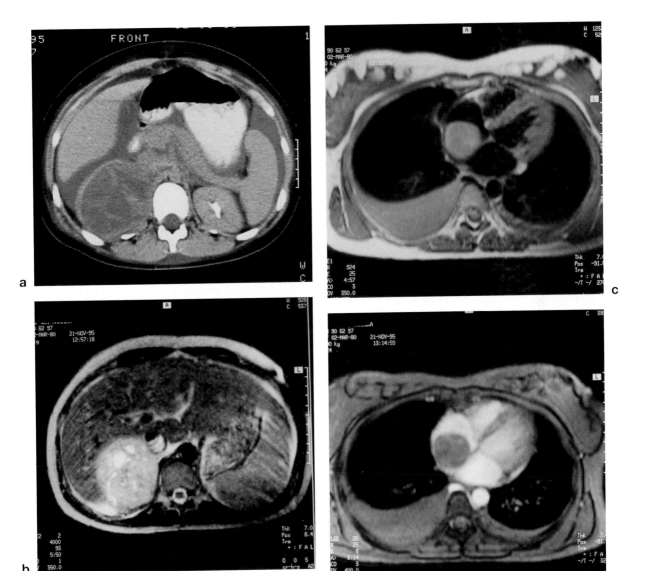

Fig. 11.8 a–d. Patient with a right adrenocortical carcinoma. **a** On CT there is a large inhomogeneous tumor enhancing after i.v. injection of contrast material. **b** MRI demonstrates increased intensity on T2-weighted images. There is extension in the vena cava. **c** Cardiac gated T1-weighted SE imaging and **d** breath-hold turbo FLASH imaging with fat saturation demonstrate extension of the tumor thrombus into the right atrium

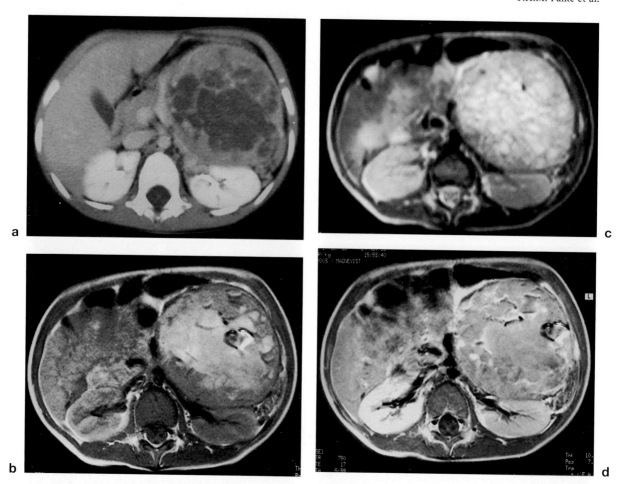

Fig. 11.9 a–d. Left adrenocortical carcinoma in a child. **a** CT after i.v. contrast material enhancement shows an adrenal tumor. **b** The mass has a low intensity on T1-weighted images and **c** an increased intensity on T2-weighted images. **d** T1-weighted MRI after intravenous injection of 0.1 mmol/kg body weight

also play a major role in monitoring tumor response during chemotherapy and the detection of complications associated with op'DDD treatment, such as the development of cysts or cystic tumors of the ovaries (LUTON et al. 1990).

11.7.2.2
Adrenal Myelolipomas

Adrenal myelolipomas are benign tumors comprising fat and bone marrow elements (NOBLE et al. 1982). A myelolipoma containing macroscopic quantities of nonfatty material (such as blood, calcium, or myeloid tissue) may have a nonspecific appearance if fat is not predominantly detectable in the lesion.

Clinical symptoms are usually consequent to large tumors, giving rise to abdominal pain. There are numerous reports of endocrine abnormalities associated with myelolipoma and these include morbid obesity, hermaphroditism, pseudohermaphroditism, pluriglandular insufficiency, Addison's disease, splanchnomegaly without acromegaly, intersex syndrome, Nelson's syndrome, Cushing's disease, and Conn's syndrome. Adrenal myelolipomas may occur in conjunction with adrenal adenoma (WHALEY et al. 1985). In cases of myelolipoma a confident diagnosis can be made on MRI based on the high signal intensity on T1-weighted images, in contradistinction to the appearance of adenomas (FALKE et al. 1987). Signal intensity can be reduced with fat suppression techniques.

11.7.2.3
Cysts

Cysts may be of any size and in most instances are unilateral. Large cysts may be complicated by hemorrhage and consequent onset of acute symptoms.

Pathologic substrates include epithelial, endothelial, and parasitic cysts, and also pseudocysts. Endothelial cyst is the most common type, representing 45% of reported adrenal cysts. The pseudocyst results from degenerative necrosis of tumors or represents a sequela of hemorrhage and exceptionally pseudocyst from the pancreas (KREFT et al. 1990). Cystic masses productive of an endocrine syndrome have occasionally been reported. Functionality of a cyst can be proven by determination of hormone levels in aspirated cyst fluid if no contraindications to percutaneous puncture exist. On MRI cysts have a homogeneous appearance of low intensity on T1-weighted images before and after i.v. injection of contrast medium and an increased intensity on T2-weighted images (Fig. 11.10). Following hemorrhage, increased intensity can be expected on T1-weighted images.

11.7.2.4
Abscesses

Abscesses are observed as a rare complication of adrenal hemorrhage in neonates (ATKINSON et al. 1985) or adrenal cysts, in tuberculosis in immunosuppressed patients, and in generalized histoplasmosis. The clinical symptoms and findings on a sectional imaging modality usually suggest the correct diagnosis.

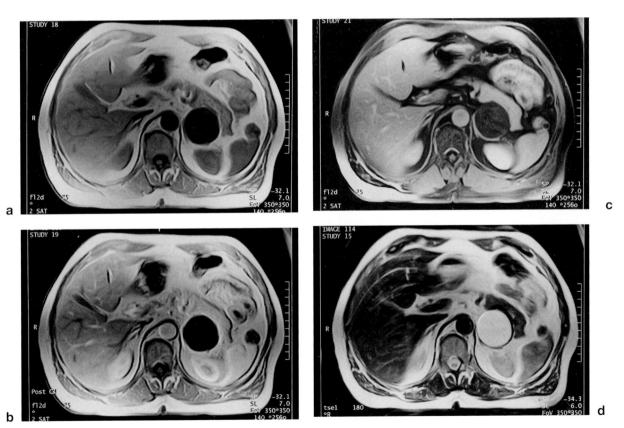

Fig. 11.10 a–d. Patient with a left adrenal cyst on MRI. **a** Before and **b** after i.v. injection of contrast material there is no enhancement of the lesion on T1-weighted FLASH 2D images. **c** Fat-suppressed FLAST 2D imaging confirms the absence of contrast enhancement. **d** On T2-weighted TSE there is a homogeneously increased signal relative to the liver

11.7.2.5
Lymphomatous Disease

Involvement of the adrenals in lymphomatous disease is quite common, with an incidence of 25% in a reported autopsy series of patients with known lymphoma (JAFRI et al. 1983). In less extensive disease, the normal shape of the adrenals may be preserved, in which case differentiation from hyperplasia may be difficult on a sectional imaging technique.

11.7.2.6
Hemangiomas

Hemangiomas are extremely rare lesions (BORASCHI et al. 1995). Cases demonstrate a rounded mass of soft tissue density with central calcifications. The findings on MRI are nonspecific and cannot be differentiated from adrenocortical carcinoma, neuroblastoma, tuberculosis, pheochromocytoma, or metastasis. Marked intravenous contrast material enhancement and detection of phleboliths are suggestive of the diagnosis.

Bilateral adrenal enlargement may occur in agnogenic myeloid metaplasia due to extramedullary hematopoiesis (KING et al. 1987). The adrenals may show focal enlargement due to hemorrhage. Extramedullary hematopoiesis resembles adrenal myelolipoma except for the absence of considerable amounts of fat.

11.7.2.7
Hemorrhage

Extensive adrenal hemorrhage may occur at any age and under various circumstances (LING et al. 1983; WILMS et al. 1987; KOCH and CORY 1986; WILLEMSE et al. 1989; ITOH et al. 1988; EKLOF et al. 1986; OUDKERK and FALKE 1981; WOLVERSON and KANNEGIESSER 1984; LUNDSTROM and CHEN 1985; ROWINSKY et al. 1986; SOLOMON and SUMKIN 1988; MIGEON et al. 1967; KORNBLUTH et al. 1990). It is usually associated with severe stress as in surgery,

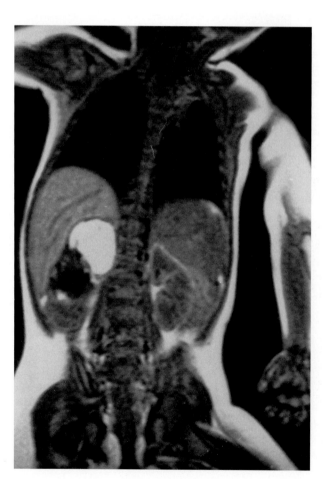

Fig. 11.11. Neonate with a right adrenal hemorrhage on T1-weighted MRI. (From GROSS et al. 1992)

sepsis, burns, hypotension, trauma (including complication from adrenal venography and liver transplantation), hemorrhagic diathesis, and underlying conditions such as tumor, cyst, and extramedullary hematopoiesis. Bilateral adrenal hemorrhage is seldom associated with acute adrenal insufficiency although others have found evidence of adrenal insufficiency in all patients with "massive" and bilateral adrenal hemorrhage.

Adrenal hematomas usually remain undiagnosed unless incidentally detected on an imaging modality. Hematomas of the adrenal, incidentally found on an imaging modality, have to be differentiated from malignant tumors. Although primary adrenal neoplasms, such as adrenocortical carcinomas, pheochromocytomas, myelolipomas, and cysts, have been reported to cause massive (sometimes subclinical) hemorrhage, this complication has only very rarely been associated with neoplasms metastatic to the adrenal gland (ROWINSKY et al. 1986).

Neonatal adrenal hemorrhage may be complicated by simultaneous renal vein thrombosis and perirenal hemorrhage (KOCH and CORY 1986). On MRI there is a mass lesion with increased intensity on T1-weighted sequences, depending on the age of the bleeding (Fig. 11.11). Additional T1-weighted sequences with spectral fat suppression may distinguish between high signal from fat and from hemorrhage. Concomitant neonatal hemorrhage and neuroblastoma is rare but has to be excluded in all neonatal extrarenal masses (OUDKERK and FALKE 1981). The determination of urinary catecholamine metabolites is of crucial significance and an essential part of the investigation. Contrast-enhanced MRI plays a role in the detection of adrenal hemorrhage and associated complications such as renal vein thrombosis, in the differentiation of adrenal masses from renal masses, and in the provision of confirmatory evidence for the presence of an underlying tumor in selected cases.

11.8
Disorders Associated with Decreased Hormonal Activity

11.8.1
Acute Hemorrhage

When a hypoadrenal crisis due to hemorrhage occurs it may be fulminant and fatal if not promptly recognized. An imaging technique may be used to confirm the presence of a bilateral hematoma whenever Addison's disease develops suddenly in a patient who was previously fit and well (WOLVERSON and KANNEGIESSER 1984). A diagnosis of acute adrenal hemorrhage should also be considered in patients treated with ACTH who develop unexplained acute abdominal flank pain. When an imaging modality demonstrates an ACTH-induced adrenal hemorrhage, ACTH medication has to be stopped and corticosteroid therapy maintained (KORNBLUTH et al. 1990). In the neonate, extensive adrenal hemorrhage may be seen following prolonged and difficult delivery associated with considerable trauma and hypoxia. The neonatal adrenal is predisposed to hemorrhage because of its size, vascular architecture, and frequent coexisting prothrombin deficiency (WILLEMSE et al. 1989). Adrenal hemorrhage may also occur as the result of overwhelming septicemia. Adrenal hemorrhage associated with bacteremic infections can lead to adrenal insufficiency whereas adrenal insufficiency rarely occurs in other causes of neonatal adrenal hemorrhage (MIGEON et al. 1967).

11.8.2
Chronic Primary Hypoadrenalism

Chronic primary hypoadrenalism is a rare condition and in Western countries is usually caused by so-called idiopathic atrophy (autoimmune adrenalitis) (WHEATLEY et al. 1985; VITA et al. 1985). Until the 1950s destruction of the adrenal cortex by tuberculosis was the most common cause. Miliary tuberculosis should still be suspected in elderly patients with a low-grade fever, weakness, anorexia, and weight loss. Other causes of chronic primary hypoadrenalism are metastatic cancer, Hodgkin's disease, sarcoidosis, amyloidosis, hemorrhage, hemochromatosis, acquired immunodeficiency syndrome, and fungal infection. In contrast to idiopathic atrophy and long-standing tuberculosis, most of these causes are associated with adrenal enlargement. Clinical manifestations only become apparent when more than 90% of functioning cells have been destroyed. The main role of imaging techniques in patients with chronic primary hypoadrenalism is to detect potentially treatable diseases (BAKER et al. 1988; HAUSER and GURRET 1986). Duration of adrenal disease, adrenal size, and the presence of calcifications are useful clues to the cause of the chronic hypoadrenalism. The presence of adrenal calcifications excludes idiopathic adrenal atrophy. Small glands generally indicate either idiopathic atrophy of long-standing tuberculosis, and enlarged glands are indicative of early tuberculosis or, exceptionally, other potentially treatable diseases described above. If clinical evidence of tuberculosis or metastatic disease is absent, the discovery of grossly enlarged glands on an imaging technique usually warrants further evaluation with percutaneous biopsy (HALVORSEN et al. 1982).

Exceptional causes of congenital adrenal insufficiency include Wolman's disease, adrenoleukodystrophy, XXXY or XXXX syndrome, and congenital lipoid adrenal hyperplasia (OGATA et al. 1988; KUMAR et al. 1987).

References

Abrams HL, Spiro R, Goldstein N (1950) Metastases in carcinoma: analysis of 1000 autopsied cases. Cancer 3:74–85

Algra P, Bloem J, Falke THM (1991) MRI and bone scintigraphy in the detection of vertebral metastases. Radiographics 11:219–235

Atkinson GO Jr, Kodroff MB, Gay BB Jr, Ricketts RR (1985) Adrenal abscess in the neonate. Radiology 155:101–104

Baker DE, Glazer GM, Francis IR (1988) Adrenal magnetic resonance imaging in Addison's disease. Urol Radiol 9:199–203

Baker EL, Gore RM, Moss AA (1982) Retroperitoneal pulmonary sequestration: computed tomographic findings. AJR 138:956–957

Berdon WE, Ruzal-Shapiro C, Abramson SJ, et al. (1992) Diagnosis of neuroblastoma: relative roles of ultrasonography, CT and MRI. Urol Radiol 14:252–259

Berliner L, Bosniak MA, Megibow A (1982) Adrenal pseudotumors on computed tomography. J Comput Assist Tomogr 6:281–285

Bilbey JH, McLoughlin RF, Kurkjian PS, Wilkins GEL, Chan NHL, Schmidt N, Singer J (1995) MR imaging of adrenal masses; value of chemical-shift imaging for distinguishing adenomas from other tumors. AJR 164:637–642

Boraschi P, Campatelli A, di Vito A, Perri G (1995) Hemorrhage in cavernous hemangioma of the adrenal gland: US, CT and MRI appearances with pathologic correlation. Eur J Radiol 21:41–43

Brady TM, Gross BH, Glazer GM, Williams DM (1985) Adrenal pseudomasses due to varices: angiographic-CT-MRI-pathologic correlations. AJR 145:301–304

Cuesta MA, Bonjer HJ, van Mourik JC (1996) Endoscopic adrenalectomy: the adrenals under the scope. 349–351

Doppman JL, Loughlin T, Miller DL, et al. (1987) Identification of ACTH-producing intrathoracic tumors by measuring ACTH levels in aspirated specimens. Radiology 163:501–503

Doppmann JL, Nieman L, Miller DL, et al. (1989) Ectopic adrenocorticotropic hormone syndrome: localization studies in 28 patients. Radiology 172:115–124

Dunnick NR, Doppman JL, Gill JR, Strott CA, Keiser HR, Brennan MF (1982) Localization of functional adrenal tumors by computed tomography and venous sampling. Radiology 142:429–433

Ehman RL, McNamara MT, Brasch RC, Felmlee JP, Gray JE, Higgins CB (1986) Influence of physiologic motion on the appearance of tissue in MR images. Radiology 159:777–782

Dklof O, Mortensson W, Sandstedt B (1986) Suprarenal haematoma versus neuroblastoma complicated by haemorrhage; a diagnostic dilemma in the newborn. Acta Radiol (Diagn) 27:3–10

Falke THM, Sandler MP (1994) Classification of silent adrenal masses: time to get practical. Nucl Med 35:1152–1154

Falke THM, te Strake L, Sandler MP, Kulkarni MV, Partain CL, Nieuwenhuizen-Kruseman AC, James AE Jr (1986a) MR imaging of the adrenals: correlation with computed tomography. J Comput Assist Tomogr 10:242–253

Falke THM, van Seters AP, Schaberg A, Moolenaar AJ (1986b) Computed tomography in untreated adults with virilising congenital adrenal cortical hyperplasia. Clin Radiol 37:155

Falke THM, te Strake LB, Sandler MP, Shaff MI, Page DL (1987) Magnetic resonance imaging of the adrenal glands. Radiographics 7:343–370

Falke THM, Peetoom JJ, de Roos A, van de Velde CJH, Mazer M (1988) Gadolinium-DTPA enhanced MR imaging of intravenous extension of adrenocortical carcinoma. J Comput Assist Tomogr 12:331–334

Falke THM, van Gils APG, van Seters AP, Sandler MP (1990) Magnetic resonance imaging of functioning paragangliomas. Magn Reson Q 6:35–64

Glazer GM, Francis IR, Woolsey EJ, et al. (1986) Adrenal tissue characterization using MR imaging. Radiology 158:73–79

Gross MD, Falke THM, Shapiro B (1992) Adrenal glands. In: Sandler MP, Gross M, Shapiro B, Falke THM (eds) Endocrine imaging. Appelton & Lange, Norwalk, CT, pp 271–349

Groth H, Vetter W, Stimpel M, Greminger P, Tenschert W, Klaiber E, Vetter H (1985) Adrenalectomy in primary aldosteronism: a long-term follow-up study. Cardiology 72 (Suppl 1):107–116

Gruss LP, Newhouse JH (1996) Eight echo T2 measurements of adrenal masses: limitations of differential diagnosis by relaxation time determination. J Comput Assist Tomogr 20:792–797

Halvorsen RA Jr, Heaston DK, Johnston WW, Ashton PR, Burton GM (1982) CT guided thin needle aspiration of adrenal blastomycosis. J Comput Assist Tomogr 6:389–391

Hauser H, Gurret JP (1986) Miliary tuberculosis associated with adrenal enlargement: CT appearance. J Comput Assist Tomogr 10:254–256

Howlett TA, Drury PL, Perry L, Doniach I, Rees LH, Besser GM (1986) Diagnosis and management of ACTH-dependent Cushing's syndrome: comparison of the features in ectopic and pituitary production. Clin Endocrinol 24:699–713

Itoh K, Yamashita K, Satoh Y, Sawada H (1988) MR imaging of bilateral adrenal hemorrhage. J Comput Assist Tomogr 12:1054–1056

Jacobsen TF, Laniado M, van Beers BE, et al. (1996) Oral Magnetic particles (Ferristene) as a contrast medium in abdominal magnetic resonance imaging. Acad Radiol 3:571–580

Jaffe N (1976) Neuroblastoma: review of the literature and an examination of factors contributing to its enigmatic character. Cancer Treat Rev 3:61–82

Jafri SZH, Francis IR, Glazer GM, Bree RL, Amendola MA (1983) CT detection of adrenal lymphoma. J Comput Assist Tomogr 7:254–256

Kenney PJ, Robbins GL, Ellis DA, Spirt BA (1985) Adrenal glands in patients with congenital renal anomalies: CT appearance. Radiology 155:181–182

Kier R, McCarthy S (1989) MR characterization of adrenal masses: field strength and pulse sequence considerations. Radiology 171:671–674

King BF, Kopecky KK, Baker MK, Clark SA (1987) Extramedullary hematopoiesis in the adrenal glands: CT characteristics. J Comput Assist Tomogr 11:342–343

Koch KJ, Cory DA (1986) Simultaneous renal thrombosis and bilateral adrenal hemorrhage: MR demonstration. J Comput Assist Tomogr 10:681–683

Kornbluth AA, Salomon P, Sachar DB, et al. (1990) ACTH-induced adrenal hemorrhage: a complication of therapy masquerading as an acute abdomen. J Clin Gastroenterol 12:371–377

Korobkin M, Lombardi TJ, Aisen AM, et al. (1995) Characterization of adrenal masses with chemical shift and gadolinium-enhanced MR imaging. Radiology 197:411–418

Korobkin M, Giordano TJ, Brodeur FJ, et al. (1996a) Adrenal adenomas: relationship between histologic lipid and CT and MR findings. Radiology 200:743–747

Korobkin M, Brodeur FJ, Francis IR, Quint LE, Dunnick NR, Goodsitt M (1996b) Delayed enhanced CT for differentiation of benign from malignant adrenal masses. Radiology 200:737–742

Kreft B, Harder TH, Winter P (1990) Pseudozyste der Nebenniere. Fortschr Roentgenstr 152:231–232

Krestin GP, Steinbrich W, Friedmann G (1989) Adrenal masses: evaluation with fast gradient-echo MR imaging and Gd-DTPA-enhanced dynamic studies. Radiology 171:675–680

Krestin GP, Friedman G, Fischback R, Neufang KFR, Allolio B (1991) Evaluation of adrenal masses in oncologic patients: dynamic contrast-enhanced MR vs CT. J Comput Assist Tomogr 15:104–110

Kumar AJ, Rosenbaum AE, Naidu S, Wener L (1987) Adrenoleukodystrophy: correlating MR imaging with CT. Radiology 165:497–504

Langman J (1969) Medical embryology. Williams and Wilkins, Baltimore

Lee MJ, Hahn PF, Papanicolaou N, et al. (1991) Benign and malignant adrenal masses: CT distinction with attenuation coefficients, size, and observer analysis. Radiology 179:415–418

Lee MJ, Mayo-Smith WW, Hahn PF, Goldberg MA, Boland GW, Saini S, Papanicolaou N (1994) State of the art MR imaging of the adrenal gland. Radiographics 14:1015–1029

Leroy-Willig A, Bittoun T, Luton TP, et al. (1987) In vitro adrenal cortex lesions characterization by NMR spectroscopy. Magn Reson Imaging 5:339–344

Ling D, Korobkin M, Silverman PM, Dunnick NR (1983) CT demonstration of bilateral adrenal hemorrhage. AJR 141:307–308

Lundstrom GK, Chen PS (1985) Bilateral adrenal hemorrhage associated with prior steroid use: CT diagnosis. J Can Assoc Radiol 36:58–60

Luton J-P, Cerdas S, Bilaud L, et al. (1990) Clinical features of adrenocortical carcinoma, prognostic factors, and the effect of mitotane therapy. N Engl J Med 322:1195–1201

Ma JT, Wang C, Lam KS, et al. (1986) Fifty cases of primary hyperaldosteronism in Hong Kong Chinese with a high frequency of periodic paralysis: evaluation of techniques for tumor localization. Q J Med 61:1021–1037

Madsen B (1980) Selective adrenal angiography: a study of adrenal and related arteries in normal and pathological conditions. (Thesis). Kobenhaven, FADL's Forlag

Mayo-Smith WW, Lee MJ, McNicholas MMJ, Hahn PF, Boland GW (1995) Characterization of adrenal masses (<5 cm) by use of chemical shift MR imaging: observer performance versus quantitative measures. AJR 165:91–95

Melby JC (1985) Diagnosis and treatment of primary aldosteronism and isolated hypoaldosteronism. Clin Endocrinol Metab 14:977–995

Migeon CJ, Kenney FM, Hung W, Voorness ML (1967) Study of adrenal function in children with meningitis. Pediatrics 40:163–183

Miller DL, Doppman JL, Nieman LK, et al. (1990) Petrosal sinus sampling: discordant lateralization of ACTH-secreting pituitary microadenomas before and after stimulation with corticotropin-releasing hormone. Radiology 176:429–431

Mitchell DG (1992) Benign disease of the uterus and ovaries: applications of magnetic resonance imaging. Radiol Clin North Am 30:777

Mitchell DG, Crovello M, Matteucci T, Petersen RO, Miettinen MM (1992) Benign adrenocortical masses: diagnosis with chemical shift MR imaging. Radiology 185:345–351

Mitchell DG, Outwater EK, Matteucci T, Rubin DL, Chezmar JL, Saini S (1995) Adrenal gland enhancement at MR imaging with Mn-DPDP. Radiology 194:783–787

Mitchell DG, Stolpen AH, Siegelman ES, Bollinger L, Outwater EK (1996) Fatty tissue on opposed-phase MR images: paradoxical suppression of signal intensity by paramagnetic contrast agents. Radiology 198:351–357

Moon KL, Hricak H, Crooks LE, et al. (1983) Nuclear magnetic resonance imaging of the adrenal gland: a preliminary report. Radiology 14:155–160

Muehler A, Platzek J, Raduechel B, et al. (1995) Characterization of a gadolinium-labeled cholesterol derivate as an organ-specific contrast agent for adrenal MR imaging. J Magn Reson 5:7–10

Najeau BB, Siles S, Panuel JU, et al. (1992) Value of MRI and MIBG-I123 scintigraphy in the diagnosis of spinal bone marrow involvement in neuroblastoma in children. Pediatr Radiol 22:443

Nelson DH (1980) The adrenal cortex: physiological function and disease. Saunders, Philadelphia, pp 48–64

Neville AM, O'Hara HJ (1985) Histopathology of the human adrenal cortex. Clin Endocrinol Metab 14:791–820

Noble MJ, Montague DK, Levin HH (1982) Myelolipoma: an unusual surgical lesion of the adrenal gland. Cancer 49:952–958

Ogata T, Ishikawa K, Kohda E, Matsuo N (1988) Computed tomography in the early detection of congenital lipoid adrenal hyperplasia. Pediatr Radiol 18:360–361

Oudkerk M, Falke THM (1981) Chemodectoma, multiple localization: neck and mediastinum. ROFO 6:601–732

Outwater EK, Mitchell DG (1994) Differentiation of adrenal masses with chemical shift imaging. Radiology 193:875–876

Outwater EK, Siegelman ES, Huang AB, et al. (1996) Adrenal masses: correlation between CT attenuation value and chemical shift ratio at MR. Radiology 200:749–752

Reinig JW (1992) MR imaging differentiation of adrenal masses: has the time finally come? Radiology 185:339–340

Reinig JW, Doppman JL, Dwyer AJ, Johnson AR, Knop RH (1986) Adrenal masses differentiated by MR. Radiology 158:81–84

Roberts L Jr, Dunnick NR, Thompson WM, Foster WL Jr, Halvorsen RA, Gibbons RG, Feldman JM (1985) Primary aldosteronism due to bilateral nodular hyperplasia: CT demonstration. J Comput Assist Tomogr 9:1125–1127

de Roos A, Doornbos J, Baleriaux D, Bloem HL, Falke THM (1988) Clinical applications of Gd-DTPA in MRI. In: Kressel HY (ed) Magnetic resonance annual 1988. Raven Press, New York, pp 113–145

Rowinsky EK, Jones RJ, Abeloff MD (1986) Massive adrenal hemorrhage secondary to metastatic lung carcinoma. Med Pediatr Oncol 14:234–237

Roy E, Sandler MP, Falke THM (1994) MRI of Carney's triad. South Med J 87:951–955

Schwartz LH, Panicek DM, Koutcher JA, Brown KT, Getrajdman GI, Heelan RT, Burt M (1995) Adrenal masses in patients with malignancy: prospective comparison of echo-planar, fast spin-echo, and chemical shift MR imaging. Radiology 197:421–425

Schwartz LH, Macari M, Huvos AG, Panicek DM (1996) Collision tumors of the adrenal gland: demonstration and characterization at MR imaging. Radiology 201:757–760

Semelka RC, Shoenut JP, Lawrence PH, Greenberg HM, Maycher B, Madden TP, Kroeker MA (1993) Evaluation of adrenal masses with gadolinium enhancement and fat-suppressed MR imaging. J Magn Reson Imaging 3: 337–343

Silverman PM (1986) Gastric diverticulum mimicking adrenal mass: CT demonstration. J Comput Assist Tomogr 10:709–711

Silverman SG, Mueller PR, Pinkney LP, Koenker RM, Seltzer SE (1993) Predictive value of image-guided adrenal biopsy: analysis of results of 101 biopsies. Radiology 187:715–718

Solomon N, Sumkin J (1988) Right adrenal gland hemorrhage as a complication of liver transplantation: CT appearance. J Comput Assist Tomogr 12:95–97

St John Sutton MG, Sheps SG, Lie JT (1981) Prevalence of clinically unsuspected pheochromocytoma. Review of a 50-year autopsy series. Mayo Clin Proc 56:354–360

Symington T (1969) Functional pathology of the human adrenal gland. Churchill Livingstone, Edinburgh, pp 13–21

Taylor L, Ayers JWT, Gross MD, Peterson EP, Menon KMJ (1986) Diagnostic considerations in virilization: iodomethyl-norcholesterol scanning in the localization of androgen secreting tumors. Fertil Steril 46:1005–1010

Telenius-Berg M, Berg B, Hamberger B, Tibblin S (1987) Screening for early asymptomatic pheochromocytoma in MEN 2. Henry Ford Hosp Med J 35:110–114

Tsushima Y, Ishizaka H, Matsumoto M (1993) Adrenal masses: differentiation with chemical shift, fast low-angle shot MR imaging. Radiology 186:705–709

van Erkel AR, van Gils APG, Lequin M, Kruitwagen C, Bloem JL, Falke THM (1994) CT and MR distinction of adenomas and non-adenomas of the adrenal gland. J Comput Assist Tomogr 18:432–438

van Gils APG, Falke THM, van Erkel AR, van de Velde CJH, Pauwels EKJ (1990) Non-invasive imaging of functioning paragangliomas (including phaeochromocytomas). Front Eur Radiol 7:1–38

van Gils APG, Falke THM, van Erkel AR, Hoogma RPLM (1991) MR imaging and MIBG scintigraphy of pheochromocytomas and extra-adrenal functioning paragangliomas. Radiographics 11:37–57

van Gils APG, van den Berg R, Falke THM, et al. (1994) MR diagnosis of paraganglioma of the head and neck: value of contrast enhancement. AJR 152:147–153

Vita JA, Silverberg SJ, Goland RS, Austin JHM, Knowlton AI (1985) Clinical clues to the cause of Addison's disease. Am J Med 78:461–466

Shaley D, Becker S, Presbrey T, Shaff MI (1985) Adrenal myelolipoma associated with Conn syndrome: CT evaluation. J Comput Assist Tomogr 9:959–960

Wheatley T, Gallagher S, Dixon AK (1985) Adrenal insufficiency and bilateral adrenal enlargement demonstration by computed tomography. Br J Postgrad Med 61:435–438

Willemse APP, Coppes MJ, Feldberg MAM, et al. (1989) Magnetic resonance appearance of adrenal hemorrhage in a neonate. Pediatr Radiol 19:210–211

Wilms GE, Baert AL, Marcal G, Goddeeris PG (1979) Computed tomography of normal adrenal glands: correlative study with autopsy specimens. J Comput Assist Tomogr 3:467–469

Wilms GE, Marchal G, Baert A, Adisoejoso B, Mangkuwerdojo S (1987) CT and ultrasound features of post-traumatic adrenal hemorrhage. J Comput Assist Tomogr 11:112–115

Wolverson MK, Kannegiesser H (1984) CT of bilateral adrenal hemorrhage with acute adrenal insufficiency in the adult. AJR 142:311–314

12 Kidneys

W. Luboldt and G.P. Krestin

12.1
Introduction

The kidneys receive 20% (1200 ml/min) of the cardiac output and achieve a filtration rate of 10%–20% (120–150 ml/min). The process of filtration can be separated into four phases, the capillary (cortical), the early tubular, the ductal, and the excretory phase, each of which can be monitored by dynamic contrast-enhanced magnetic resonance imaging (MRI). Thereby morphologic information can be complemented by functional information in order to delineate and characterize kidney diseases.

In comparison to computed tomography (CT), MRI offers the advantage of multiplanar imaging and has the potential to provide increased tissue

contrast as well as increased temporal and spatial resolution in the foreseeable future. However, presently MRI of the kidneys is technically challenging, given the inherent respiratory-induced motion of the kidneys and the limited contrast between normal and abnormal renal tissues on conventional spin-echo images. Rapid imaging techniques, respiratory compensation algorithms, fat suppression, chemical shift imaging, phased array surface coils, and paramagnetic contrast media have enhanced MRI of the kidneys and made it competitive with CT. Furthermore, the possibility of procuring supplementary information by means of MR angiography (MRA), MR urography, dynamic perfusion imaging, blood oxygenation level dependent (BOLD) functional MRI, blood flow measurements, spectroscopy, or stress renography has made MRI more attractive, not least for research purposes.

12.2
Imaging Strategies

Magnetic resonance imaging of the kidneys has to be tailored to the clinical questions, i.e., evaluation of mass lesions, staging of renal carcinoma, characterization of retroperitoneal and peritransplant fluid collections, and assessment of vascular patency.

12.2.1
Standard Protocol

1. Axial T1-Weighted Images

Due to the demarcating character of fat, T1 weighting is used for anatomic orientation in axial planes (Fig. 12.1a). The images also provide precontrast baseline. T1-weighted sequences can be achieved using either spin-echo (SE) sequences with motion compensation techniques (ROPE, flow compensa-

W. Luboldt, MD, MSC Department of Diagnostic Radiology, University Hospital Zurich, Rämistrasse 100, CH-8091 Zurich, Switzerland
G.P. Krestin, MD, Department of Diagnostic Radiology, University Hospital Zurich, Rämistrasse 100, CH-8091 Zürich, Switzerland

tion) (Table 12.1) or gradient recalled echo (GRE) sequences during suspended respiration (FLASH, SPGR, FFE).

2. Axial T2-Weighted Images

T2-weighted sequences (Table 12.1) may help to differentiate cystic from hemorrhagic and solid lesions (Fig. 12.1b). Fast or turbo spin echo (FSE/TSE) sequences (hybrid-RARE) with motion compensation, T2-weighted GRE sequences with small flip angles (10°–15°) or single shot FSE (SSFSE / HASTE (Half Fourier Acquired Single Shot Turbo Spin Echo) sequences with an echo time (TE) between 40 and 90 ms are suitable for this purpose. The later sequences can be performed in a breath-hold interval and are insensitive to bowel peristalsis. Fat saturation may help to visualize peri- and pararenal extension of disease. Acquisition of these images in the axial plane allows direct comparison with the nonenhanced T1-weighted sequence.

3. Coronal Contrast-Enhanced Dynamic Sequence

The exact extent of a space-occupying lesion should be visualized in an additional plane. The best orientation, with simultaneous demonstration of both kidneys at their maximum lengths, is provided by a coronal or coronal oblique projection. Rapid fat-saturated T1-weighted imaging based on spoiled GRE (SPGR) sequences (Table 12.1) prior to as well as in a series following bolus administration of a gadolinium compound helps demarcation, delineation and characterisation of renal pathologies (Fig. 1c-f). Additionally it provides functional information regarding renal perfusion and filtration.

4. Axial, Fat-Saturated T1-Weighted Images

For the evaluation of late perfusion effects, the perirenal extent of renal masses, and interstitial contrast uptake, T1-weighted fat-suppressed images may be performed in the same plane as images obtained before contrast administration. The use of fat saturation increases the sensitivity for contrast uptake. Comparison of the precontrast non fat-saturated and postcontrast fat-saturated examinations then permits both, detection of pathological enhancement and prove of fat content.

12.2.2
Targeted Protocols

Assessment of the renal vasculature

Coronal contrast enhanced dynamic sequences already provide information about the renal vasculature. However, for better delineation of the renal arteries and, in particular, veins in patients with malignant renal tumors, axial 2D time of flight (TOF) sequences with flow compensation are mandatory (Table 12.1).

In case fast gradient systems (maximum gradient amplitude: 22 mT/m, slew rate: 120 mT/m/ms) are available, contrast-enhanced 3D MRA (Table 12.1) is recommended for the assessment of the renal arteries. Based on an ultrashort TR, the technique allows for imaging within a comfortable breathold interval. Using macromolecular blood pool contrast agents (STILLMAN et al. 1996, ANZAI et al. 1997), instead of the low molecular gadolinium compounds also the renal veins can also be imaged in a quality similar to that obtained for the renal arteries. It should be noted that the advantages of blood pool contrast agents in venous imaging is offset by

Table 12.1.

Sequence	Plane	Options	TR/TE/Flip	matrix	Section/Gap
SE (T1w)	axial	FC + RC	300–400/min/–	256 × 192/224	8/2
FSE (T2w)	axial	FC + RT + FS	3500–5000/106/–	256 × 192/224	8/2
+ i.v. bolus of a gadolinium compound (0.1 mmol/kg BW)					
(3D-SPGR)*	coronal	0.5/0.75 NEX	2–4/1–2/40°	256/384 × 192	2–2.4
SPGR (dyn)	coronar-oblique	FS	100–150/min/60°	256 × 192/160	8
(GR (TOF))**	axial	FC	<30/<15/<30°	256 × 192/160	5
SE (T1w)	axial	FC + RC + FS	300–400/min/–	256 × 192/224	8/2

min = minimum, FC = Flow Compensation, RC = Respiratory Compensation, RT = Respiratory Trigger, FS = Fat Saturation
* for the assessment of renal arteries, ** for the assessment of renal veins and vena cava

sacrificing clarity due to superimposition of arterial and venous vessels which possible requires further efforts in the analysis of multiplanar reformats. In contrast to blood pool enhanced MRA, gadolinium enhanced MRA has to be performed at the first pass of the gadolinium prior to distribution over the intravascular space and before the renal elimination as well as diffusion of contrast into the interstitial space lowers its intravascular concentration. For maximum signal intensity the injection of gado-

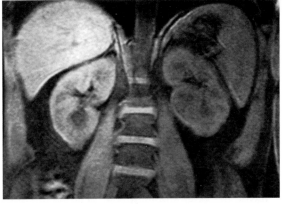

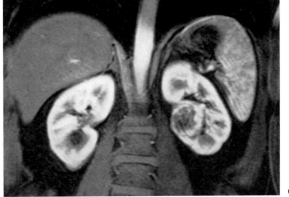

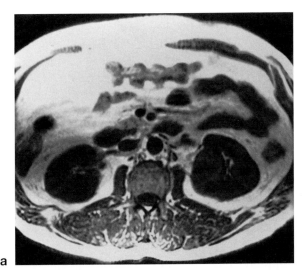

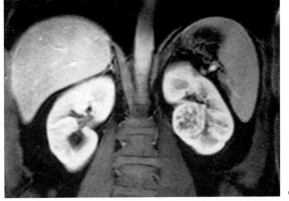

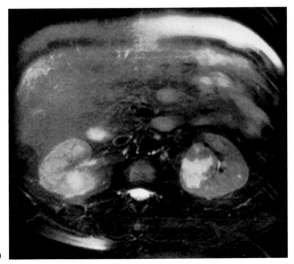

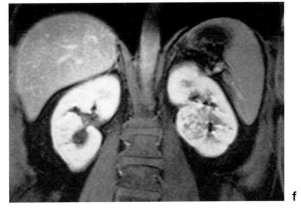

Fig. 12.1 a–f. Parapelvic cyst in the right kidney; renal cell carcinoma in the left kidney. **a** T1-weighted axial imaging shows homogeneous, low signal intensity of the cyst and heterogeneous signal intensity of the solid tumor. **b** T2-weighted axial imaging reveals hyperintense signal for both lesions. **c–f** The precontrast image (**c**) and images obtained 30 s (**d**), 60 s (**e**), and 240 s (**f**) following administration of Gd-DPTA (0.1 mmol/kg body weight) show no enhancement of the cyst, and heterogeneous enhancement of the RCC with delineation of a capsule

linium has to be timed in a manner that allows acquisition of the central k-space lines during the bolus
maximum, whereas for optimal spatial resolution
the bolus has to be maintained over the whole scan
period. Therefore, the mode of contrast administration determines the quality of MRA. Timing is
crucial in order to achieve a coincidence between
scanning and arrival of the contrast bolus. The delay
time can be individually determined with the help of
a test bolus (1 ml gadolinium followed by a saline
flush) and subsequent measurement of the intensity-
time course in the aorta. The time to peak enhancement, the scan duration, the gadolinium dose
(maximum 0.3 mmol/kg body weight), and the time
interval at which the central k-line is acquired
(which depends on the sequence design) are the parameters determining the injection mode (scan delay
and injection rate). Automated start triggering, using either the absolute signal intensity or the slope of
the intensity increase, will replace the prebolus technique and help to standardize the gadolinium injection for routine contrast-enhanced MRA.

Assessment of Renal Function and Perfusion

Following a bolus application of gadolinium a series
of images can be performed in the same position in
order to visualize the contrast dynamics. Using a 2D
spoiled GRE sequence in single-slice mode a temporal resolution of approximately 2 s can be achieved.
T2-weighted echo planar imaging (EPI) helps to increase the temporal resolution, but at the cost of
spatial resolution.

Assessment of the Collecting System

A rapid acquisition with a relaxation enhancement
(RARE) sequence is used for MR urography
(FRIEDBURG et al. 1987; AERTS et al. 1996). The
method requires no contrast material and is independent of renal function. Nevertheless, it does have
certain disadvantages: the necessity for a static dilated urine-containing system or the application of
furosemide (ROTHPEARL et al. 1995), the inability to
directly image a calculus, and the inability to distinguish between vesicoureteric reflux and obstructive
megaureter (SIGMUND et al. 1991). MR urography
may be considered when there is a contraindication
to intravenous urography, such as allergic reaction
to contrast material, severe renal failure, or pregnancy (ROY et al. 1994).

12.3
Contrast Dynamics of the Kidneys

Vascular insufficiency, glomerular and tubuloin-
terstitial disorders, and obstructive uropathies may
lead to functional disturbances without any morphologic correlate. Therefore, in diffuse disease functional
evaluation has to supplement morphologic imaging.

Rapid MRI coupled with the administration of
renally eliminated contrast material allows monitoring of the renal passage. The cortex of the kidney
enhances strongly as early as 10–20 s after the bolus
injection whereas the medulla shows no significant
enhancement. The delayed enhancement of the medulla is due to its blood supply, which accounts for
only 1%–6.5% of the entire renal perfusion. Depending on the bolus geometry and circulation time,
maximum cortical enhancement is reached after 20–
50 s. With ongoing filtration of gadolinium into the
Bowman capsule and following passage through
the tubules, the signal increase is transferred from
the cortex to the outer or inner medulla, respectively.
Due to the urine concentrating process, maximum
enhancement of the medulla is reached 10–20 s
after maximum enhancement of the cortex. Concentration of the urine in the collecting ducts (50- to
100-fold) results in such a high gadolinium concentration that the T2 (T2*)-shortening effects of
gadolinium become dominant. Therefore, the signal
intensity on unspoiled GRE images (FFE, FISP,
GRASS) drops in the medullary pyramids to values
similar to those on the precontrast images (VON
SCHULTHESS 1989; KRESTIN et al. 1987, 1988;
KIKINIS et al. 1987; CARVLIN et al. 1987; MUNECHIKA
et al. 1991).

Contrast dynamics can be quantitatively evaluated
by plotting the signal intensity values in the cortex
and medulla as a function of time (VON SCHULTHESS
et al. 1991). The obtained intensity-time curves
provide information about renal perfusion, filtration, and excretion for the differentiation between
pre-, intra-, and postrenal disorders.

12.4
Vascular Disorders

12.4.1
Renal Artery Stenosis

Renal artery stenoses can be caused by atheromatous
lesions or congenital fibromuscular dysplasia and
explain 2%–3% of the cases with arterial hyperten-

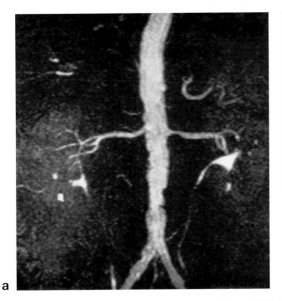
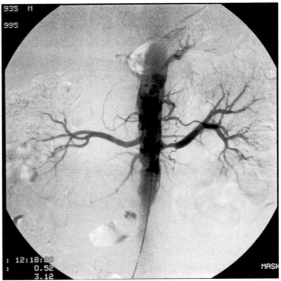

a   b

Fig. 12.2 a,b. Renal artery stenosis. Contrast-enhanced MRA (**a**) demonstrates a proximal stenosis of the left renal artery as clearly as does digital subtraction angiography (**b**)

sion. The diagnosis of a renal artery stenosis is important because it represents one of the few entities responsible for arterial hypertension in which causal treatment is feasible. Whereas the atheromatous lesions are mostly located near the ostium, in the proximal part of the renal artery, fibromuscular dysplasia manifests in the more distal part of the renal artery and presents typically as a "string of beads" predominately in young woman.

Despite providing only two-dimensional data, catheter angiography is still the gold standard for the diagnosis of renal artery stenosis. Although suffering from flow artifacts, TOF as well as phase-contrast MRA have shown promising results for the screening of renal arteries (YUCEL et al. 1993; SERVOIS et al. 1994; DEBATIN et al. 1991). Due to its insensitivity to flow dynamics and directions, contrast-enhanced MRA appears superior to these techniques in the evaluation of renovascular pathologies. In contrast to conventional angiography, MRA provides three-dimensional data, thereby permitting multiplanar/curved reconstruction of variable thickness as well as maximum intensity projections (Fig. 12.2) from any desired perspective. Furthermore, MRA overcomes the disadvantages of conventional angiography, i.e., the invasiveness, the radiation exposure, and the use of nephrotoxic contrast material. Therefore, MRA is favored for screening of the renal arteries.

In addition to the morphologic classification of a stenosis, MRI also allows evaluation of the hemo-

dynamic significance of a stenosis by phase encoded velocity measurements. These measurements yield valid information when the flow through the vessel is laminar and the vessel does not move (DEBATIN et al. 1994, 1995). The flow profile over the cardiac cycle itself or in relation to that of the aortic flow profile (branching ratio of flow) or contralateral kidney might provide useful information. However, the clinical impact of MR flow quantification is still under investigation.

12.4.2
Ischemia/Infarction

Acute infarction is usually caused by thromboemboli and is seen as a well-defined wedge-shaped defect in the renal outline. On both T1- and T2-weighted images the signal intensities of the infarcted areas are usually lower than that of the noninfarcted parenchyma. Differences in renal blood flow between the kidneys can be best appreciated on serial dynamic MRI following a bolus injection of gadolinium (LAISSY et al. 1994). The signal intensity-versus-time plots of kidneys with significant postischemic changes show a less steep increase in signal intensity in the cortex and a steeper increase in signal intensity in the medulla than do those of normal kidneys (VOSSHENRICH et al. 1996). Postcontrast T1-weighted images are useful to demonstrate the extent of infarction (KIM et al. 1992). Complete renal ischemia leads to poor corticomedullary differentiation in Gd-DTPA-enhanced turbo FLASH MRI. Diffusion-weighted imaging also shows promise for the provision of information concerning the renal microcirculation that is not otherwise available (LORENZ et al. 1992).

12.4.3
Renal Vein Thrombosis

For the diagnosis of acute renal vein thrombosis, MRI is considered the method of choice. Gradient-echo MRI provides accurate information regarding renal vein patency and aneurysms (CHOYKE and POLLACK 1988; SPRITZER et al. 1988; HRICAK et al. 1985). Renal veins are generally well visualized on the coronal images of the dynamic examination (Fig. 12.3). If the renal veins cannot be assessed on the coronal images, an axial TOF sequence focused on the veins with a thinner slice thickness should additionally be performed.

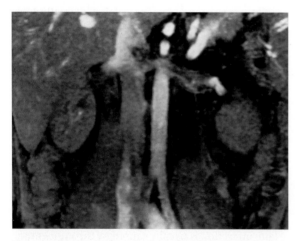

Fig. 12.3. Renal vein thrombosis. A clot in the left renal vein is visualized on a coronal GRE image after administration of contrast material

12.5
Functional Disorders

12.5.1
Hydronephrosis

Most cases of acute obstruction of the urinary tract are caused by stones whereas chronic hydrone-

phrosis results from ureteral strictures, neoplastic masses, retroperitoneal fibrosis, or retroperitoneal or pelvic inflammatory disease. In general, obstruction results in urinary stasis which prolongs the tubular phase on contrast-enhanced dynamic MRI. Preliminary reports indicate that acute obstruction can be distinguished from chronic obstruction (KRESTIN et al. 1988; KRESTIN 1990; SEMELKA et al. 1990; FRANK et al. 1991; VON SCHULTHESS et al. 1991). In acutely obstructed kidneys (onset of obstruction within 3 days), MRI reveals cortical enhancement similar to and medullary enhancement higher than that in normal kidneys, whereas chronically obstructed kidneys can be recognized by their decreased cortical enhancement in conjunction with a diminished or even absent ductal phase. The underlying pathophysiology of the contrast behavior revealed by MRI in hydronephrosis is still unclear because various factors, such as the patient's hydration status, the renal contrast perfusion (hemodynamics), contrast filtration, stasis, and concentrating ability are involved in a complex manner. Also, the change in the surrounding environment of gadolinium during its renal passage in conjunction with the non-linearity in the relationship between gadolinium concentration and its signal complicates analysis of the renal contrast dynamics.

12.5.2
Renal Insufficiency/Failure

The etiology of renal insufficiency/failure can be divided according to prerenal, intrarenal and post-renal causes. MRI is valuable for depicting conditions such as renal artery stenosis, renal infarction, renal vein thromboses, hydronephrosis and focal disorders. In case of renal insufficiency, gadolinium enhanced MRI can be still performed (SCHUHMANN et al. 1991, BELLIN et al. 1992, HAUSTEIN et al. 1992) where CT with iodinated contrast material is contraindicated. In patients of acute renal failure, laborchemically defined by creatinine values greater than 2.5 mg/dl, MRI without or with contrast can be the method of choice if ultrasonography proves equivocal. Regardless of the underlying cause, a serum creatinine value greater than 3.0 mg/dL results in loss of corticomedullary differentiation on T1-weighted fat suppressed spin echo imaging, whereas the serum creatinine value must be higher (>8.5 mg/dL) for corticomedullary differentiation to be lost on dynamic gadolinium-enhanced studies

(SEMELKA et al. 1994). The end-stage of renal failure is reflected morphologically by parenchymal atrophy, absence of corticomedullary differentiation, and increased lipomatosis. Due to interstitial fibrosis, nonfunctioning kidneys show low signal intensity on T2-weighted MR images.

12.6
Focal Disorders

On nonenhanced MR images, both solid and cystic renal and pararenal masses often present with signal intensities similar to those of bland cysts (Fig. 12.1a,b) and adjacent normal renal tissue. Therefore, detection of focal lesions is based only on visible intrarenal displacements or alteration of the outer contour (CHOYKE 1988) (Fig. 12.1). Contrast administration helps to delineate renal lesions from normal surrounding tissue. Additional fat suppression increases the sensitivity for contrast enhancement, allowing demonstration hyperperfused solid masses of small cysts or with a diameter of <1 cm (SEMELKA et al. 1991, 1992).

12.6.1
Benign Lesions

12.6.1.1
Renal Cysts

Cysts can be subdivided into simple cortical or parapelvine cysts, complicated cysts, and cysts associated with autosomal dominant diseases such as polycystic disease, tuberous sclerosis, and von Hippel-Lindau disease.

Simple cysts (Fig. 12.4) are the most common renal lesions. Frequently they are multiple and bilateral. Classically they are located in the renal cortex and are characterized by sharp and regular margins. Their content of water-equivalent fluid results in low signal on T1-weighted and high signal on T2-weighted images. Simple cysts are homogeneous in their signal pattern and display a thin, usually nonenhancing wall (Fig. 12.4).

Complicated cysts (Fig. 12.5) are characterized by septa, hemorrhage, and subsequent calcification. Due to the hemorrhage, signal intensity may be intermediate to high on T1-weighted images (Fig. 12.5a). Hemorrhagic cysts may resemble angiomyolipomas (Fig. 12.9). However, use of fat suppression (Fig. 12.5b) aids in the differentiation between hemorrhagic cysts and angiomyolipoma (Fig. 12.9b). Hemorrhage and enhancement after contrast administration can make complicated cysts indistinguishable from cystic renal cell carcinoma. Neither the existence of a fluid-fluid level nor the MR signal of the fluid itself helps to differentiate between infected, hemorrhagic, and malignant cysts. Nevertheless, contrast-enhanced MRI appears to be superior to contrast-enhanced CT in the classification of renal cysts (WURSTLIN et al. 1993).

Polycystic kidney disease is a slowly progressing disease leading to chronic renal failure (it is the third most prevalent cause of the latter). It is associated with saccular (berry) aneurysms of cerebral arteries

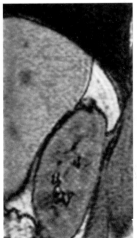 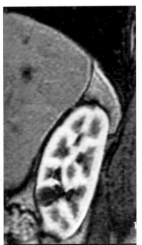 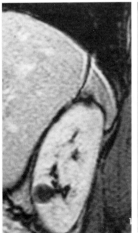 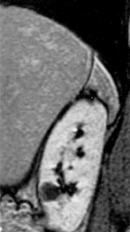

Fig. 12.4. Simple renal cyst with sharp margins, without enhancement following gadolinium administration

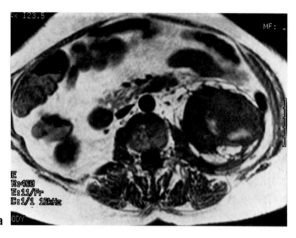

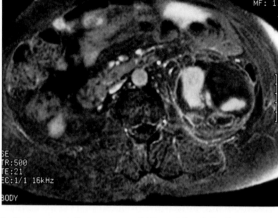

a

b

Fig. 12.5 a,b. Hemorrhagic cyst. **a** Precontrast T1-weighted SE image showes a low signal intensity mass with high signal intensity inclusions (hemorrhage) and areas of low signal intensity (hemosiderin) within the perirenal fascia.

b Postcontrast fat-suppressed T1-weighted SE image. The fluid in the cyst and perirenal space does not enhance; the hemorrhagic inclusions show high signal intensity and thus can be well differentiated from perirenal fat

(in 10%–30% of cases) and additional cysts, mainly in the liver (in 25%–50% of cases).

Tuberous sclerosis and *von Hippel-Lindau disease* are both neurocutaneous autosomal dominant disorders associated with renal cysts. Whereas in tuberous sclerosis the incidence of angiomyolipomas (see 12.6.1.5) is increased (ZIMMERHACKL et al. 1994), in von Hippel-Lindau disease there is an increased incidence of adenomas and carcinomas.

12.6.1.2
Hematoma

Hematoma can occur following trauma, surgery, percutaneous intervention, or shock-wave lithotripsy (RUIZ and SALTZMAN 1990). Therefore, the diagnosis is usually provided by the patients' history. Spontaneous development of hematoma should arouse suspicion of an underlying renal mass (ZERHOUNI et al. 1984; KENDALL et al. 1988) (present in 57%–63% of cases), vascular disease (present in 18%–26% of cases), or coagulopathy (FISHMAN et al. 1984). Hematomas can be subcapsular or perirenal. Subcapsularly located hematomas show a typical lenticular shape, compressing the renal parenchyma medially while causing the renal capsule to bulge laterally. Acute (within 72 h of bleeding) hematomas show signal intensities similar to or less than that of the renal cortex on T1-weighted images whereas subacute (after 3–7 days) and chronic hematomas show hyperintense areas due to the paramagnetic effect of the decomposition products of hemoglobin.

12.6.1.3
Inflammation/Abscess

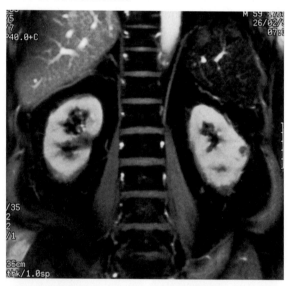

Fig. 12.6. Abscess. Contrast-enhanced T1-weighted spoiled GRE image demonstrates bulging of the lateral aspect of the left kidney, with a small hypovascular central area

The spectrum of inflammatory disease of the kidney ranges from acute, uncomplicated pyelonephritis, usually undetectable with imaging methods, to intrarenal or perinephric abscess, with focal bacterial nephritis as an intermediate state. Global renal enlargement due to edema or focal blurring of the corticomedullary junction may be the only visible sign of inflammation on nonenhanced MR images. Following i.v. administration of gadolinium, focal bacterial infectious lesions demonstrate poor enhancement and therefore can be detected as blurred low signal areas in the renal parenchyma. Infiltration of perirenal fat or thickening of the perinephric fascia (Gerota's fascia) may be an additional sign of inflammation (Fig. 12.6). Fully developed renal abscesses are characterized by a central fluid collection (Fig. 12.6) and a rimlike enhancement (HAUSER et al. 1992; BROWN et al. 1996).

12.6.1.4
Renal Oncocytoma

Renal oncocytomas (synonyms: proximal tubular adenoma, benign oxyphilic adenoma) account for 2%–14% of renal tumors. Usually they appear well demarcated with a pseudocapsule, and 30% display a central stellate scar. On conventional angiography they show a spoke wheel-like configuration in 80% of cases. On T1-weighted images oncocytomas present as low-intensity homogeneous masses with increased signal intensity on T2-weighted images (Fig. 12.7) (HARMON et al. 1996). These MRI findings differ somewhat from those of renal cell carcinomas, which typically show intermediate to high signal on T1- and T2-weighted sequences and usually

contain areas of either hemorrhage or necrosis. Characteristic central scars or spoke wheel-like enhancement may be seen after injection of contrast material but these appearances are not pathognomonic. In contrast to the aggressively growing renal carcinomas, most oncocytomas allow renal-sparing surgery.

12.6.1.5
Angiomyolipoma

Renal angiomyolipomas (AMLs) are rare benign mesenchymal tumors which are associated with tuberous sclerosis in 20% of cases (ZIMMERHACKL et al. 1994). The tumor is composed of fat tissue intermixed with smooth muscle and thick-walled blood vessels (Fig. 12.8). Due to the easy access to

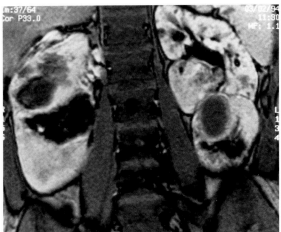

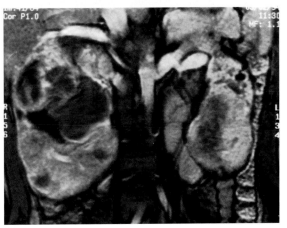

Fig. 12.8 a,b. Multiple angiomyolipomas in tuberous sclerosis. These postcontrast GRE images reveal multiple inhomogeneous masses in both kidneys with areas of low signal intensity due to dephasing between fat and water protons in the lipid-containing lesions

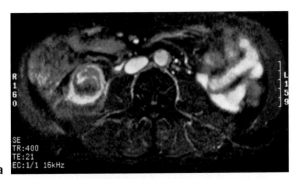

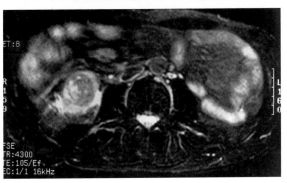

Fig. 12.7 a,b. Oncocytoma. T1-weighted postcontrast fat-suppressed SE (a) and T2-weighted fat-suppressed fast SE (b) imaging reveals an inhomogeneous lesion at the lower pole of the right kidney, which is indistinguishable from a RCC

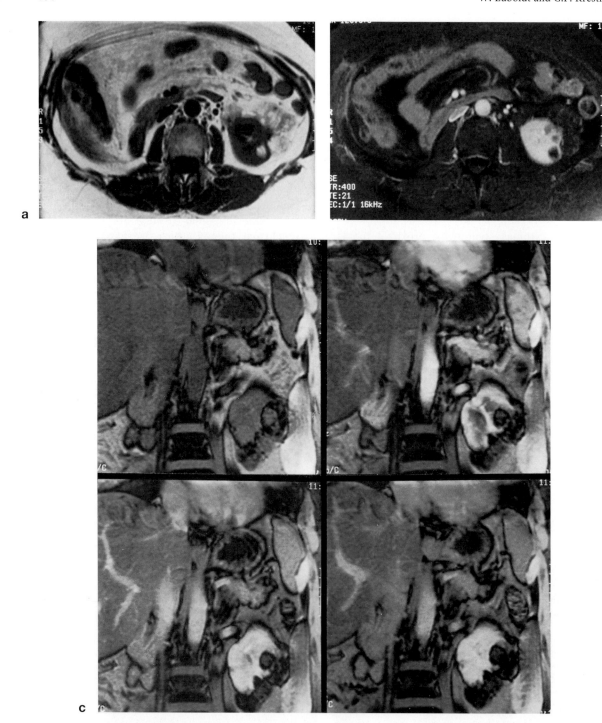

Fig. 12.9 a–c. Angiomyolipoma. **a** A T1-weighted SE image showes high signal intensity lesions in the left kidney. **b** T1-weighted, fat-saturated postcontrast SE image; the previously hyperintense lesions show an overall signal void and lack of enhancement. **c** Dynamic contrast-enhanced GRE images obtained before (*top left*) and 30 s (*top right*), 60 s (*bottom left*), and 240 s (*bottom right*) after injection of contrast material. The lesions display a low signal intensity due to dephasing between fat and water protons; there is no visible enhancement

modern imaging techniques, AMLs are increasingly being detected incidentally during diagnostic evaluation of common urologic diseases before they become symptomatic (the most common symptoms being flank pain and hematuria). The presence of a highly echodense renal mass on ultrasonography and the detection of even small amounts of fat on CT usually establish the diagnosis of AML. If these procedures provide equivocal results, angiography and MRI may become necessary. Due to their fatty component, angiomyolipomas show a hyperintense signal on T1-weighted images (Fig. 12.9a) which is typically suppressed when fat saturation is used (Fig. 12.9b). The sharp margin of angiomyolipomas, intensified by the chemical shift artifact, reflects their benign, noninfiltrative growth character (Fig. 12.8c). Angiomyolipomas show only minimal enhancement. Because of iron-containing blood derivatives and dephasing between fat and water, angiomyo-lipomas appear hypointense on GRE images (Figs. 12.8, 12.9).

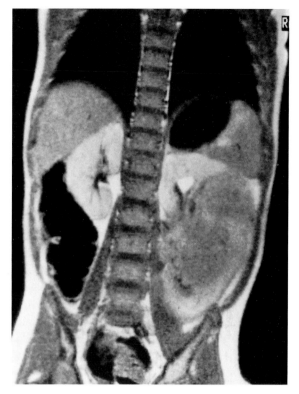

Fig. 12.10. Wilms' tumor. MRI reveals the extension of a Wilms' tumor in the left kidney for surgical planning

12.6.2
Malignant Lesions

12.6.2.1
Wilms' Tumor

Wilms' tumor (synonym: nephroblastoma) is the most common malignant abdominal neoplasm in children aged 1–8 years. Occurrence after adolescence is very rare. The incidence in childhood (peak age 2.5–3 years) in conjunction with the morphology (average size of 12 cm, sharp margination, partially cystic structure with focal hemorrhage and necrosis) (Fig. 12.10) is almost pathognomonic for Wilms' tumor. Ultrasonography is the primary method for imaging pediatric abdominal tumors (MÜLLER et al. 1993). However, pretherapeutic evaluation and planning of surgical procedures often require additional information. While the results of CT are limited by the lack of retroperitoneal fat in children and the use of ionizing radiation, MRI, with its high tissue contrast, is well suited for the assessment of Wilms' tumor (DIETRICH and KANGARLOO 1986). Due to its cystic-necrotic structure intermixed with hemorrhage, Wilms' tumor has a very heterogeneous presentation of MR images. MRI aids in confirmation and staging of Wilms' tumor (demonstrating venous involvement and lymph node metastasis).

12.6.2.2
Renal Cell Carcinoma

Renal cell carcinoma (RCC; synonyms: renal adeno-carcinoma, hypernephroma) arises from proximal tubular cells. RCC is histologically subdivided into clear cell carcinoma (95%) and papillary adenocarcinoma (5%). Whereas clear cell carcinoma is hypervascular and aggressive, papillary carcinoma is hypovascular, slowly growing, well encapsulated, and metastasizes late. Renal adenoma cannot be differentiated from RCC. Small adenomas (>2 cm) should be considered as RCCs of low metastatic potential.

Usually RCC is solid, solitary, and unilateral. Multiple or bilateral presentation occurs in less than 5% of cases. RCC without hemorrhage or necrosis tends to be isointense to normal renal parenchyma on both T1- and T2-weighted images. Since RCC is typically hypervascular, it shows on dynamic contrast enhanced imaging a rapid signal increase in the early perfusion phase followed by a relatively early onset of signal decrease (wash out of contrast) (Fig. 12.11). The contrast perfusion/uptake pattern typically consists of hyperintense ill-defined margins and heterogeneous inner enhancement due to necrosis or deposit of hemosiderin. Since small, homogeneously enhancing RCCs can be overlooked when they are located in the similarly enhancing cortex, a dynamic or a more delayed (interstitial phase) examination is mandatory for better exclusion of RCCs in the renal cortex.

Renal cell carcinoma shows locally aggressive growth, infiltrating adjacent tissues (Figs. 12.11, 12.12) and vessels (Fig. 12.13). It metastasizes into the bones, the liver, and the lungs. Accurate preoperative staging helps to establish the appropriate therapeutic management, the optimal surgical technique, and the prognosis (HOLLAND 1973; LIEBER et al. 1981). Staging criteria (ROBSON et al. 1969; AMENDOLA et al. 1990; McCLENNAN 1991) include tumor size, the perinephric fat and perinephric fascial invasion, direct invasion of adjacent organs, intravascular extension, and number of metastic lymph nodes (Tab. 2a). Because nephron-

sparing treatment has been proposed for small RCCs (SOKOLOFF et al. 1996; LERNER et al. 1996; STEINBACH et al. 1995; MARSH and LANGE 1995), accuracy in staging of RCC is becoming increasingly important. At present morphologic criteria indicating tumor enucleation include a tumor diameter of less than 4 cm, stage I–II tumor (confined to the renal capsule) with a pseudocapsule, and a peripheral location. Because satellite carcinomas are found even in low-stage RCCs (with an incidence of 3.75%), intraoperative ultrasonography is recommended (OYA et al. 1995) to exclude satellite lesions if nephron-sparing surgery is intended.

Magnetic resonance imaging is superior to CT in assessing local extension of renal cancers arising from the upper pole (SEMELKA et al. 1993). Chemical shift imaging (GRE sequences with a multiple of 2.1 ms used as the TE at 1.5 T) artificially accentuates the renal contours (KRESTIN et al. 1987) and thus facilitates the assessment of the capsule integrity for the purpose of staging (Fig. 12.12). If tumor tissue has infiltrated perirenal fat, the signal from water-containing tumor cells will negatively interfere with

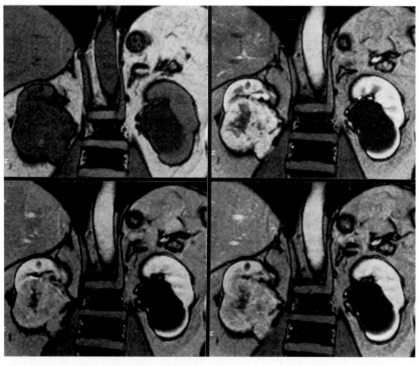

Fig. 12.11. Renal cell carcinoma (RCC) in the right kidney and parapelvic cyst in the left kidney. Coronal dynamic contrast-enhanced GRE images obtained before (*top left*) and 30 s (*top right*), 60 s (*bottom left*), and 240 s (*bottom right*) following administration of contrast material. The RCC shows an inhomogeneous rapid enhancement followed by a relatively early decrease in signal. The infiltration of the psoas muscle (stage T4) is well documented. The cyst in the left kidney is a simple cyst without contrast uptake

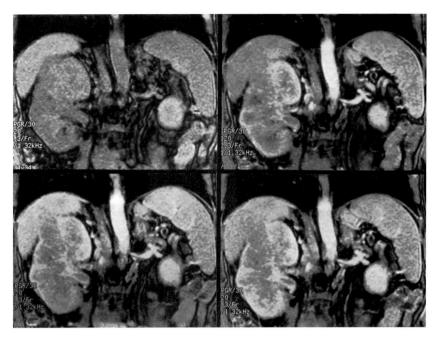

Fig. 12.12. RCC in the right kidney. Coronal dynamic contrast-enhanced GRE images obtained before (*top left*) and 30 s (*top right*), 60 s (*bottom left*), and 240 s (*bottom right*) following administration of contrast material. A large inhomogeneous mass is demonstrated in the right kidney with infiltration into the lower surface of the liver (stage T4)

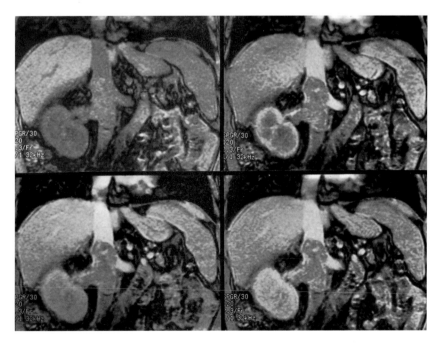

Fig. 12.13. RCC of the right kidney. Coronal dynamic contrast-enhanced GRE images obtained before (*top left*) and 30 s (*top right*), 60 s (*bottom left*), and 240 s (*bottom right*) following administration of contrast material. Enhancing tumor thrombus is demonstrated in the renal vein and inferior vena cava below the diaphragm (stage T3b)

Table 12.2.

TNM-Classification of renal cell carcinoma

T1	Tumor size ≤ 7 cm; limited to the kidney
T2	Tumor size > 7 cm; limited to the kidney
T3a	invades adrenal gland / perinephrotic tissue, but not beyond Gerota's fascia
T3b	grossly extends into renal vein or vena cava below diaphragm
T3c	grossly extends into renal vein or vena cava above diaphragm
T4	Tumor invades beyond Gerota's fascia
N1	solitar metastic lymph node
N2	more than one metastic lymph node
M1	distant metastasis

that of fat on opposed phase imaging, resulting in a loss of signal intensity on the image (KRESTIN 1990; KRESTIN et al. 1992). However, similar alterations can be observed simply as a result of lymphatic or venous edema around the kidneys. In such cases, detection of perirenal invasion can be improved using fat-suppressed contrast-enhanced images. Enhancement of the previously low signal intensity areas in perirenal tissue is indicative of extrarenal tumor invasion (CHOYKE 1988; SEMELKA et al. 1991).

Renal cell carcinoma is an angioinvasive tumor with the propensity not only to invade the renal vein but also to propagate into the inferior vena cava as a tumor thrombus (Fig. 12.13). MRI, with its capability for multiplanar slice acquisition, has supplanted other imaging techniques for the staging of tumor thrombi in renal cell carcinoma (HOCKLEY et al. 1990). Furthermore, MRI allows differentiation between a tumor thrombus and a bland thrombus: (MYNENI et al. 1991) by the use of dynamic contrast-enhanced GRE sequences. A bland thrombus has low signal because of the presence of hemosiderin and shows no enhancement, whereas a tumor thrombus reveals a higher signal (isointense to the primary tumor) and contrast uptake.

Distinction between lymph nodes and surrounding structures is rendered difficult by pulsation and breathing artifacts. On SE images, lymph nodes are sometimes difficult to differentiate from bowel loops (Fig. 12.14) or enlarged collateral veins. Using GRE images, retroperitoneal lymphadenopathy may be detected as accurately as with CT or ultrasonography. The intermediate signal intensity of the nodes allows clear differentiation from high signal intensity flowing blood as well as from low signal muscles (crus of diaphragm). Although bowel loops

also may be identified on such images, additional administration of an oral contrast agent may facilitate differentiation in some cases. However, as with CT or ultrasonography, the only criterion for diagnosis of malignant involvement remains the measurement of lymph node size; therefore, the sensitivity and specificity of MRI for N-staging presently do not exceed those of the aforementioned methods (EILENBERG et al. 1990). Research in differentiation between normal and metastatic lymph nodes is continuing. Presently a lymphotropic MRI-contrast agent (dextran-coated, ultrasmall super-paramagnetic iron oxide) which physiologically accumulates in the reticuloendothelial system of lymph nodes is under investigation. This method defines malignant non-functioning lymph nodes through the lack of contrast uptake. Benefiting from the high sensibility of T2* weighted sequences to iron induced changes in susceptibility, MR lymphography may become a useful technique for lymph-node staging in the future (ANZAI et al. 1997).

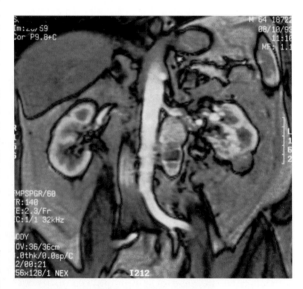

Fig. 12.14. RCC of the left kidney. Postcontrast GRE image showing a large para-aortic lymph node metastasis

12.6.2.3
Renal Metastases and Lymphoma

Metastases represent the most common malignant lesions of the kidneys. Usually they are derived from carcinoma of the lung, breast, or stomach. Due to their hematogenous spread, metastases are normally

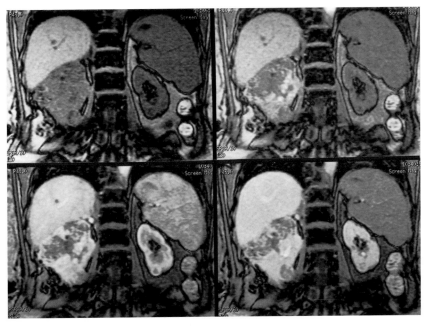

Fig. 12.15. Multiple, bilateral metastases. Coronal dynamic contrast-enhanced GRE images obtained before (*top left*) and 30 s (*top right*), 60 s (*bottom left*), and 240 s (*bottom right*) following administration of contrast material. Metastases, typically located in the cortical zone, are best delineated by contrast-enhanced dynamic imaging

located in the highly perfused renal cortex (Fig. 12.15). In the peripheral zone they are rarely symptomatic (CHOYKE et al. 1987). Most metastases are small and multifocal and/or bilateral (Fig. 12.15). Mostly they cannot be differentiated from other solid lesions of the kidneys unless an extrarenal primary tumor and/or hematogenous spread to other organs suggests the presence of metastatic involvement of the kidneys.

Due to the lack of intrarenal lymphoid tissue, lymphomatous involvement of the kidneys is based on hematogenous spread of lymphoid cells or on contiguous growth from retroperitoneal lymph nodes. Lymphoma in the kidney may appear as diffuse infiltration, as a focal rounded mass, or in conjunction with large para-aortic retroperitoneal masses with extension into the renal hilum or the subcapsular space. Lymphomas presenting as a large para-aortic mass often show diminished renal cortical perfusion of the involved kidney. Lymphomas have low to intermediate signal intensity on T1- and T2-weighted images. Enhancement of lymphomatous tissue is mildly heterogeneous and minimal on the early images, and remains minimal on the late images after gadolinium administration (HAUSER et al. 1992). In contrast to renal cell carcinoma, lymphomas show neither central necrosis nor renal vein thrombus. Infiltration of perinephric fat and thickening of the perinephric fascia may occur in lymphoma, similar to inflammatory diseases.

12.6.3
Pitfalls

The differential diagnosis of RCC includes complicated cysts, adenoma, angiomyolipoma, and renal abscess. In cases of relatively acute or organizing hemorrhage, cysts may have low signal on T2-weighted images and thus mimic RCC. The lack of gadolinium uptake helps in the differentiation. Adenoma cannot be differentiated from RCC by imaging; only the rapid growth of a lesion can be used as a criterion of malignancy. Angiomyolipoma may have a similar appearance to RCC when the vascular part predominates and may require biopsy for definitive diagnosis. A renal abscess can also resemble a RCC and differentiation from cystic renal cell carcinoma can only be achieved on the basis of clinical symptoms.

12.7
Renal Transplant

After renal transplantation various complications may arise, usually producing unspecific symptoms and signs such as oliguria, high levels of serum creatinine, fever, and pain at the site of the graft. These complications may be based on macroscopic causes such as obstruction, leakage, peritransplant fluid collections, and vascular problems such as vascular stenosis or thrombosis, arteriovenous fistula, and pseudoaneurysm. MRI, with its capability for multiplanar imaging, appears well suited for the evaluation of renal transplants. T2 weighting supports the visualization of perirenal fluid collections, dynamic contrast-enhanced imaging provides functional information, and MRA or MR urography helps to detect vascular or urethral complications.

Microscopic causes of allograft transplant dysfunction such as rejection, acute tubular necrosis, drug toxicity, infection, inflammation, or the development of recurrent disease are frequently associated with nonspecific imaging findings. Therefore allograft biopsy is necessary for definitive diagnosis. Differentiation between acute rejection and acute tubular necrosis (ATN) in transplanted kidneys is very important in order to avoid unnecessary immunosuppression in cases of ATN. Acute vascular rejection sometimes can be differentiated from other functional disturbances by a characteristic enhancement pattern (VESTRING et al. 1992). However, MRI, supplemented by MRA (GEDROYC et al. 1992), MR flow quantification (MYERS et al. 1994), or spectroscopy (GRIST et al. 1991), offers many possibilities in the morphologic and functional evaluation of renal transplants.

12.8
Conclusion

Magnetic resonance imaging allows imaging tailored to a pathology, provides morphologic and functional information, and is not limited by nephrotoxic contrast media or ionizing radiation. Contrast-enhanced MRI coupled with multiplanar and chemical shift imaging helps to assess large retroperitoneal masses and to classify them as intra- or extrarenal.

Magnetic resonance imaging is equivalent or slightly superior to CT for the detection and characterization of small renal tumors and for the preoperative staging of RCC (SEMELKA et al. 1992,

1993). Due to its flexibility in the choice of contrast and sensitivity to contrast perfusion/interstitial uptake, MRI may surpass CT in the differentiation between benign and malignant mass lesions.

References

Aerts P, Van Hoe L, Bosmans H, Oyen R, Marchal, Baert AL (1996) Breath hold MR urography using the HASTE technique. AJR 166:543–545

Amendola MA, King LR, Pollack HM, Gefter W, Kressel HY, Wein AJ (1990) Staging of renal carcinoma using magnetic resonance imaging at 1.5 Tesla. Cancer 66:40–44

Anzai Y, Prince MR, Chenevert TL, Maki JH, Londy F, London M, McLachlan SJ. MR angiography with an ultrasmall superparamagnetic iron oxide blood pool agent (1997) J Magn Reson Imaging 7:209–214

Anzai Y, Prince MR (1997). Iron oxide-enhanced MR lymphography: the evaluation of cervical lymph node metastases in head and neck cancer. J Magn Reson Imaging 7:75–81.

Bellin MF, Deray G, Assogba U, et al. (1992) Gd-DOTA: evaluation of its renal tolerance in patients with chronic renal failure. Magn Reson Imaging 10:115–118

Brown ED, Brown JJ, Kettritz U, Shoenut JP, Semelka RC (1996) Renal abscesses: appearance on gadolinium enhanced magnetic resonance images. Abdom Imaging 21:172–176

Carvlin MJ, Arger PH, Kundel HL, Axel L, Dougherty L, Kassab EA, Moore B (1987) Acute tubular necrosis: use of Gadolinium-DTPA and fast MR imaging to evaluate renal function in the rabbit. J Comput Assist Tomogr 11:488–495

Choyke PL (1988) MR imaging in renal cell carcinoma. Radiology 169:572–573

Choyke PL, Pollack HM (1988) The role of MRI in diseases of the kidney. Radiol Clin North Am 26:617–631

Choyke PL, White EM, Zeman RK, Jaffe MH, Clark LR (1987) Renal metastases: clinicopathologic and radiologic correlation. Radiology 162:359–363

Debatin JF, Spritzer CE, Grist TM, Beam C, Svetkey LP, Newman GE, Sostman HD (1991) Imaging of the renal arteries: value of MR angiography. AJR 157:981–990

Debatin JF, Ting RH, Wegmuller H, et al. (1994) Renal artery blood flow quantitation with phase contrast MR imaging with and without breath holding. Radiology 190:371–378

Debatin JF, Leung DA, Wildermuth S, Holtz D, McKinnon GC (1995) Advances in vascular echoplanar imaging. Cardiovasc Intervent Radiol 18:277–287

Dietrich RB, Kangarloo H (1986) Kidneys in infants and children: evaluation with MR. Radiology 159:215–221

Eilenberg SS, Lee JKT, Brown JJ, Mirowitz SA, Tartar VM (1990) Renal masses: evaluation with gradient-echo Gd-DTPA-enhanced dynamic MR imaging. Radiology 176:333–338

Fishman MC, Pollack HM, Arger PH, Banner MP (1984) Radiographic manifestations of spontaneous renal sinus hemorrhage. AJR 142:1161–1164

Frank JA, Choyke PL, Austin HA, Girton ME (1991) Functional MR of the kidney. Magn Reson Med 22:319–323

Friedburg HG, Hennig J, Frankenschmidt A (1987) RARE MR urography: a fast nontomographic imaging procedure for demonstrating the efferent urinary pathways using nuclear magnetic resonance. Radiologe 27:45–47

Gedroyc WM, Negus R, al Kutoubi A, Palmer A, Taube D, Hulme B (1992) Magnetic resonance angiography of renal transplants. Lancet 339:789–791

Grist TM, Charles HC, Sostman HD (1991) Renal transplant rejection: diagnosis with 31P MR spectroscopy. AJR 156: 105–112

Gylys Morin V, Hoffer FA, Kozakewich H, Shamberger RC (1993) Wilms tumor and nephroblastomatosis: imaging characteristics at gadolinium enhanced MR imaging. Radiology 188:517–521

Harmon WJ, King BF, Lieber MM (1996) Renal oncocytoma: magnetic resonance imaging characteristics. J Urol 155: 863–877

Hauser M, Krestin GP, Brennan RP, Burger HR, Fuchs WA (1992) Cross-sectional imaging for differentiation of bilateral solid multifocal intrarenal and perirenal lesions. Radiology 185 (P):344

Haustein J, Niendorf HP, Krestin G, Louton T, Schuhmann Giampieri G, Clauss W, Junge W (1992) Renal tolerance of gadolinium DTPA/dimeglumine in patients with chronic renal failure. Invest Radiol 27:153–156

Hockley NM, Foster RS, Bihrle R, Steidle CP, Kopecky KK (1990) Use of magnetic resonance imaging to determine surgical approach to renal cell carcinoma with vena caval extension. Urology 36:55–60

Holland JM (1973) Proceedings: cancer of the kidney – natural history and staging. Cancer 32:1030–1042

Hricak H, Amparo E, Fisher MR, Crooks LE, Higgins CB (1985) Abdominal venous system: assessment using MR. Radiology 156:415–422

Kendall AR, Senay BA, Coll ME (1988) Spontaneous subcapsular renal hematoma: diagnosis and management. J Urol 139:246–250

Kikinis R, von Schulthess GK, Jäger P, Dürr R, Bino M, Kuoni W, Kübler O (1987) Normal and hydronephrotic kidney: evaluation of renal function with contrast-enhanced MR imaging. Radiology 165:837–842

Kim SH, Park JH, Han JK, Han MC, Kim S, Lee JS (1992) Infarction of the kidney: role of contrast enhanced MRI. J Comput Assist Tomogr 16:924–928

Krestin GP (1990) Morphologic and functional MR of the kidneys and adrenal glands. Field & Wood, Philadelphia

Krestin GP (1994) Magnetic resonance imaging of the kidneys: current status. Magn Reson Q 10:2–21

Krestin GP, Friedmann G, Steinbrich W, Bunke J (1987) Fast MR imaging of renal and adrenal tumors: the value of dynamic studies with Gd-DTPA. Radiology 165(P): 272

Krestin GP, Friedmann G, Heindel W, Steinbrich W, Linden A (1988) Rapid Gd-DTPA-enhanced dynamic MR versus radionuclide nephrography for the assessment of renal function. Radiology 169(P):192

Krestin GP, Gross-Fengels W, Marincek B (1992) Bedeutung der Magnetresonanztomographie (MRT) für die Diagnostik und Stadieneinteilung des Nierenzellkarzinoms. Radiologe 32:121–126

Laissy JP, Faraggi M, Lebtahi R, et al. (1994) Functional evaluation of normal and ischemic kidney by means of gadolinium DOTA enhanced TurboFLASH MR imaging: a preliminary comparison with 99Tc MAG3 dynamic scintigraphy. Magn Reson Imaging 12:413–419

Lerner SE, Hawkins CA, Blute ML, Grabner A, Wollan PC, Eickholt JT, Zincke H (1996) Disease outcome in patients with low stage renal cell carcinoma treated with nephron sparing or radical surgery. J Urol 155:1868–1873

Leung DA, McKinnon GC, Davis CP, Pfammatter T, Krestin GP, Debatin JF (1996) Breath hold, contrast enhanced, three dimensional MR angiography. Radiology 200:569–571

Lieber MM, Tomera FM, Taylor WF, Farrow GM (1981) Renal adenocarcinoma in young adults: survival and variables affecting prognosis. J Urol 125:164–168

Lorenz CH, Powers TA, Partain CL (1992) Quantitative imaging of renal blood flow and function. Invest Radiol 27(Suppl 2):109–114

Marsh CL, Lange PH (1995) Rationale for total nephrectomy for suspected renal cell carcinoma. Semin Urol Oncol 13:273–280

McClennan BL (1991) Oncologic imaging. Staging and follow up of renal and adrenal carcinoma. Cancer 67(Supple 4): 1199–1208

Müller M, Krestin GP, Willi U (1993) Abdominale Tumoren beim Kind: Vergleich zwischen Magnetresonanztomographie (MRT) und Ultrasonographie (US). Fortschr Röntgenstr 158:9–14

Munechika H, Sullivan DC, Hedlund LW, Beam CA, Sostman HD, Herfkens RJ, Pelc NJ (1991) Evaluation of acute renal failure with magnetic resonance imaging using gradient-echo and Gd-DTPA. Invest Radiol 26:22–27

Myers BD, Sommer FG, Li K, et al. (1994) Determination of blood flow to the transplanted kidney. A novel application of phase contrast, cine magnetic resonance imaging. Transplantation 57:1445–1450

Myneni L, Hricak H, Carroll PR (1991) Magnetic resonance imaging of renal carcinoma with extension into the vena cava: staging accuracy and recent advances. Br J Urol 68: 571–578

Oya M, Nakamura K, Baba S, Hata J, Tazaki H (1995) Intrarenal satellites of renal cell carcinoma: histopathologic manifestation and clinical implication. Urology 46:161–164

Powers TA, Lorenz CH, Holburn GE, Price RR (1991) Renal artery stenosis: in vivo perfusion MR imaging. Radiology 178:543–548

Prince MR, Narasimham DL, Stanley JC, Chenevert TL, Williams DM, Marx MV, Cho KJ (1995) Breath hold gadolinium enhanced MR angiography of the abdominal aorta and its major branches. Radiology 197:785–792

Robson CJ, Churchill BM, Anderson W (1969) The results of radical nephrectomy for renal cell carcinoma. J Urol 101: 297–301

Rothpearl A, Frager D, Subramanian A, et al. (1995) MR urography: technique and application. Radiology 194:125–130

Roy C, Saussine C, Jahn C, et al. (1994) Evaluation of RARE MR urography in the assessment of ureterohydronephrosis. J Comput Assist Tomogr 18:601–608

Ruiz H, Saltzman B (1990) Aspirin-induced bilateral renal hemorrhage after extracorporeal shock wave lithotripsy therapy: implications and conclusions. J Urol 143:791–792

Schuhmann-Giampieri G, Krestin G (1991) Pharmacokinetics of Gd DTPA in patients with chronic renal failure. Invest Radiol 26:975–979

Semelka RC, Hricak H, Tomei E, Floth A, Stoller M (1990) Obstructive nephropathy: evaluation with dynamic Gd-DTPA-enhanced MR imaging. Radiology 175:797–803

Semelka RC, Hricak H, Stevens SK, Finegold R, Tomei E, Carroll PR (1991) Combined Gadolinium-enhanced and fat-saturation MR imaging of renal masses. Radiology 178:803–809

Semelka RC, Shoenut JP, Kroeker MA, MacMahon RG, Greenberg HM (1992) Renal lesions: controlled comparison between CT and 1.5T MR imaging with nonenhanced and gadolinium enhanced fat suppressed spin echo and breath hold FLASH techniques. Radiology 182:425–430

Semelka RC, Shoenut JP, Magro CM, Kroeker MA, MacMahon R, Greenberg HM (1993) Renal cancer staging: comparison of contrast enhanced CT and gadolinium enhanced fat suppressed spin echo and gradient echo MR imaging. J Magn Reson Imaging 3:597–602

Semelka RC, Corrigan K, Ascher SM, Brown JJ, Colindres-RE (1994) Renal corticomedullary differentiation: observation in patients with differing serum creatinine levels. Radiology 190:149–152

Servois V, Laissy JP, Feger C, et al. (1994) Two dimensional time of flight magnetic resonance angiography of renal arteries without maximum intensity projection: a prospective comparison with angiography in 21 patients screened for renovascular hypertension. Cardiovasc Intervent Radiol 17:138–142

Sigmund G, Stoever B, Zimmerhackl LB, et al. (1991) RARE MR urography in the diagnosis of upper urinary tract abnormalities in children. Pediatr Radiol 21:416–420

Sokoloff MH, deKernion JB, Figlin RA, Belldegrun A (1996) Current management of renal cell carcinoma. CA Cancer J Clin 46:284–302

Spritzer CE, Sussman SK, Blinder RA, Saeed M, Herfkens RJ (1988) Deep venous thrombosis evaluation with limited-flip-angle, gradient-refocused MR imaging: preliminary experience. Radiology 166:371–375

Steinbach F, Stockle M, Hohenfellner R (1995) Clinical experience with nephron sparing surgery in the presence of a normal contralateral kidney. Semin Urol Oncol 13:288–291

Stillman AE, Wilke N, Li D, Haacke M, McLachlan S (1996). Ultrasmall superparamagnetic iron oxide to enhance MRA of the renal and coronary arteries: studies in human pa-

tients. J Comput Assist Tomogr 20:51–55

Vestring T, Dietl KH, Fahrenkamp A, et al. (1992) Cortical necrosis of the transplanted kidney. MR tomographic confirmation of the diagnosis? ROFO Fortschr Geb Rontgenstr Neuen Bildgeb Verfahr 156:507–512

von Schulthess GK (1989) Morphology and function in MRI. Springer, Berlin Heidelberg New York

von Schulthess GK, Kuoni W, Gerig G, Wüthrich R, Duewell S, Krestin GP (1991) Semiautomated ROI analysis in dynamic MR studies. II. Application to renal function examination. J Comput Assist Tomogr 15:733–741

Vosshenrich R, Kallerhoff M, Grone HJ, et al. (1996) Detection of renal ischemic lesions using Gd-DTPA enhanced turbo FLASH MRI: experimental and clinical results. J Comput Assist Tomogr 20:236–243

Wurstlin S, Arlart IP, Guhl L, Nagler Reus N, Edelman RR (1993) Magnetic resonance tomographic identification and characterization of renal space occupying lesions using GE sequences with application of Gd-DTPA. ROFO Fortschr Geb Rontgenstr Neuen Bildgeb Verfahr 158:518–524

Yucel EK, Kaufman JA, Prince M, Bazari H, Fang LS, Waltman AC (1993) Time of flight renal MR angiography: utility in patients with renal insufficiency. Magn Reson Imaging 11:925–930

Zerhouni EA, Schellhammer P, Schaefer JC, et al. (1984) Management of bleeding renal angiomyolipomas by transcatheter embolization following CT diagnosis. Urol Radiol 6:205–209

Zimmerhackl LB, Rehm M, Kaufmehl K, Kurlemann G, Brandis M (1994) Renal involvement in tuberous sclerosis complex: a retrospective survey. Pediatr Nephrol 8:451–457

13 Lymphatic System

R.H. Oyen

CONTENTS

13.1
Introduction

Magnetic resonance imaging (MRI) is noninvasive, well tolerated, rather simple to perform, and capable of direct imaging of the retroperitoneal area, including retroperitoneal nodal areas. Theoretically MRI has several advantages, including the ability to display vascular anatomy without the need for intravascular contrast agents. Other general advantages of MRI include multiplanar imaging capability and superior soft tissue contrast resolution. Poorer spatial resolution may, however, compromise the visualization of normal structures (e.g., differentiation of normal lymph nodes from bowel loops and vessels). Oral contrast agents for MRI are not yet routinely used, and differentiating lymphadenopathy from bowel loops is a challenge. Continuous technical improvements, however, are reducing the acquisition times needed for imaging, improving resolution, and decreasing artifacts from patient movement and peristaltic and respiratory motion. Finally, the availability of MRI is increasing. For these reasons MRI will attract greater interest for the evaluation of the retroperitoneal space and retroperitoneal disease processes. In this chapter only more frequent diseases of the retroperitoneal lymphatic system will be discussed.

13.2
Retroperitoneal Cystic Lymphangioma

Retroperitoneal cystic lymphangioma is a rare benign neoplasm of the lymphatic system. It consists of various numbers of cyst-like cavities filled with a serous, serosanguinous, or chylous fluid with high signal intensity on T2-weighted sequences (Fig. 13.1). The pathogenesis of cystic lymphangioma is still unclear. Cystic lymphangioma most commonly occurs in the neck (75%) and in the axillary region (20%); it is rare in the retroperitoneum. It is also rare in the mediastinum, mesentery, omentum, colon, pelvis, groin, spleen, bone, and skin. Although retroperitoneal cystic lymphangioma is a benign lesion, it may cause significant morbidity due to its large size and its often invasive character, with a strong tendency to secondary infection. Cystic lymphangioma can grow very large from the mediastinum through the retroperitoneum to the groin (FISHER and HILLER 1994). Multiplanar MRI is best suited to evaluate the exact extent of these lesions (BONHOMME et al. 1997). Rarely multiple cystic lymphangiomas at different sites have been reported (GRAF et al. 1993). The treatment of choice is surgical excision; needle aspiration and tuberculostatic therapy have also been used successfully (FISHER and HILLER 1994). A case has been described of a rare localization of the disease originating in the left lower extremity and extending into the retroperitoneum and mediastinum in a 16-year-old female (MUHLE et al. 1992). MRI contributed to the diagnosis and the exact determination of the extent. Investigation 1.5 years later revealed that the lymphangiomas in the left thigh had reduced and the proliferation of lymphangioma in the retroperitoneum and mediastinum had stagnated. Symptomatic or infected collections may be effectively drained by percutaneous radiologic techniques.

R.H. OYEN, MD, PhD, Department of Radiology, University Hospitals K.U. Leuven, Herestraat 49, B-3000 Leuven, Belgium

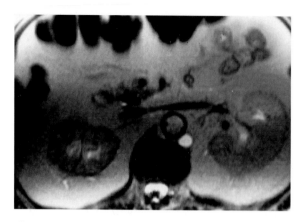

Fig. 13.1. Axial MR shows a small lymphangioma (retroperitoneal lymphatic cyst) displaying high signal intensities on this HASTE sequence

13.3
Renal Peripelvic Lymphatic Cysts

Renal peripelvic lymphatic cysts (in fact they should be considered lymphangiomas) are usually seen as an isolated finding. They appear as multiple mass lesions with low attenuation on computed tomography (CT) and show no contrast enhancement. The lesions have low signal intensity on T1-weighted images and high signal intensity on T2-weighted images (YOUNATHAN and KAUDE 1992).

13.4
Lymph Node Disease

Lymph node enlargement is the only criterion for abnormality when using MRI. In the abdomen and pelvis lymph nodes larger than 1.5 cm in cross-sectional diameter are considered abnormal whereas retrocrural nodes are considered abnormal if larger than 6 mm. Enlarged lymph nodes are most readily identified in patients who have abundant pelvic and retroperitoneal fat. The detection of nodal enlargement in thin adults is often considerably more difficult because of lack of perivascular and retroperitoneal fat. Another problem interfering with the diagnosis of retroperitoneal lymph nodes is that fluid-filled bowel loops can mimic adenopathy and may be difficult to differentiate. In general transverse scans are sufficient for the detection of lymphadenopathy. Coronal or sagittal imaging does not add substantial diagnostic information.

Lymph nodes have a T1 relaxation time similar to that of muscle and longer than that of fat. Therefore lymph nodes are readily distinguished from surrounding fat on predominantly T1-weighted image sequences. T2-weighted images can distinguish lymph nodes from surrounding muscle but may decrease the conspicuity of lymph nodes surrounded by fat. Nodes that are calcified, necrotic, or filled with lymphangiographic contrast may be heterogeneous and become indistinguishable from surrounding fat. One report indeed suggested that because certain lymphangiographic contrast agents may reduce the T1 time and prolong the T2 relaxation time of opacified lymph nodes, abnormal lymph nodes may be indistinguishable from surrounding fat on standard spin-echo MR pulse sequences (BUCKWALTER et al. 1992).

13.4.1
Benign Lymphadenopathy

Benign lymphadenopathies seldom occur in the retroperitoneal cavity. They represent only 6% of all lymph node enlargement (DEUTCH et al. 1987). A variety of inflammatory and granulomatous diseases may demonstrate retroperitoneal lymphadenopathy. Tuberculosis, sarcoidosis, mastocytosis, rheumatoid arthritis, Crohn's disease, Whipple's disease, and amyloidosis have to be considered as a potential cause of benign retroperitoneal lymph node enlargement. A rare cause of lymphadenopathy is sinus histiocytosis with massive lymphadenopathy, which is seen predominantly in the first two decades of life (MERINE et al. 1987). Finally, lymph node enlargement has also been described as a late complication of renal transplantation, occasionally even in the form of bulky disease (FRICK et al. 1984). Lymphography will probably continue to play an important role in the staging of lymphatic malignancy in centers with great expertise.

Reactive lymph nodes can reach a size of more than 2 cm, especially in immunosuppressed patients. Documentation of enlarged lymph nodes can be of importance in patients without malignancies, revealing a target for diagnostic biopsies or sources of cultures as, for example, in patients with fever of unknown origin. Unfortunately, MRI is not able to distinguish benign from malignant lymph nodes. It has been shown in animal studies (rabbits) that reactive lymph node hyperplasia induced by interstitial egg yolk injection and lymph node metastases secondary to implantation of VX2 tumors (squamous cell carcinoma) cannot be differentiated by standard MRI (these models therefore may serve for testing the efficacy of lymphographic techniques in MRI) (WAGNER 1994). Consequently malignant lymphomas and lymph node metastases must be considered in the diagnosis of benign lymphadenopathy. Percutaneous needle biopsy of enlarged lymph nodes may be important in these cases to establish a histologic diagnosis. Differentiation between benign and malignant lymphadenopathy is particularly important in patients with AIDS, in which lymphadenopathy may represent lymphoma, Kaposi's sarcoma, tuberculosis, or benign reactive disease. Opportunistic infections in AIDS patients are often caused by *Mycobacterium avium-intracellulare*. The most common manifestation is retroperitoneal and mesenteric lymphadenopathy, sometimes with necrotic areas in larger lymph nodes (FEDERLE et al. 1988). With *Pneumocystis carinii* infections, calcifications may be expected (RADIN et al. 1990).

13.4.2
Castleman's Disease

Castleman's disease is a benign disease characterized by lymph node enlargement due to hyperplasia of abnormal lymphoid follicles and paracortical lymphocytic hyaline vascular stroma or plasmacytosis (MENKE et al. 1996). There is a wide variety of nonspecific radiologic findings (FIELDS et al. 1995). Coexistence of Hodgkin's disease and Castleman's disease is well documented in the literature (ABDEL-REHEIM et al. 1996). Precise staging is important to separate the widespread from the localized form of the disease, as the localized form may be successfully treated surgically. On CT, significant enhancement with intravenous contrast is indicative of Castleman's disease. Calcifications may be found. On T1-weighted images the masses have intermediate or high signal intensity with areas of low signal intensity due to vessels and calcification. On T2-weighted images, the masses are of high signal intensity (MOON et al. 1994; YAMASHITA et al. 1993). Rarely origin from lymphoid tissue is not obvious. This explains why extranodal forms of Castleman's disease have been reported. An example is a case with an extralymphatic para-adrenal manifestation where coronal MRI contributed in demonstrating the extraadrenal location of the mass. The signal characteristics in this patient were similar to those in cases with typical cervical, mediastinal, or retroperitoneal locations (YAMAKITA et al. 1992). Such signal characteristics, however, are not specific for this benign condition; rather, the findings are similar to those in

lymphadenopathy, lymphoma, or metastases. Moreover, association with lymphoma has been reported (ABDEL-REHEIM et al. 1996). In tumors or masses with the above characteristics in areas where lymphoid tissue is normally present, Castleman's disease should be added to the differential diagnosis.

13.4.3
Lymphoma

The malignant lymphomas are primary neoplasms of the lymphatic system. These tumors first involve lymph node groups and eventually spread to other organ systems. The staging and follow-up of lymphomas varies among institutions. Abdominal and pelvic CT scanning is the most frequently used technique for assessment of the retroperitoneal and pelvic lymph nodes in patients with Hodgkin's disease and non-Hodgkin's lymphoma. Evaluation of other subdiaphragmatic lymph node sites (mesentery, splenic hilus, porta hepatis, celiac axis) with CT and probably with MRI is relatively insensitive in patients with Hodgkin's disease. In contrast, the frequently (50%) enlarged nodes at these sites in patients with non-Hodgkin's lymphomas are more readily detected by CT scans. However, when such abnormality is detected, these patients generally have known evidence of disease at other subdiaphragmatic sites, so that this incremental information rarely impacts on patient management or stage. Recent studies indicate that MRI has the same potential as CT for detection of retroperitoneal and intraperitoneal lymph nodes in patients with lymphoma (CASTELLINO 1991) (Fig. 13.2). One of the major limitations of MRI is its difficulty in differentiating masses from bowels and blood vessels. Attempts are being made to use nonbiodegradable superparamagnetic particles, in plain and viscous aqueous suspensions, as oral contrast medium (LONNEMARK 1991). Such paramagnetic particles at a concentration of 0.5 g/l displayed a good contrast effect at 0.5 T, and permitted differentiation of bowels from adjacent structures, resulting in improved diagnostic accuracy.

In general, it is felt that MRI does not improve on the diagnostic accuracy compared with CT imaging (ELLIS 1984). A comparative study of CT and MRI in the initial assessment of lymphoma suggested that MRI (0.15 T; no contrast enhancement), although more sensitive than CT, was less specific, yielding more false-positive findings (SKILLINGS et al. 1991). In another series the authors concluded that MRI

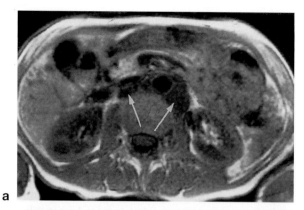

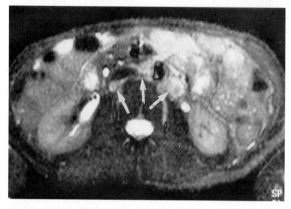

Fig. 13.2 a,b. Retroperitoneal lymphadenopathies in a patient with lymphoma. The lymph nodes are hypointense on the T1-weighted image (*arrows* in **a**) and are heterogeneously hyperintense on the T2-weighted image (*arrows* in **b**). Note that in this thin patient it is difficult to distinguish lymph nodes from bowel loops

mass is inactive (MONTALBAN et al. 1992) (Fig. 13.2). This is consistent with signal characteristics obtained in patients with histologically proven retroperitoneal fibrosis (VAN HOE et al. 1995; AMISS 1991; ARRIVE et al. 1989). Benign retroperitoneal fibrosis has a low signal intensity on both T1- and T2-weighted images. When a mass displays high signal intensity on T2-weighted images, however, differentiation between malignant retroperitoneal fibrosis and benign yet immature fibrosis is impossible.

The role of MRI in predicting relapse in residual masses after treatment of lymphoma has been investigated in several studies (HILL et al. 1993). MRI has a high specificity (90%), positive predictive value (71%), and negative predictive value (75%), but poor sensitivity (45%). Comparison with other investigations (i.e., CT, gallium-67 single-photon emission CT, erythrocyte sedimentation rate) showed that it was the only investigation to allow the prediction of relapse.

As mentioned above, lymph node enlargement has also been described in AIDS patients as part of systemic disease. Malignant degeneration is possible in such cases. The most common type of AIDS-related lymphoma is non-Hodgkin's lymphoma, but Burkitt's lymphoma and Hodgkin's lymphoma are also seen (KUHLMAN et al. 1991). In general these lymphomas have a somewhat greater predilection for extranodal sites, and non-Hodgkin's lymphoma may be the first manifestation of AIDS before other AIDS-related diseases or opportunistic infections. Kaposi's sarcoma usually manifests as bulky adenopathy and tumor infiltrating the retroperitoneum.

and CT may be equivalent in the detection of nodal involvement, but that MRI has advantages in its ability to diagnose bone marrow involvement (HOANE et al. 1994).

Signal intensities reflect gross histologic characteristics and cannot be considered specific, especially in the first 6 months after the initiation of therapy. Tumor size changes and signal intensity changes are not parallel in all cases. Therefore it has been proposed that MRI may only have a role in monitoring masses in patients with lymphoma (RAHMOUNI et al. 1993). Others, however, found that low signal intensity on T2-weighted sequences matched residual fibrous masses, whereas high signal intensity was seen in both fibrous and tumor masses (COHEN-HAGUENAUER et al. 1993; MONTALBAN et al. 1992). Progressive disease or relapse is more likely to occur in patients with high signal intensity on T2-weighted images; hypointensity therefore suggests that the

13.4.4
Metastatic Lymphadenopathy

Metastatic retroperitoneal tumors are usually lymph node metastases from a pelvic, testicular, lung, or gastrointestinal malignancy. The N-staging in patients with known malignancy relies on the size of the lymph nodes (Figs. 13.3, 13.4). As mentioned earlier, in the abdomen and pelvis, lymph nodes larger than 1.5 cm in cross-sectional diameter are considered abnormal. A solitary pelvic or abdominal lymph node between 1 and 1.5 cm in size is regarded with suspicion, and a cluster of multiple small nodes is also suspect. Nevertheless, size should not be the only criterion. In a prospective study of patients with prostatic carcinoma it has been shown that asymmetry is an important additional criterion, too (OYEN et al. 1994). Certainly, the presence of enlarged retro-

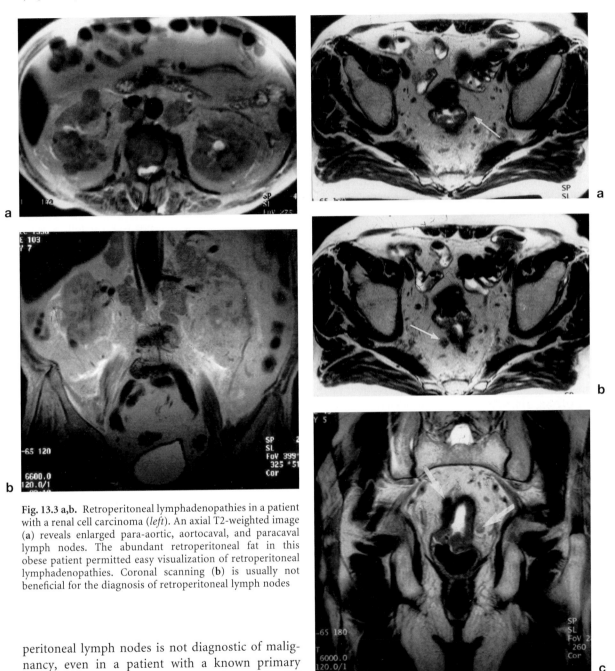

Fig. 13.3 a,b. Retroperitoneal lymphadenopathies in a patient with a renal cell carcinoma (*left*). An axial T2-weighted image (**a**) reveals enlarged para-aortic, aortocaval, and paracaval lymph nodes. The abundant retroperitoneal fat in this obese patient permitted easy visualization of retroperitoneal lymphadenopathies. Coronal scanning (**b**) is usually not beneficial for the diagnosis of retroperitoneal lymph nodes

Fig. 13.4 a–c. Rectal carcinoma with pararectal lymphadenopathies (*arrows*). **a,b** Axial and **c** coronal T2-weighted sequences. Although the lymph nodes are only 1 cm in diameter, they should be considered as metastatically involved in a patient with rectal carcinoma

peritoneal lymph nodes is not diagnostic of malignancy, even in a patient with a known primary tumor. In one study which compared CT with MRI in the evaluation of metastatic retroperitoneal adenopathy from testicular carcinoma it was found that the two modalities were comparable (ELLIS 1984). It should be mentioned that in these patients, after successful therapy, residual fibrosis or necrosis can result in para-aortic masses that, with CT, are indistinguishable from recurrent or residual tumor (Soo et al. 1981). With MRI the low signal of fibrosis on T2-weighted images may serve as a criterion to distinguish it from tumor and edema, which show a high signal intensity.

In the imaging of metastatic lymphadenopathy, MRI suffers from the following drawbacks. First, it has limited ability to differentiate lymphadenopathy from bowels and blood vessels (Fig. 13.3). Second, there are no specific signal characteristics to distinguish enlarged metastatic lymph nodes from enlarged reactive lymph nodes. Third, it is not possible to detect micrometastases in lymph nodes of normal size. Some authors have used dynamic contrast-enhanced single-section turbo fast low-angle shot (FLASH) images to identify metastatic lymph nodes in patients with bladder carcinoma (BARENTSZ et al. 1996). It is known that on CT lymph nodes enhance after intravenous administration of iodinated contrast medium; Barentsz et al. observed similar enhancement of metastatic nodes with MRI. All metastatic lymph nodes that were depicted with this technique showed enhancement as early as or even slightly earlier than the bladder tumor. The authors reported that this technique was even sensitive enough to depict metastases in nodes of a normal size (11 × 6 × 5mm). It is questionable, however, whether this single-section technique allows the consistent depiction of normal-sized lymph nodes. Moreover, BARENTSZ et al. reported that in two patients with benign lymph nodes (one enlarged, one of normal size) early enhancement was demonstrated (false-positive enhancement). This is not really surprising since hyperemia is expected in reactive lymph nodes. Therefore the value of this technique requires further investigation.

The same authors have used three-dimensional T1-weighted magnetization-prepared rapid gradient echo (MP-RAGE) imaging (BARENTSZ et al. 1996). Multiplanar reconstruction was performed with these MP-RAGE data in which the pelvic lymph nodes were optimally visible. The authors reported a high accuracy of the combination of the three-dimensional MP-RAGE and the dynamic technique in the staging of lymph nodes in patients with bladder carcinoma (93%). It is important to emphasize that the difference between unenhanced and enhanced images in terms of accuracy for nodal staging did not appear to be significant.

13.4.5
Future Perspectives

Several studies are ongoing to find lymph node-specific contrast agents. In an animal study (in rats) differentiation between normal and metastatic lymph nodes improved when diethylene triamine penta-acetic acid (DTPA) conjugated with a polyglucose-associated macrocomplex (PGM) was administered intravenously (dose 2, 10, or 20mmol gadolinium per kilogram of tissue) (HARIKA et al. 1996). When labeled with Gd-DTPA, the PGM-based graft co-polymer significantly increased signal intensity on MR images of normal but not of metastatic lymph nodes without causing distortion artifacts.

BENGELE et al. (1994) investigated the use of the ultrasmall superparamagnetic iron oxide colloid BMS 180549, which accumulates in lymph nodes following either subcutaneous or intravenous injection. With a subcutaneous injection in the front extremities, the axillary and brachial nodes attained the highest accumulations of the agent. With a subcutaneous injection in the rear extremities, the popliteal, iliac, and axillary lymph nodes attained the highest accumulations. With intravenous injection, the iliac, mediastinal, and mesenteric nodes attained the highest accumulations.

Superparamagnetic iron oxide nanoparticles (AMI-227) showed regional specificity with significant enhancement of nodal structures and demonstrated potential as an interstitial MR lymphographic agent (TANOURA et al. 1992). According to another study (in rats) AMI-227 uptake may help differentiate tumor-bearing from non-tumor-bearing lymph nodes (VASSALO et al. 1994). In the latter study the signal intensity of hyperplastic nodes was lower than on unenhanced images. This T2 effect was a result of active uptake of particles by macrophages in the lymphatic sinuses. In this way, even small metastases (3mm in diameter) were discernible when using the optimal examination time (12h after interstitial administration) and with proton density weighted spin-echo sequences (HAMM et al. 1992; TAUPITZ et al. 1993a,b). At higher doses the tumor itself consistently showed increased signal intensity on T1-weighted images. This T1 effect probably resulted from particles leaking into the interstitial spaces of the tumor and probably indicates altered capillary permeability in tumor (GUIMARAES et al. 1994; OKUHATA 1992).

The utility of a monocrystalline iron oxide nanoparticle as a contrast agent in MRI of lymph nodes was investigated by WEISSLEDER et al. (1994) in rabbits. It was shown that nodal accumulation occurred primarily after extravasation of the agent into the interstitial space and subsequent trapping by lymph node macrophages.

Experimental results in an animal model (rabbit) have indicated that inhalational administration of iron colloid agents can deliver them to the pulmonary lymphatic system and has potential for lung hilar and mediastinal MR lymphography (OKUHATA et al. 1994; CASE et al. 1992).

References

Abdel-Reheim FA, Koss W, Rappaport ES, Arber DA (1996) Coexistence of Hodgkin's disease and giant lymph node hyperplasia of plasma-cell type. Arch Pathol Lab Med 120:91–96

Amis ES (1991) Retroperitoneal fibrosis. Am J Roentgenol 157:321–329

Arrive L, Hricak H, Tavares NJ, Miller TR (1989) Malignant versus non-malignant retroperitoneal fibrosis: differentiation with MR imaging. Radiology 172:139–143

Barentsz JO, Jager GJ, van Vierzen PBJ, et al. (1996) Staging urinary bladder cancer after transurethral biopsy: value of fast dynamic contrast-enhanced MR imaging. Radiology 201:185–193

Bengele HH, Palmacci S, Rogers J, Jung CW, Crenshaw J, Josephson L (1994) Biodistribution of an ultrasmall superparamagnetic iron oxide colloid, BMS 180549, by different routes of administration. Magn Reson Imaging 12:433–442

Bonhomme A, Broeders A, Oyen RH, Stas M, De Wever I, Baert AL (1997) Cystic lymphangioma of the retroperitoneum: case report. Br J Radiol (to be published)

Buckwalter KA, Ellis JH, Baker DE, Borello JA, Glazer GM (1992) Pitfall in MR imaging of lymphadenopathy after lymphangiography. Radiology 161:831–832

Case TC, Unger E, Bernas MJ, et al. (1992) Lymphatic imaging in experimental filariasis using magnetic resonance. Invest Radiol 27:293–297

Castellino RA (1991) Diagnostic imaging evaluation of Hodgkin's disease and non-Hodgkin's lymphoma. Cancer 67:1177–1180

Cohen-Haguenauer O, Brice P, Gaci M, et al. (1993) Gallium-67 scintigraphy in malignant lymphoma. Press Med 22:521–525

Deutch SJ, Sandler MA, Alpern MA (1987) Abdominal lymphadenopathy in benign diseases: CT detection. Radiology 163:335–338

Ellis HH (1984) Comparison of NMR and CT imaging in the evaluation of metastatic retroperitoneal lymphadenopathy from testicular carcinoma. J Comput Assist Tomogr 8:709–719

Federle MP, Nyberg DA, Hulnick DH, Jeffrey RB (1988) Malignant neoplasms: Kaposi's sarcoma, lymphoma, and other diseases with similar radiographic features. In: Federle MP, Megibow AJ, Naidich DP (eds) Radiology of AIDS. Raven Press, New York, p 107

Fields S, Bar-Ziv J, Portnoy O, Sasson T, Sherman Y, Libson E (1995) Radiologic spectrum of localized Castleman's disease. Isr J Med Sci 31:660–669

Fisher D, Hiller N (1994) Case report: giant tuberculous cystic lymphangioma of posterior mediastinum, retroperitoneum and groin. Clin Radiol 49:215–216

Frick MP, Salomonowitz E, Hanto DW, Gedgaudas-McClees K (1984) CT of abdominal lymphoma after renal transplantation. Am J Roentgenol 142:97–99

Graf D, Pfister J, Streuli HK (1993) Multiple retroperitoneal and mediastinal lymph cysts in primary ectatic lymph vessels. Helv Chir Acta 60:27–30

Guimaraes R, Clement O, Bittoun J, Carnot F, Frija G (1994) MR lymphography with supermagnetic iron nanoparticles in rats: pathologic basis for contrast enhancement. Am J Roentgenol 162:201–207

Hamm B, Taupitz M, Hussmann P, Wagner S, Wolf KJ (1992) MR lymphography with iron oxide particles: dose response studies and pulse sequence optimization in rabbits. Am J Roentgenol 158:183–190

Harika L, Weissleder R, Poss K, Papisov MI (1996) Macromolecular intravenous contrast agent for MR lymphography: characterization and efficacy studies. Radiology 198:365–370

Havard AC, Collins DJ, Guy RL, Husband JE (1992) Magnetic resonance behaviour of lipiodol. Clin Radiol 45:198–200

Hill M, Cunningham D, MacVicar D, et al. (1993) Role of magnetic resonance imaging in predicting relapse in residual masses after treatment of lymphoma. J Clin Oncol 11:2273–2278

Hoane BR, Shields AF, Porter BA, Borrow JW (1994) Comparison of initial lymphoma staging using computed tomography and magnetic resonance imaging. Am J Hematol 47:100–105

Kuhlman JE, Browne D, Shermak M, Hamper UM, Zerhouni EA, Fishman EK (1991) Retroperitoneal and pelvic CT of patients with AIDS: primary and secondary involvement of the genitourinary tract. Radiographics 11:473

Lonnemark M (1991) Superparamagnetic particles as oral contrast medium in MR imaging of malignant lymphoma. Acta Radiol 32:232–238

Menke DM, Tiemann M, Camoriano JK, et al. (1996) Diagnosis of Castleman's disease by identification of an immunophenotypically aberrant population of mantle zone B lymphocytes in paraffin-embedded lymph node biopsies. Am J Clin Pathol 105:268–276

Merine D, Fishman EK, Siegelman SS (1987) Renal xanthogranulomatosis: radiological, clinical and pathological features in two cases. J Comput Assist Tomogr 11:785–789

Montalban C, Rodriguez-Garcia JL, Mazairas L, Ayala I, Marcos-Robles J (1992) Magnetic resonance imaging for the assessment of residual masses after treatment of non-Hodgkin's lymphomas. Postgrad Med J 68:643–647

Moon WK, Im JG, Han MC (1994) Castleman's disease of the mediastinum: MR imaging features. Clin Radiol 49:466–468

Muhle C, Asmus R, Spielmann RP (1992) Magnetic resonance tomographic characteristics and follow-up observation in a case of cystic lymphangiomas in the left lower extremity, the retroperitoneum and the mediastinum. Aktuel Radiol 2:159–161

Nuzzo G, Lemmo G, Trischitta MM, Boldrini G, Giovannini I (1996) Retroperitoneal cystic lymphangioma. J Surg Oncol 61:234–237

Okuhata Y (1992) An experimental study on MR lymphography with various iron colloid agents. Nippon Igaku Hoshasen Gakkai Zasshi 25:1148–1160

Okuhata Y, Xia T, Urahashi S (1994) Inhalation MR lymphography: a new method for selective enhancement of the lung hilar and mediastinal lymph nodes. Magn Reson Imaging 12:1135–1138

Oyen RH, Van Poppel HP, Ameye FE, Van de Voorde WA, Baert AL, Baert LV (1994) Lymph node staging of localized prostatic carcinoma with CT and CT-guided fine-needle aspiration biopsy: a prospective study of 285 patients. Radiology 190:315–322

Radin DR, Baker EL, Klatt EC (1990) Visceral and nodal calcifications in patients with AIDS-related Pneumocystis carinii infection. Am J Roentgenol 154:27

Rahmouni A, Tempany C, Jones R, Mann R, Yang A, Zerhouni E (1993) Lymphoma: monitoring tumor size and signal intensity with MR imaging. Radiology 188:445–451

Skillings JR, Bramwell V, Nicholson RL, Prato FS, Wells G (1991) A prospective study of magnetic resonance imaging in lymphoma staging. Cancer 67:1838–1843

Soo CS, Bernardino ME, Chuang VP, Ordonez N (1981) Pitfalls of CT findings in post-therapy testicular carcinoma. J Comput Assist Tomogr 5:39–41

Tanoura T, Bernas M, Darkazanli A, Elam E, Unger E, Witte MH, Green A (1992) MR lymphography with iron oxide compound AMI-227: studies in ferrets with filariasis. Am J Roentgenol 159:875–881

Taupitz M, Wagner S, Hamm B, Binder A, Pfefferer D (1993a) Interstitial MR lymphography with iron particles: results in tumor-free and VX2 tumor-bearing rabbits. Am J Roentgenol 161:193–200

Taupitz M, Wagner S, Hamm B, Dienemann D, Lawaczeck R, Wolf KJ (1993b) MR lymphography using iron oxide particles. Detection of lymph node metastases in the VX2 rabbit tumor model. Acta Radiol 34:10–15

Van Hoe L, Oyen R, Gryspeerdt S, Baert AL, Bobbaers H, Baert L (1995) Pseudotumoral pelvic retroperitoneal fibrosis associated with orbital fibrosis. Case report. Br J Radiol 68:421–423

Vassallo P, Matei C, Heston WD, McLachlan SJ, Koutcher JA, Castellino RA (1994) AMI-227-enhanced MR lympho-graphy: usefulness for differentiating reactive from tumor-bearing lymph nodes. Radiology 193:501–506

Wagner S (1994) Benign lymph node hyperplasia and lymph node metastases in rabbits. Animal models for magnetic resonance lymphography. Invest Radiol 29:364–371

Weissleder R, Heautot JF, Schaffer BK, Nossiff N, Papisov MI, Bogdanov A Jr, Brady TJ (1994) MR lymphography: study of a high-efficiency lymphotropic agent. Radiology 191:225–230

Yamakita N, Sugimoto M, Takeda N, et al. (1992) Pseudo-adrenal incidentaloma: magnetic resonance imaging in a patient with para-adrenal Castleman's disease. Urol Int 49:171–174

Yamashita Y, Hirai T, Matsukawa T, Ogata I, Takahashi M (1993) Radiological presentations of Castleman's disease. Comput Med Imaging Graph 17:107–117

Younathan CM, Kaude JV (1992) Renal peripelvic cysts (lym-phangiomas) associated with generalized lymphan-giomatosis. Urol Radiol 14:161–164

14 Stomach, Duodenum, and Small Bowel

H.-J. Brambs

CONTENTS

14.1
Introduction

At present, magnetic resonance imaging (MRI) does not have an established role in the diagnostic evaluation of gastrointestinal disease. However, the development of fast and powerful gradient coils, artifact suppression techniques, and rapid pulse sequences has improved image quality and reduced image degradation from respiratory- and peristalsis-induced motion artifacts. These refinements have essentially facilitated gastrointestinal MRI, and recent studies have shown the utility of MRI in the assessment of gastrointestinal disorders.

Endoscopy and double contrast barium studies are the primary means for establishing the diagnosis of a pathology of the upper gastrointestinal tract. MRI is at present not routinely used for the gastrointestinal tract for a variety of reasons which are based on economic grounds (high costs and availability) and diagnostic strategies which favor endoscopic examinations over cross-sectional imaging in gastrointestinal disease. Exceptions to the rule are alterations of the small bowel, where the endoscopic approach is limited. Complications which occur predominantly extraluminally cannot be detected endoscopically, and the development of strictures makes endoscopy more difficult or impossible.

Basically, MRI of the gastrointestinal tract is a source of numerous pitfalls and misinterpretations. Retained food within the gastrointestinal lumen can simulate a mass. Depending on the contents (air, fluids, lipids, proteinaceous material), the gastrointestinal tract can show a variety of signal intensity patterns which hamper diagnosis. Particularly air within the bowels can create significant susceptibility artifacts. Nondistension of the gastrointestinal tract can simulate focal or diffuse thickening of a bowel segment appearing to represent inflammatory or neoplastic disease. Small bowel loops usually demonstrate a signal intensity similar to that of soft tissue. Therefore such loops cannot be differentiated from enlarged lymph nodes or other abdominal masses. Peristaltic gastric and bowel motion results in blurring of the gastrointestinal wall. These types of artifacts are particularly severe on T2-weighted images.

14.2
Oral Contrast Agents

One of the rationales for developing intraluminal gastrointestinal contrast agents for MRI is to distinguish bowel loops from other abdominal structures such as the pancreas (Brasch 1992). Oral contrast agents will be used in a similar manner to the oral contrast agents used with computed tomography (CT) scanning. As with CT scanning, it can be difficult to distinguish collapsed bowel from adjacent disease and it can be impossible to identify intrinsic bowel abnormalities on MR images acquired without an oral contrast agent.

A remarkably wide variety of compounds with varying properties have been introduced as potential

H.-J. Brambs, MD, Professor, Director, Department of Diagnostic Radiology, Radiologische Universitätsklinik und Poliklinik, Steinhövelstrasse 9, D-89075 Ulm, Germany

gastrointestinal contrast agents for MRI. These contrast agents can be classified as positive, such as Gd-DTPA and oil emulsions (KAMINSKY et al. 1991; HAMED et al. 1992; MIROWITZ 1993), or negative, such as superparamagnetic iron oxides, perflubron, and barium (HAHN et al. 1990; OKSENDAL et al. 1991; MATTREY et al. 1994). These contrast agents can be further classified as miscible or immiscible with water. Miscible agents mix with the bowel contents and alter their signal intensity, whereas immiscible agents mark the bowel lumen by replacing the bowel contents.

There are some theoretical advantages and disadvantages to both positive and negative bowel contrast agents (BROWN 1996). It depends particularly on the clinical problem whether it is preferable to increase or decrease the intraluminal signal. At present, there is no consensus regarding which oral contrast agent is ideal. In the future, several compounds will be available with different properties, and the radiologist will be asked to select the agent most appropriate for the clinical problem being investigated.

For evaluating intrinsic abnormalities of the bowel wall, administration of an intravenous gadolinium chelate is useful. In these cases a negative oral contrast agent should be used.

Optimal bowel contrast is achieved when the marking is uniform throughout the bowel and adequate contrast between the bowel loop and the surrounding structures can be achieved. The volume of oral contrast agent used and the timing of imaging must be tailored to the abdominal region being investigated.

14.3
MR Technique

14.3.1
Stomach and Duodenum

As with CT, optimal delineation of the gastric and duodenal wall is achieved by distension of the lumen. For this purpose a substantial volume of contrast medium has to be administered. As with CT, the most common diagnostic dilemma in gastric MRI is the need to differentiate mural thickening that is truly pathologic from a circumscribed area of incomplete distension. With adequate distension the symmetrical distribution of the gastric folds can be clearly seen. After intravenous gadolinium the stomach wall enhances significantly on immediate

postcontrast images and a severely enhancing inner zone (mucosa and submucosa) can be differentiated from a less enhancing outer zone (muscle layer) (HAMED et al. 1992; MIROWITZ 1993). The combination of contrast enhancement and fat-suppressed sequences can be advantageous in demonstrating gastric abnormalities.

The normal duodenal wall is usually thinner than the stomach wall, measuring approximately 1–2 mm in thickness. Incomplete distension of the duodenum may simulate diseases of the duodenum or adjacent organs and structures such as the pancreas and the ligaments.

14.3.2
Small Bowel

A critical element in adequate MR examinations is having the bowel loops empty to reduce gut motility and prevent misinterpretations due to bowel contents. MRI can be markedly improved using oral contrast agents (Fig. 14.1). Particularly negative contrast agents combined with intravenous contrast enhancement are useful in the evaluation of small bowel disease.

One of the major problems of the oral administration of contrast agents is inhomogeneous distribution of contrast material and lack of contrast material in the area of interest (KAMINSKY et al. 1991; GOURTSOYIANNIS et al. 1993). Several techniques have been proposed to achieve an adequate contrast filling of the small bowel loops, including (a) hydro-MRI, using about 1000 ml of a 2.5% mannitol solution which the patient has to drink prior to the MR examination (SCHUNK et al. 1997), and (b) administration of dilute barium contrast, using about 1350 ml of 2% barium (LOW and FRANCIS 1997).

In selected cases optimal conditions can be achieved when MRI is performed immediately after a small bowel enema (BRAMBS et al. 1993; ASCHOFF et al. 1997). The enteroclysis is performed as described previously to obtain double contrast images of the small intestine (HERLINGER 1978). The methylcellulose solution (ca. 1400 ml) is blended with 100 ml of gadopentate-dimeglumine (Magnevist enteral, Schering) as a positive agent or 100 ml of Oral Magnetic Particles (Abdoscan, Nycomed) as a negative contrast agent (RIEBER et al. 1997). Additionally, 20–40 mg N-butylscopolamine is given intravenously in order to suppress peristalsis and to delay passage of the intraenteric contrast material. This procedure

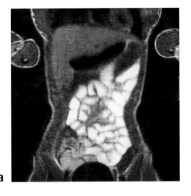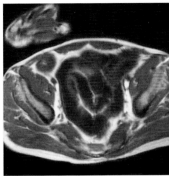

a   b

Fig. 14.1. **a** Coronal section of the abdomen following administration of a positive oral contrast agent (gadolinium). **b** Transverse section following administration of a negative oral contrast agent (superparamagnetic iron oxide)

has the advantage that the complete filling and distension of the bowel loops can be monitored fluoroscopically. The combination of a regular enteroclysis and small bowel MRI provides additional information about transmural and extraluminal pathology. Furthermore, it can be assumed that with the combination of the fluoroscopic and the MRI technique the radiation dose of the enteroclysis can be markedly reduced (Rieber et al. 1997).

14.4
Gastrointestinal Pathology

14.4.1
Gastric Tumors

Magnetic resonance imaging is of limited interest in the detection, characterization, and staging of gastric carcinoma. As in CT scans, gastric carcinoma most frequently appears as an area of localized or diffuse mural thickening (Fig. 14.2). This finding is nonspecific and can be observed in numerous conditions, for example in gastritis, where mural thickening can be impressive and exceed 1–2 cm. Mural thickening strongly suggests neoplasm when it is associated with adjacent adenopathy, liver metastases, or infiltration in the adjacent ligaments and fat tissue. MRI is sensitive in the detection of peritoneal spread of disease on gadolinium-enhanced fat-suppressed images (Oi et al. 1997). The ability of MRI to detect enlarged lymph nodes is comparable to that of CT and reflects on the size of the nodes.

Sagittal and coronal images are suggested to be potentially helpful to assess tumor extension to other organs (Scatarige and Disantis 1989). However, no relevant reports have been published on the accuracy of MRI in the staging of gastric tumors.

14.4.2
Small Bowel Cancer

Only 1%–5% of gastrointestinal cancers occur within the small bowel, although this bowel segment constitutes over 75% of the length of the alimentary tract. Duodenum and proximal jejunum are the most frequent sites. These tumors have a nonspecific presentation and there is a long delay in diagnosis from onset of symptoms to diagnosis. Radiologic misinterpretation or false-negative examination are major causes of this delay (Maglinte et al. 1991).

Metastases are the most common malignancies found in the small bowel. Malignant carcinoid tumors are the most frequent primary small bowel tumors. Adenocarcinomas account for about one-quarter of primary small bowel malignancies.

14.4.3
Lymphoma

Lymphoma can affect any portion of the alimentary tract. The stomach is the segment most frequently involved (Fig. 14.3). Non-Hodgkin's lymphoma is the most common type and gastrointestinal localizations are observed in 10%–20% of patients with this tumor type. Primary intestinal lymphoma arises from mural lymphoid tissue which is highly concentrated within the terminal ileum.

Lymphomas may be well localized or may diffusely infiltrate a long segment of bowel loops. Multiple lesions may be seen in one-third of patients, a feature that can help distinguish lymphoma from adenocarcinoma. In rare cases lymphoma of the small bowel may present as an intussuscepting mass.

Until now, CT has been the most important cross-sectional imaging method. However, MRI could be able to overtake the role of CT imaging: to contribute

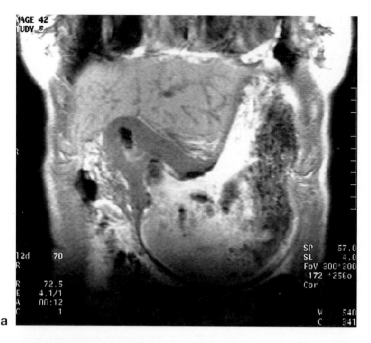

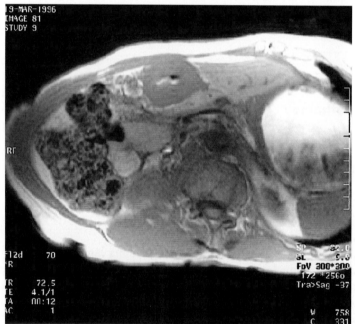

Fig. 14.2 a–c. Adenocarcinoma of the gastric antrum. **a** T1-weighted coronal section with marked circumferential thickening of the gastric wall. **b** T1-weighted transverse section. **c** Significant increase in signal intensity of the tumor after intravenous administration of Gd-DTPA

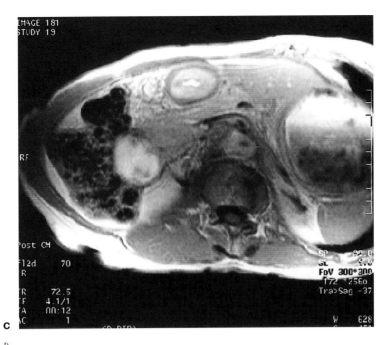

Fig. 14.2 (*Continued*)

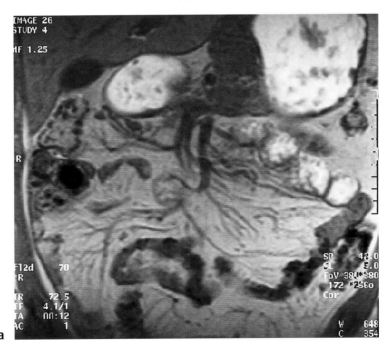

Fig. 14.3a,b. Primary lymphoma of the stomach. **a** Hypointense tumor mass at the mid portion of the stomach, associated with multiple enlarged lymph nodes in the retroperitoneum (**b**)

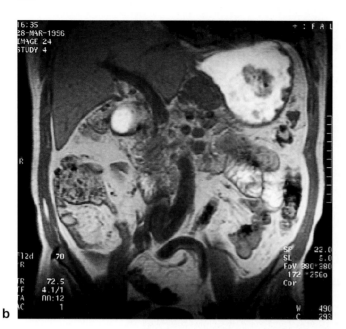

b

Fig. 14.3 (*Continued*)

to the positive diagnosis, to stage the disease before treatment, and to follow the tumoral response in patients under treatment. MRI seems to be superior to CT in the characterization of residual tumor masses under treatment because residual scars can be distinguished from viable lymphomas by virtue of the lower intensity of fibrotic tissue on T2-weighted images (NEGENDANK et al. 1990; MONTALBAN et al. 1992).

14.4.4
Intestinal Ischemia

Magnetic resonance imaging recognizes changes in tissue water content, and several authors have demonstrated increased intensity within 6 h of intestinal ischemia. In an animal model, PARK et al. (1993) could show that MRI can differentiate ischemic from nonischemic bowel 24 h after ischemic injury. In another model, KLEIN et al. (1996) could demonstrate that signal to noise and contrast to noise differed significantly between experimental and control groups in T1-weighted and proton density images. In ischemic segments the bowel wall did not show contrast enhancement. Intramural gas or portal venous gas usually cannot be demonstrated with MRI, which represents a deficit of MRI. However, compared with CT, MRI has the advantage of showing changes in tissue water occurring in bowel wall ischemia (KLEIN et al. 1996).

14.4.5
Inflammatory Bowel Disease

Crohn's disease is the most common chronic inflammatory disorder to affect the small bowel and is characterized by involvement of the mucosa, the bowel wall, and the surrounding mesentery. Thirty percent of patients with Crohn's disease have exclusively small bowel involvement. The current diagnostic procedures are enteroclysis, ileocolonoscopy, ultrasound, and CT. Endoscopy of the terminal segment of the ileum can be achieved only in a relatively low percentage of patients and assesses only superficial mucosal changes. The transmural component of the inflammatory process cannot be estimated by either enteroclysis or endoscopy.

Magnetic resonance imaging has a lot of potential in evaluating Crohn's disease: it demonstrates wall thickening and assesses the degree of contrast enhancement, it shows extraintestinal alterations such as inflammatory infiltration of the surrounding tissue, it demonstrates enlarged lymph nodes, and it detects complications such as fistulas and abscess formation.

As with CT, mural disease is shown by circumferential and symmetric bowel wall thickening (Figs. 14.4, 14.5) which is often discontinuous. Mural contrast enhancement, wall thickness, and length of diseased bowel correlate with clinical indexes of disease activity (Figs. 14.6–14.8). Therefore, MRI may be useful in evaluating the severity of Crohn's disease

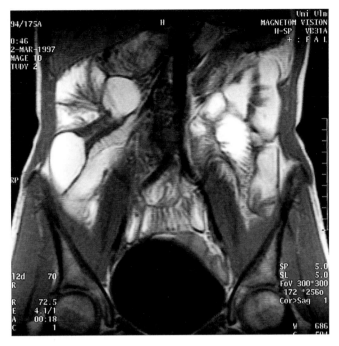

Fig. 14.4. Crohn's disease with segmental small bowel wall thickening and stricture in the terminal ileum. T1-weighted imaging with positive contrast following enteroclysis

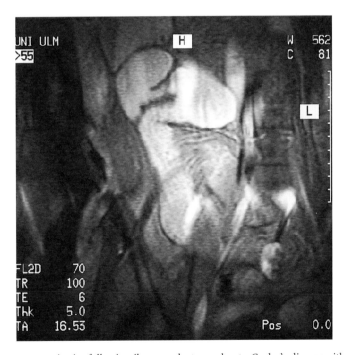

Fig. 14.5. Stricture at the anastomotic site following ileoascendostomy due to Crohn's disease with only discrete bowel wall thickening. T1-weighted imaging with positive oral contrast

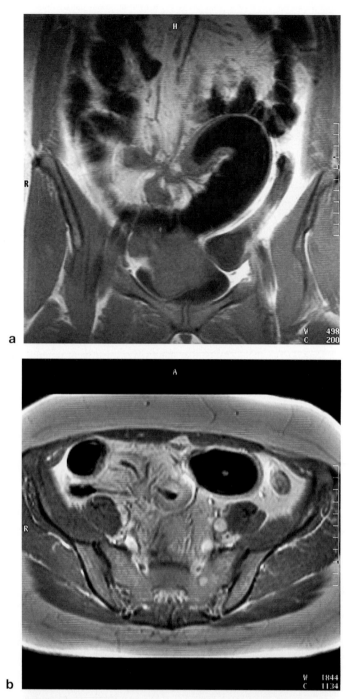

Fig. 14.6 a,b. Dilatation of a small bowel loop filled with negative contrast agent following enteroclysis. At the segment with
bowel wall thickening adjacent bowel loops are stuck together
and show fistulous communications (**a**). Following intravenous administration of Gd-DTPA significant contrast enhancement can be observed (**b**)

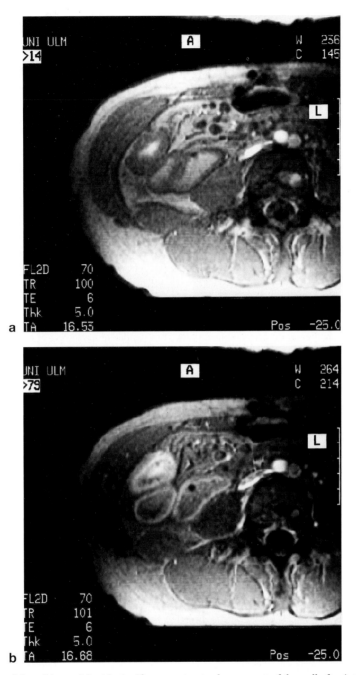

Fig. 14.7. Thickened small bowel loops (**a**) with significant contrast enhancement of the wall after intravenous administration of gadolinium (**b**)

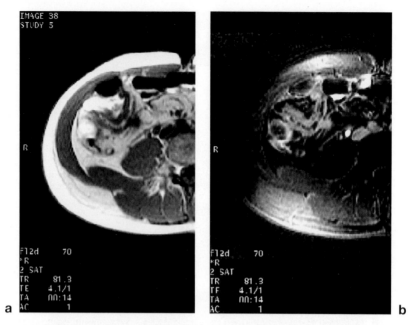

Fig. 14.8. a Inflammatory thickening of the terminal ileum loop with significant narrowing of the bowel lumen. **b** Following intravenous Gd-DTPA there is marked contrast enhancement which is underlined using a fat suppression technique

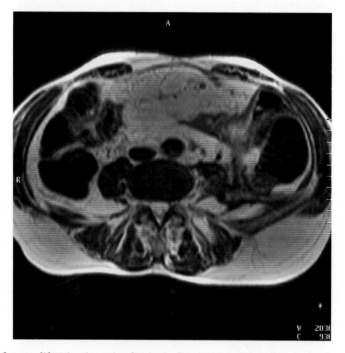

Fig. 14.9. Extensive fibrofatty proliferation (creeping fat sign) adjacent to chronic inflammatory bowel disease

and may provide information complementary to clinical evaluation (SHOENUT et al. 1994; KETTRITZ et al. 1995).

The most common mesenteric abnormality is fibrofatty proliferation (creeping fat), which results in an increased distance of the bowel loops in double contrast examinations (Fig. 14.9). This unspecific sign can also be caused by extreme bowel wall thickening or by interenteric abscess formation. These conditions can be clearly differentiated by MRI.

Furthermore, MRI can demonstrate fistulas (Fig. 14.10), particularly when they communicate with the abdominal wall, retroperitoneal muscles, spine, or adjacent organs such as bladder, vagina, prostate, or seminal vesicles. Heavily T2-weighted images have been shown to demonstrate the anatomy of fistulous tracts better than CT scanning. The fluid in the tract appears as a high signal, well contrasted by the surrounding tissue on these images (HAGGETT et al. 1995).

About 10%–20% of patients with Crohn's disease eventually develop intra-abdominal abscesses, which are most frequently associated with small bowel disease or ileocolitis. These abscesses usually result from fistulas, perforation, or surgical operations for Crohn's disease. An intra-abdominal abscess may be difficult to diagnose on clinical grounds in patients with Crohn's disease because symptoms may be inconspicuous. On MRI abscesses usually appear as circumscribed fluid-filled masses which usually show a peripheral contrast enhancement (Figs. 14.11, 14.12). With MRI it is possible to confirm the diagnosis and define the full extent and location of the abscess cavity.

Magnetic resonance imaging is assumed to monitor the early treatment response by showing decrease in bowel edema and reduction of signal intensity in postcontrast imaging (MADSEN et al. 1997).

14.4.6
Acute Appendicitis

Ultrasound is the primary imaging method in the evaluation of acute appendicitis, with a sensitivity ranging from 75% to 90%, and a specificity of 75% to near 100%. Whereas a normal appendix is usually not visible with MRI (Fig. 14.13), the inflamed appendiceal wall gives an intense contrast following administration of gadolinium. A recent study has shown that fat-suppressed contrast-enhanced MRI is very helpful in the detection of the acute disease and in particular can be used when ultrasound is nondiagnostic in cases of acute disease (INCESCU et al. 1997).

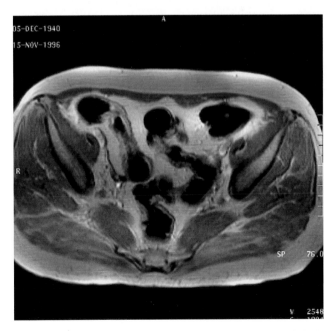

Fig. 14.10. T1-weighted imaging. Interenteric fistula in the right lower abdomen. Segmental thickening of adjacent small bowel loops filled with a negative contrast agent

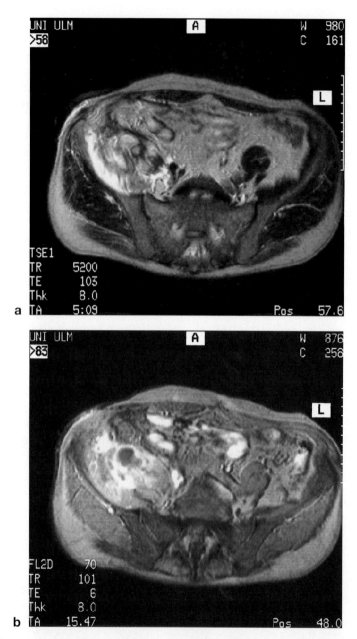

Fig. 14.11 a,b. Extensive retroperitoneal abscess formation in Crohn's disease. Since the bowel loops are filled with a positive contrast agent, precise delineation of the hyperintense abscess wall is hampered

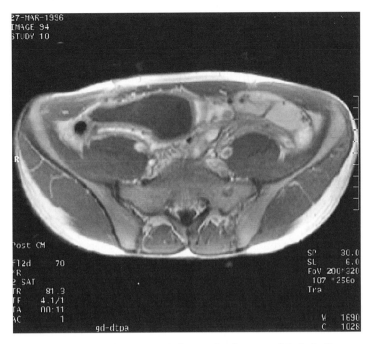

Fig. 14.12. Interenteric abscess in a patient following surgical operation because of Crohn's disease

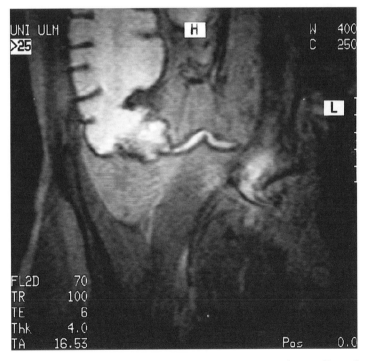

Fig. 14.13. By means of MR enteroclysis using a positive oral contrast agent a normal appendix can be demonstrated

14.5
Summary

With faster scanning times, better contrast agents, and improved spatial resolution, the indications for MRI of the gastrointestinal tract will no doubt expand.

Magnetic resonance imaging lacks the ability to assess depth of neoplastic involvement within gastric and bowel wall and is not able to diagnose metastatic tumor foci in normal-sized lymph nodes. Because of the low accuracy for assessing early tumor stages, neither MRI nor CT is recommended for routine use in preoperative staging.

Cross-sectional imaging plays a prominent role in assessing inflammatory disease of the gastrointestinal tract, particularly to define associated complications such as abdominal fistulas and abscesses. Furthermore, MRI appears to have particular potential in defining the extent and severity of inflammatory bowel disease. In combination with enteroclysis, additional information can be achieved and probably the radiation dose of the fluorocopic method can be reduced.

References

Aschoff AJ, Zeitler H, Merkle EM, Reinshagen M, Brambs HJ, Rieber A (1997) MR-Enteroklyse zur kernspintomographischen Diagnostik entzündlicher Darmerkrankungen mit verbesserter Darmkontrastierung. Fortschr Röntgenstr 167:387–391

Brambs HJ, Laniado M, Arndt E, Duda SH, Damman F, Jenss H, Cornelius I (1993) MRI performed with oral Gd-DTPA after enteroclysis in Crohn disease. Eur Radiol (Suppl) 3:150

Brasch RC (1992) New directions in the development of MR imaging contrast media. Radiology 183:1–11

Brown JJ (1996) Gastrointestinal contrast agents for MR imaging. MRI Clin North Am 4:25–35

Gourtsoyiannis NC, Bays D, Papaioannou N, Theotokas J, Barouxis G, Karabelas T (1993) Benign tumors of the small intestine: preoperative evaluation with a barium infusion technique. Eur J Radiol 16:115–125

Haggett PJ, Moore NR, Shearman JD, Jewell DP, Mortensen NJ (1995) Pelvic and perineal complications of Crohn's disease: assessment using magnetic resonance imaging. Gut 36:407–410

Hahn PF, Stark DD, Lewis JM, et al. (1990) First clinical trial of a new superparamagnetic iron oxide for use as an oral gastrointestinal contrast agent in MR imaging. Radiology 175:695–700

Hamed MM, Hamm B, Ibrahim ME, et al. (1992) Dynamic MR imaging of the abdomen with gadopentate dimeglumine: normal enhancement pattern of liver, spleen, stomach, and pancreas. Am J Roentgenol 158:303–307

Herlinger H (1978) A modified technique for the double contrast small bowel enema. Gastrointest Radiol 2:397–400

Incesu L, Coskun A, Selcuk MB, Akan H, Sozubir S, Bernay F (1997) Acute appendicitis: MR imaging and sonographic correlation. Am J Roentgenol 168:669–674

Kaminsky S, Laniado M, Gogoll M, Kornmesser W, Clauß W, Felix R (1991) Gadopentetate dimeglumine as a bowel contrast agent: safety and efficacy. Radiology 178:503–508

Kettritz U, Isaacs K, Warshauer DM, Semelka RC (1995) Pilot study comparing MRI of the abdomen with clinical evaluation. J Clin Gastroenterol 21:249–253

Klein HM, Klosterhalfen B, Kinzel S, et al. (1996) CT and MRI of experimentally induced mesenteric ischemia in a porcine model. J Comput Assist Tomogr 20:254–261

Low RN, Francis IR (1997) Double contrast MR imaging of the gastrointestinal tract with iv Gd-DTPA and dilute barium oral contrast compared to computed tomography. 97th Annual Meeting of the American Roentgen Ray Society, Boston

Madsen SM, Thomsen HS, Munkholm P, Schlichting P, Davidsen B (1997) Magnetic resonance imaging of Crohn disease: early recognition of treatment response and relapse. Abdom Imaging 22:164–166

Maglinte DDT, O'Connor K, Besette J, et al. (1991) The role of the physician in the late diagnosis of primary malignant tumors of the small intestine. Am J Gastroenterol 86:304–308

Mattrey RF, Trambert MA, Brown JJ, et al. (1994) Perflubron as an oral contrast agent for MR imaging: results of a phase III clinical trial. Radiology 191:841–848

Mirowitz SA (1993) Contrast enhancement of the gastrointestinal tract on MR images using intravenous gadolinium-DTPA. Abdom Imaging 18:215–219

Montalban C, Rodriguez-Garcia JL, Mazairas L, et al. (1992) Magnetic resonance imaging of assessment of residual masses after treatment of non-Hodgkin's lymphomas. Postgrad Med J 68:643–647

Negendank WG, Al-Katib AM, Karanes C, et al. (1990) Lymphomas: MR imaging contrast characteristics with clinical-pathologic correlations. Radiology 177:209–216

Oi H, Matsushita M, Nakamura H (1997) Dynamic MR imaging for extraserosal invasion of advanced gastric cancer. Abdom Imaging 22:35–40

Oksendal AN, Jakobsen TF, Gundersen HG, Rinck PA, Rummeny E (1991) Superparamagnetic particles as an oral contrast agent in abdominal magnetic resonance imaging. Invest Radiol 26:67–70

Park A, Towner RA, Langer JC (1993) Diagnosis of intestinal ischemia in the rat using magnetic resonance imaging. J Invest Surg 6:177–183

Rieber A, Wruk D, Tomczak R, Merkle E, Aschoff A, Zeitler H, Brambs HJ (1997) MRT bei Dünndarmerkrankungen: Einsatz positiver und negativer Kontrastmittel in Kombination mit der Enteroklyse. Fortschr Röntgenstr 166:S10

Scatarige JC, Disantis DJ (1989) CT of the stomach and duodenum. Radiol Clin North Am 27:687–707

Schunk K, Metzmann U, Kersjes W, et al. (1997) Verlaufskontrolle des Morbus Crohn: Kann die Hydro-MRT die fraktionierte Magen-Darm-Passage ersetzen? Fortschr Röntgenstr 166:389–396

Shoenut JP, Semelka RC, Magro CM, Silverman R, Yaffe CS, Micflikier AB (1994) Comparison of magnetic resonance imaging and endoscopy in distinguishing the type and severity of inflammatory bowel disease. J Clin Gastroenterol 19:31–35

15 Colon and Rectum

J. Scheidler, M. Steinborn, and A. Heuck

CONTENTS

15.1 Introduction

With the development of techniques to limit respiratory and bowel motion, attenuate high signal of adjacent fat, and decrease susceptibility artifacts, magnetic resonance (MR) imaging has joined computed tomography (CT) as a diagnostic modality for the evaluation of the colon and rectum. Nevertheless, despite the inherent strengths of MR imaging,

J. Scheidler, MD, Department of Diagnostic Radiology, Klinikum Großhadern, Ludwig-Maximilians University, Marchioninistrasse 15, D-81377 München, Germany
M. Steinborn, MD, Department of Diagnostic Radiology, Klinikum Großhadern, Ludwig-Maximilians University, Marchioninistrasse 15, D-81377 München, Germany
A. Heuck, MD, Department of Diagnostic Radiology, Klinikum Großhadern, Ludwig-Maximilians University, Marchioninistrasse 15, D-81377 München, Germany

specifically high soft tissue contrast and multiplanar imaging capability, controversy still exists on the clinical utility of MR imaging in comparison to other imaging modalities like helical CT and endosonography.

This chapter will describe typical MR features of congenital abnormalities and inflammatory, benign, and malignant diseases of the colon and rectum. Current MR imaging protocols including advanced techniques such as breath-hold imaging, the use of phased array and endorectal coils, and single-shot sequences will be presented. The clinical utility of various oral contrast agents will be discussed.

15.2 Technical Considerations

15.2.1 Pulse Sequences

Adequate evaluation of colorectal pathology requires both T1- and T2-weighted images. T1-weighted images provide tissue characterization (hemorrhage, fluid, fat) and are essential for the detection of lymph node metastasis. Due to limited coverage and image quality degradation by respiratory and bowel motion artifacts, standard spin-echo (SE) sequences require at least two slice stacks, respiratory compensation, and medical suppression of bowel peristalsis to achieve sufficient image quality for the evaluation of the colon. Total imaging time has been greatly reduced with the introduction of breath-hold imaging. Either spoiled gradient-recalled echo (SPGR, FLASH, FFE, spoiled FAST) or magnetization-prepared spoiled gradient-recalled echo sequences (FSPGR, turbo-FLASH, TFE) may be used for T1-weighted MR imaging of the entire colon. In combination with phased array and/or endorectal coils, these sequences provide comparable image quality to T1-weighted SE sequences and do not necessarily require medical suppression of bowel motion.

Fast spin-echo (FSE, turboSE) sequences significantly reduce acquisition time for T2-weighted imaging compared with standard SE. Respiratory compensation, however, cannot be combined with FSE sequences. Therefore, even with sufficient inhibition of peristalsis, satisfactory image quality is often not achieved with T2-weighted FSE sequences. Recently, the development of T2-weighted FSE sequences with long echo trains as well as single shot half-Fourier fast spin-echo (HASTE) has made high-quality T2-weighted imaging of the bowel possible. Advantages of these sequences include acquisition times as short as 1 s per section and low susceptibility artifacts, which is particularly important for gas-filled bowel.

Contrast-enhanced sequences (intravenous gadolinium chelates) are useful for the evaluation of bowel disease. The combination of i.v. gadolinium chelates with frequency-selective fat suppression further increases the conspicuity of abnormal contrast enhancement. No data are available on the value of other fat suppression techniques in bowel disease, e.g., frequency selective fat suppression in T2-weighted turboSE sequences, fat suppression with turbo short T1 inversion recovery (turbo-STIR) sequences, and fat suppression with the Dixon technique.

15.2.2
Transmitter and Receiver Coils

When using endorectal and/or multicoil array systems as receiver coils, the body coils serve as a transmitter of radiofrequency pulses. Endorectal and multicoil array systems, either alone or in combination, significantly improve the signal-to-noise level. High-quality breath-hold imaging with resolution and slice thickness comparable to non-breath-hold studies requires the use of multicoil array systems.

Image acquisition with endorectal coils permits the use of a smaller field of view, thus increasing image resolution in the pelvis. The endorectal coil should not be used in the presence of the following conditions: previous rectal surgery, recent radiation therapy to the pelvis, inflammatory bowel disease (ulcerative colitis or Crohn's disease), bleeding diathesis, or obstruction of the rectum or colon, including large hemorrhoids. Patient preparation (use of laxatives), coil placement, and maximum balloon distention are important factors in assuring optimal quality of MR images when using an endorectal coil.

15.2.3
Intraluminal Contrast Agents

The utility of oral MR contrast agents is still controversial. It has been shown that lesion conspicuity and diagnostic accuracy may increase after oral contrast administration. On the other hand, the induction of motion and susceptibility artifacts by oral contrast agents may neutralize their diagnostic benefits. Increased cost-consciousness has raised the question of whether there is a real need for intraluminal contrast in MR since multiplanar imaging capability and high contrast resolution do not necessarily require oral contrast as in CT. Considerable investigational and commercial activity has led to the development of three types of contrast agents, discussed below.

15.2.3.1
Positive Intraluminal Contrast Agents

Ferric ammonium citrate (FAC) was one of the first substances proposed as an oral MR contrast agent (WESBEY et al. 1983). FAC-based agents produce bright intraluminal signal intensity on T1-weighted images due to the paramagnetic properties of FAC (PATTEN et al. 1992). High signal intensity on T2-weighted images, however, is due to the high water content of the agents. Limitations of FAC-based agents are increased peristalsis-related artifacts and inconsistent bowel marking distal to the duodenum (HIROHASHI et al. 1994). Furthermore, gastrointestinal side-effects have been reported in up to 22% of patients with one FAC-based formulation (PATTEN et al. 1993).

Enteral gadopentate dimeglumine acts similarly to its intravenous counterpart: there is paramagnetic shortening of T1 and T2 relaxation with a predominant effect on T1 shortening. Mixed with mannitol to decrease dilutional effects, it effectively marks the bowel and demonstrates bowel wall thickening (KAMINSKY et al. 1991). Gadopentate dimeglumine may also improve MR imaging of the colon and rectosigmoid following rectal administration (VLAHOS et al. 1994).

15.2.3.2
Negative Intraluminal Contrast Agents

Negative bowel contrast agents can be classified into three categories: (a) superparamagnetic iron particles, (b) diamagnetic materials such as barium sulfate, and (c) materials that produce little or no MR signal such as air and Perflubron.

Superparamagnetic agents consist of ferrite-type crystalline iron oxide particles (SPIO: small particles of iron oxide). Tow SPIO-based preparations (OMP; Ferumoxsil) are on the market. At standard concentrations, dark intraluminal signal intensity is produced on both T1- and T2-weighted images. The dark signal is caused by local magnetic field heterogeneity that enhances spin dephasing, resulting in T2* shortening (RUBIN et al. 1994). It has bee shown that uniform bowel marking can be achieved with both preparations (RUBIN et al. 1993; HALDEMANN-HEUSLER et al. 1995; SCHEIDLER et al. 1997b). Potential problems are magnetic susceptibility artifacts, particularly on gradient-echo images, due to aggregation and flocculation of the particles. Additional concerns include high costs and suboptimal palatability.

Barium sulfate produces negative intraluminal contrast on MR images when administered in concentrations of 60%–90%. The signal intensity is diminished by a decreased amount of mobile protons in the suspension, and T2 shortening is caused by diamagnetic susceptibility effects of barium sulfate (LANGMO et al. 1992). Good bowel delineation has been reported with oral and rectal administration (PANACCIONE et al. 1991; ROS et al. 1991). Barium sulfate has been combined with iron oxide particles to reduce susceptibility artifacts and to improve taste (DAVIS et al. 1994).

Perflubron, previously referred to as perfluorooctylbromide or PFOB, is a tasteless, odorless, and nontoxic agent that is immiscible with water. It produces no MR signal since all hydrogen atoms have been replaced by fluorine or bromine atoms. Perflubron has been shown to be an effective bowel marker for MR imaging (BROWN et al. 1991; ANDERSON et al. 1994). Particular advantages of Perflubron are the rapid bowel transit of the agent, its resistance to concentration-dependent signal alterations due to the immiscibility, and its magnetic susceptibility similar to that of most human tissues. Perflubron, however, has not yet achieved widespread clinical use, this can be attributed to its cost, which is substantially higher than that of other MR bowel contrast agents.

15.2.3.3
Biphasic Intraluminal Contrast Agents

Biphasic agents produce high or low intraluminal signal depending on the concentration of the agent and the parameters used for imaging. Administration of a manganese chloride-containing agent results in bright signal on T1-weighted images due to the paramagnetic T1 shortening effects of the manganese ion. Additionally, dark signal intensity is found on T2-weighted sequences, presumably due to T2 shortening. First trials of the agent have shown promising results (BERNARDINO et al. 1994).

Ultrasmall iron oxide particles (USPIO) colloids, with a particle size significantly smaller (19 nm) than the particles used for the SPIO-based agents, have been found to exhibit biphasic properties. In an animal model, a USPIO-containing agent generated high signal intensity on T1-weighted images and bowel darkening on T2-weighted sequences (ROGERS et al. 1994).

15.2.4
Suggested Imaging Protocol

Imaging protocols for the colon should consist of T1- and T2-weighted transaxial studies covering the entire colon frame. Breath-hold sequences are preferable with a slice thickness not exceeding 8 mm, but this technique requires phased array coils to achieve sufficient signal-to-noise. Commonly recommended imaging protocols include: (a) precontrast transaxial T1-weighted breath-hold spoiled gradient echo, (b) transaxial or coronal T2-weighted breath-hold FSE or HASTE, and (c) gadolinium-enhanced T1-weighted breath-hold spoiled gradient echo, in either the transaxial or the coronal plane. Bowel filling or bowel contrast may especially aid in the detection of mucosal abnormalities. Suspected pathology in the rectum requires sagittal instead of coronal imaging. High-quality MR imaging of the pelvis can also be done using standard SE and FSE sequences; however, sufficient medical suppression of bowel motion is mandatory. Both glucagon (1 mg i.m.) and butylscopolamine (20 mg i.v.) significantly reduce motion artifacts (KIER et al. 1993). As an alternative, fasting for at least 5 h before scanning achieves reproducible bowel hypotonicity and is well tolerated by the patients. Fat suppression further reduces bowel and respiratory motion artifacts (MIROWITZ et al. 1994). Respiratory compensation techniques are recommended for standard SE sequences. Anterior and posterior saturation bands are also helpful to avoid ghosting artifacts due to abdominal wall movement and additionally reduce image nonuniformity when multicoil array systems are used.

15.3
Congenital Abnormalities

15.3.1
Variations in the Location of the Colon

The gastrointestinal tract can undergo nonrotation (most common form) or partial or complete malrotation because the duodenojejunal and cecocolic segments rotate independently. Failure of the third and fourth portions of the duodenum to traverse the aorta anteriorly denotes nonrotation. Malrotation is indicated by the malalignment of the superior mesenteric artery and vein on transaxial images. Other variations in colon location include interposition of the colon between the anterior surface of the liver and the anterior abdominal wall (Chilaiditi's syndrome), a lateral position of the hepatic flexure in relation to the right hepatic lobe, and a retrorenal position of the ascending colon (HOPPER et al. 1987). Occasionally, the ascending colon can also be found in the hepatorenal fossa.

15.3.2
Duplication Cysts

Duplication cysts can be found throughout the gastrointestinal tract. These uncommon malformations are usually discovered during childhood and are typically located in the mesentery. They become symptomatic due to mass effect or infection caused by stasis of intestinal contents in cysts communicating with bowel. On MR images they exhibit a well-defined, thin cystic wall with variable signal intensity. The signal intensity of the cyst content is higher than simple fluid on T1-weighted images and is high on T2-weighted sequences. After i.v. gadolinium, the cyst wall enhances, whereas the fluid-filled lumen remains of lower signal intensity, allowing for reliable distinction from solid lesions.

15.4
Inflammatory Bowel Disease

15.4.1
Ulcerative Colitis

Ulcerative colitis is a mucosal disease with a predictable distribution. In contrast to Crohn's disease, ulcerative colitis primarily affects the rectum and spreads contiguously retrograde, whereas Crohn's disease may start anywhere in the gastrointestinal tract and spreads discontinuously, skipping entire segments of the small and large bowel. The etiology of ulcerative colitis remains unknown; however, a positive family history has been reported in up to 25% of cases, indicating a genetic predisposition. The main symptoms of ulcerative colitis are intermittent diarrhea and rectal bleeding. The course of the disease is complicated by toxic megacolon with fever and abdominal pain combined with excessive dilatation of the fluid-filled colon. After longstanding disease patients are at great risk for the development of colon cancer. Failure of conservative treatment may require total colectomy.

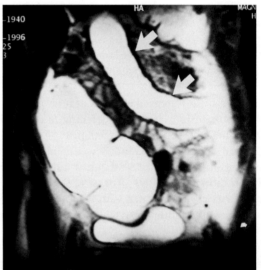

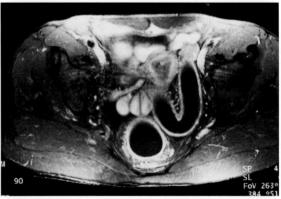

Fig. 15.1 a,b. Ulcerative colitis. The coronal T2-weighted HASTE sequence (a) after retrograde filling with aqueous methylcellulose suspension shows distension of the ascending colon and cecum. The dilated and elongated sigmoid colon shows wall thickening and loss of haustration (*arrows*). The T1-weighted fat-suppressed contrast-enhanced SE sequence (b) demonstrates thickening and enhancement of the rectal and sigmoid wall, indicating a chronic inflammatory process

The characteristic MR appearance reflects the underlying pathology. The mucosal-based process starts with cryptal microabscesses that coalesce to form mucosal ulcers. Following intravenous gadolinium, marked mucosal enhancement is seen on MR imaging that spares the submucosa. Depending on the severity of disease, enhancement of the mucosa is found beginning in the rectum and spreading contiguously retrograde to the cecum (Fig. 15.1). In 30% of patients disease is also present in the terminal ileum ("backwash ileitis"). Inflammatory tissue stranding is seen in the fat surrounding involved colon segments. Prominent vasa recta are frequently present. In toxic megacolon the disease is not limited to the level of the mucosa, but involves the entire thickened colon wall without sparing the submucosa. Patients with long-standing disease demonstrate low signal intensity from submucosal edema and lymphangiectasia. The thickened and shortened colon wall presents as a "lead pipe" colon with loss of haustral markings (Fig. 15.1).

15.4.2
Crohn's Disease

Crohn's disease is the most common inflammatory process of the small bowel. Although the term "ileitis terminalis" suggests that the disease is limited to this bowel segment, isolated terminal ileitis is present only in 30% of cases. Twenty percent of patients have isolated involvement of the colon, and in 40% disease affects both the terminal ileum and the proximal colon. Since the disease can be found anywhere within the gastrointestinal tract and the pattern of spread is discontinuous, identification of the site of involvement and the extent of bowel disease is important for the planning of surgery and the assessment of response to medical treatment.

Crohn's disease affects all layers of the bowel wall. Starting with superficial aphthous ulcers in the mucosa, progressive transmural ulcerations may lead to a network of deep transmural fissures that often extends beyond the serosa. Affected bowel segments are thickened from fibrosis and edema and are often enveloped by excess mesenteric fat. Complications of the disease include development of fistulae, sinus tracts, strictures, and abscesses.

MR imaging can distinguish ulcerative colitis from Crohn's disease on the basis of morphologic criteria (SHOENUT et al. 1994). The typical appearance of Crohn's disease on MR imaging is a thickened segment of distal ileum demonstrating intense

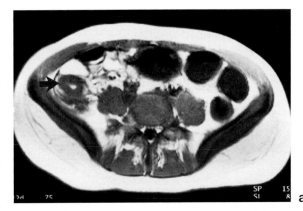

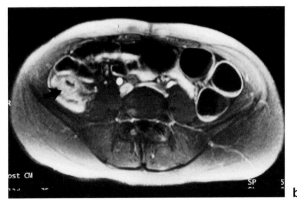

Fig. 15.2 a,b. Crohn's disease of the terminal ileum. Axial T1-weighted FLASH breath-hold sequence (**a**) shows wall thickening of the terminal ileum (*arrow*). The fat-suppressed contrast-enhanced image (**b**) reveals contrast enhancement of the ileac wall (*arrow*).

full-thickness enhancement of the bowel wall after i.v. administration of gadolinium (Figs. 15.2–15.6). Often associated with this finding is an asymmetric involvement of the cecum. Additional findings leading to the diagnosis are rectal sparing, presence of fistulae and sinus tracts, and skip lesions. Fat tissue stranding and enlarged lymph nodes can be found in the mesentery. On MR imaging, chronic disease is characterized by a wall thickness greater than 1 cm with insignificant contrast enhancement after i.v. gadolinium. Additionally, strictures with or without proximal bowel dilatation may be present.

Various authors have described a good correlation between MR imaging findings and disease activity (SHOENUT et al. 1993b, 1994; KETTRITZ et al. 1995). Assessment of disease severity is based on bowel wall thickness, degree of contrast enhancement, and length of segmental involvement. An index based on the product of these findings on gadolinium-enhanced fat-suppressed MR images has been proposed and was correlated to the clinical

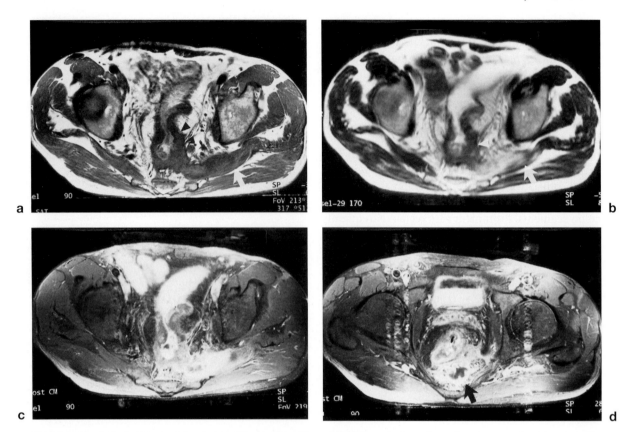

Fig. 15.3 a–d. Crohn's disease of the rectum and rectosigmoid junction. The T1-weighted SE image in the axial orientation (a) shows thickening of the rectosigmoid bowel wall (*arrowheads*) and the left piriform muscle (*arrow*). High signal intensity of the piriform muscle (*arrow*) is present on the T2-weighted HASTE sequence (b), indicating edema and inflammatory wall thickening of the sigmoid colon (*arrowhead*). The piriform muscle shows intensive contrast enhancement on the corresponding T1-weighted image with fat saturation (c). A contrast-enhanced image caudally (d) demonstrates a precoccygeal abscess formation with a thickened, strongly enhancing abscess wall and low signal intensity areas in the central portion, indicating fluid accumulation (*arrow*)

Crohn's disease activity index (KETTRITZ et al. 1995). A linear relationship was found between both indices of disease activity, suggesting the ability to assess the severity of disease by MR imaging.

15.4.3
Appendicitis

Appendicitis most often affects children and young adults. Most commonly the diagnosis is made clinically although the lack of ionizing radiation and the high contrast resolution make MR imaging well suited as a problem-solving imaging modality. Unenhanced T1-weighted images demonstrate dark inflammatory stranding in the periappendiceal fat. Contrast enhancement of the inflamed appendix is best shown on fat-suppressed images. An appendiceal abscess appears as a low signal cavity with

significant enhancement of the abscess wall after i.v. administration of gadolinium.

15.4.4
Diverticulitis

Diverticula are most commonly located in the sigmoid and the descending colon. Diverticula are demonstrated on MR imaging as signal voids against the high signal intensity of the pericolonic fat (Fig. 15.7). Early diagnostic signs of diverticulitis on unenhanced MR images may be mild wall thickening and pericolonic soft tissue stranding. Full-blown diverticulitis is characterized by intense contrast enhancement of the thickened bowel wall and the surrounding inflammatory tissue, which is best seen on T1-weighted fat-suppressed images. Contrast-enhanced fat-suppressed imaging also highlights

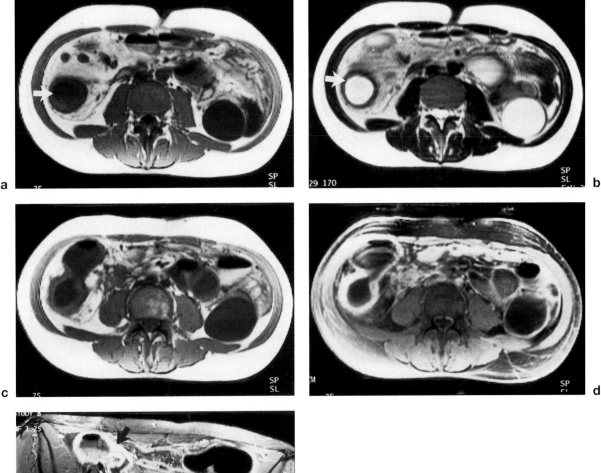

Fig. 15.4 a–e. Crohn's disease. Axial T1- (**a**) and T2-weighted (**b**) breath-hold sequences after rectal application of aqueous methylcellulose suspension demonstrate circular bowel wall thickening of the ascending colon (*arrow*). Unenhanced (**c**) and contrast-enhanced T1-weighted FLASH with fat suppression (**d**) demonstrate strong contrast enhancement of the thickened colonic wall, indicating the acute stage of disease. Fat-suppressed T1-weighted SE (**e**) clearly shows inflammation of the ileocaecal valve and the terminal ileum (*arrow*)

fistulae and sinus tracts when present. Adjacent fluid collections with an enhancing rim are indicative of abscess formation.

15.4.5
Pouchitis

The current treatment of choice for patients requiring colectomy for ulcerative colitis or familial adenomatous polyposis is ileoanal anastomosis with ileac reservoir (pouch) creation to preserve the natural pathway and sphincter function. Symptomatic inflammation of this pouch, a condition known as pouchitis, will develop in 40%–50% of patients who undergo this surgery (STAHLBERG et al. 1996). Patients will present with crampy abdominal pain, fever, rectal bleeding, and diarrhea, and they may have either acute intermittent attacks or a chronic pouchitis syndrome. Most of the reported cases of pouchitis have occurred in patients with a previous history of ulcerative colitis, whereas complications develop in only a handful of patients with familial polyposis (RUBINSTEIN and FISHER 1996).

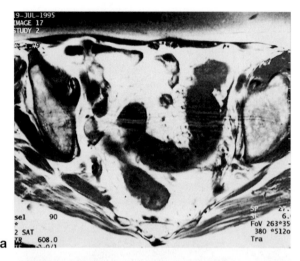

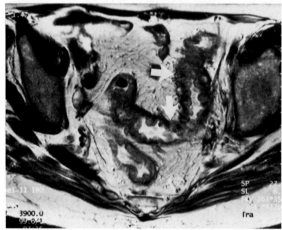

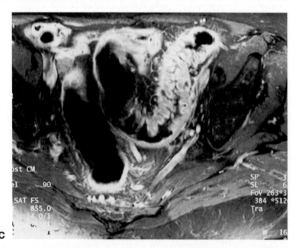

Fig. 15.5 a–c. Crohn's disease of the sigmoid. Axial T1-weighted SE (**a**) and T2-weighted TSE (**b**) sequences after rectal filling of the colon with aqueous methylcellulose suspension demonstrate circular bowel wall thickening leading to a stenosis of the sigmoid colon (*arrows* in **b**) Pseudopolypoid aspect of the enhancing thickened bowel wall on fat-suppressed images after i.v. Gd-DTPA (**c**)

The normal pouch appears as an oval to round structure. Focal wall thickening, stranding of the adjacent fat, and marked enhancement of the pouch wall on contrast-enhanced fat-suppressed T1-weighted images are findings consistent with pouchitis. Rectal contrast administration may be helpful to exclude leakage.

15.4.6
Fistulae

Various conditions (e.g., inflammatory, infectious, and neoplastic disease as well as radiation therapy) can lead to the development of fistulae resulting in a pathologic communication between the colon and other organs or skin. Fistulae of the colon are most commonly seen in the inner pelvis due to cancer invading the rectum or colorectal cancer with extracolonic spread. For perianal fistulae, however, Crohn's disease is likely to be the underlying pathology.

Magnetic resonance imaging has proven to be an effective modality for the evaluation of fistulae (HRICAK et al. 1993; OUTWATER and SCHIEBLER 1993; ANDERSON et al. 1994; CHOU et al. 1994; MYHR et al. 1994; deSOUZA et al. 1995; HAGGETT et al. 1995; HUSSAIN et al. 1996; SPENCER et al. 1996; STOKER et al. 1996). Best results have been obtained with endorectal and/or multicoil arrays in the presurgical evaluation of perianal fistulae (MYHR et al. 1994; deSOUZA et al. 1995; HAGGETT et al. 1995; HUSSAIN et al. 1996; SPENCER et al. 1996; STOKER et al. 1996). Of particular importance is the identification of fistulous tracts extending above the levator ani muscle. Any part of a fistulous tract or abscess that is above the levator ani will not adequately drain in the inferior direction. Therefore, the therapeutic approach to these fistulae requires additional drainage of supralevatoric components, either surgically or with percutaneous drainage. MR imaging allows clear identification of perianal fistulae and their anatomic relationship to the sphincter muscle (HUSSAIN et al. 1995). Endoanal MR imaging allows more accurate depiction and classification of fistula than endoanal sonography (HUSSAIN et al. 1996).

Several MR imaging patterns of fistulae have been described. Fluid-filled fistulae have high signal intensity on T2-weighted images. Gas-containing tracts are identified by a signal void. Contrast-enhanced fat-suppressed sequences show the fistula tracts as enhancing linear structures. Confident diagnosis of organ-to-organ fistulae can be made when focal

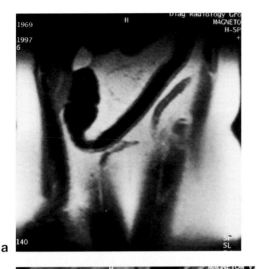

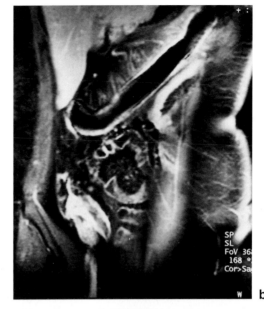

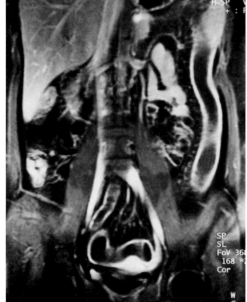

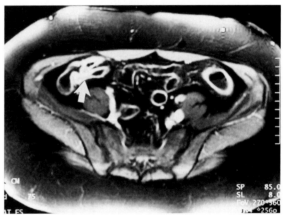

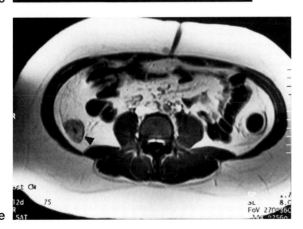

Fig. 15.6 a–e. Crohn's disease of the colon and distal ileum. The coronal T1-weighted breath-hold FLASH sequence (a) shows a smooth wall of the transverse colon with loss of haustration as a result of the chronic inflammatory process. Strong enhancement of the colon wall is indicative of a relapse of the disease (b,c; fat-suppressed contrast-enhanced FLASH). Bowel wall thickening is also present in the terminal ileum at the level of the ileocoecal valve (*arrow* on 6d) and at the coecal pole (arrowhead on 6e) as demonstrated on T1-weighted contrast-enhanced axial images (d fat-suppressed T1-weighted image; e T1-weighted image without fat suppression)

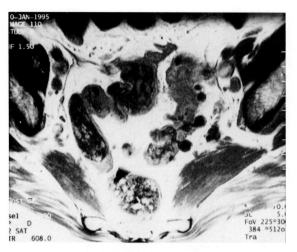

Fig. 15.7. Diverticula of the sigmoid colon. Multiple ectatic rounded gas-filled expansions of the sigmoid wall are present on this unenhanced axial T1-weighted image

discontinuity of the organ wall is demonstrated. Filling of viscerocutaneous fistulae with diluted Gd-DTPA or saline solution (for T2-weighted images) may improve the identification of their path and extent (MYHR et al. 1994).

15.5
Neoplasms

15.5.1
Benign Tumors

15.5.1.1
Polyps

Polyps most commonly occur in the colon, but they are found throughout the gastrointestinal tract. They are histologically categorized as tubular, tubulovillous, or villous. Of these types, villous adenomas have the greatest tendency to undergo malignant transformation. Three pathogenic types occur: hyperplastic, hamartomatous, and adenomatous. Adenomatous polyps carry the highest potential for malignancy. Malignant potential is also related to polyp size. Most polyps smaller than 1 cm have to be considered benign; however, malignancy has to be considered in any polyp larger than 2 cm since up to 46% of them contain cancer.

There are two syndromes in which polyposis occurs in the colon and rectum. Familial adenomatous polyposis syndrome is an autosomal dominant disease that carries a 100% risk of malignant trans-

formation to colorectal carcinoma. Diffuse adenomatous polyposis of the colon associated with bony abnormalities and soft tissue tumors is characteristic of Gardner's syndrome, an inherent autosomal dominant disease. For both entities total colectomy is warranted to prevent the development of colorectal cancer.

The MR appearance of colon polyps is dependent on their morphology. Tubular adenomas appear as sessile or pedunculated masses that arise from the colon wall and protrude into the lumen (Fig. 15.8). They are of low signal intensity on T1-weighted images and have intermediate to high signal intensity on T2-weighted sequences (Fig. 15.9). Signal intensity on T1- and T2-weighted images increases with the number of mucin-producing cells within the adenoma. Villous adenomas are hard to identify. The possibility of villous adenoma should be raised if enhancing interstices are appreciated on gadolinium-enhanced fat-suppressed MR images. Malignant transformation is almost certain if the adenoma extends beyond the colon wall.

15.5.1.2
Lipoma

Colonic lipomas are rare submucosal neoplasms (0.2%–0.3% on autopsy series) (HANCOCK and VAJCNER 1988). The most common location is near the ileocecal valve, either in the cecum/ascending colon or in the terminal ileum. Due to their fatty composition they have a pathognomonic appearance on MR images. Demonstrating homogeneous high signal intensity on T1-weighted images, frequency selective fat suppression will show a characteristic signal loss. Central necrosis and internal hemorrhage, however, are suggestive of malignancy and require further diagnostic evaluation (YOUNATHAN et al. 1991).

15.5.2
Malignant Tumors

15.5.2.1
Colorectal Carcinoma

Colorectal cancer is the most common malignancy of the gastrointestinal tract. Patients with familial polyposis, Gardner's syndrome, ulcerative colitis, and ureterosigmoidostomies are at increased risk. The most frequent sites of occurrence are the

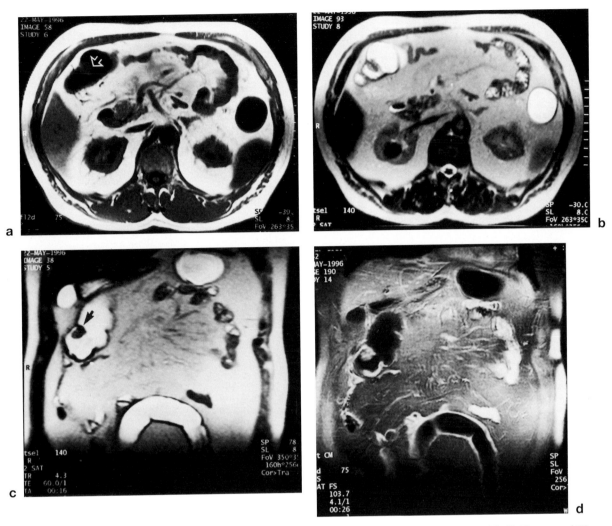

Fig. 15.8 a–d. Pedunculated polyp of the ascending colon. The T1-weighted breath-hold FLASH sequence in the transverse orientation (**a**) shows a low signal intensity structure within the lumen of the ascending colon (*arrow*). The structure is adherent to the lateral colonic wall. The T2-weighted breath-hold HASTE image (**b**) after retrograde filling with aqueous methylcellulose suspension shows an intermediate intensity structure outlined by the intraluminal fluid. The coronal T2-weighted breath-hold HASTE image (**c**) shows the pedunculated polyp adherent to the upper lateral colonic wall (*arrow*). After contrast injection the fat-suppressed coronal image (**d**) demonstrates mild heterogeneous enhancement of the polyp, especially in the central part

rectum and the sigmoid colon. Tumor shape may be polypoid, asymmetrical, or circumferential ("apple-core").

Correct tumor depiction requires colonic preparation and filling. Air insufflation, water/cellulose enemas, or oral/rectal contrast agents (SCHEIDLER et al. 1997b) are helpful to achieve sufficient bowel distention. Colorectal carcinomas have a low signal intensity comparable to skeletal muscle on T1-weighted sequences and intermediate to high signal intensity on T2-weighted images (Figs. 15.10–15.13). After i.v. gadolinium they reveal various degrees of enhancement. Since there are no specific features to distinguish malignant from benign tumors, diagnosis of malignancy has to be based on the depth of the colon wall infiltration, tumor growth beyond the serosa, and the presence of lymph node metastases.

Staging of colorectal cancer follows either Dukes' or the TNM classification (Table 15.1). TNM staging has the advantages of more closely indicating the depth of infiltration into the bowel wall and the lymph node status. Newly designed body phased array coils and/or endorectal coils have been shown to improve spatial resolution compared with standard body coils (SMITH et al. 1992; HUCH-BÖNI et al. 1996; SCHEIDLER et al. 1997a). Endorectal coil imaging

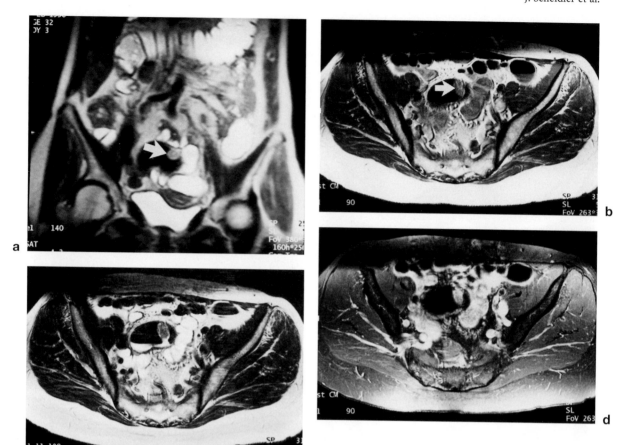

Fig. 15.9 a–d. Polyp of the sigmoid colon. The T2-weighted HASTE sequence (**a**) in the coronal orientation shows a 1.5 cm by 1 cm structure adherent to the upper wall of the sigmoid colon (*arrow*). The structure shows high signal intensity in its periphery and in the center, surrounded by a zone of low signal intensity. The axial T1-weighted SE (**b**) and T2-weighted TSE images (**c**) demonstrate an intermediate to low signal intensity mass (*arrow* in **b**) adherent to the upper anterior sigmoid wall. After contrast injection, slight peripheral enhancement is demonstrated in the T1-weighted fat-suppressed SE sequence (**d**)

Table 15.1. Surgical-pathologic staging according to the TNM classification (THOENI and ROGALLA 1994)

Astler-Coller classification (modified from Dukes)	TNM classification	Description	Approximate 5-year survival (%)
A	T1N0M0	Nodes (−), limited to submucosa	80
B1	T2N0M0	Nodes (−), limited to muscularis +/− serosa	70
B2	T3N0M0	Nodes (−), lesion transmural into adjacent tissue	60–65
C1	T2N1M0	Nodes (+), lesion into muscularis +/− serosa	35–45
C2	T3N1M0	Nodes (+), lesion transmural into adjacent	25
	T4N1M0	tissue (T3) and beyond (T4)	
D	Any T and N; M1	Any of the above + distant metastases	<25

permits reliable differentiation of the rectal wall layers (SCHNALL et al. 1994). Various imaging protocols, such as T2-weighted fat-suppressed imaging (SCHNALL et al. 1994), fast short TI recovery sequences (STIR) (MASUKO et al. 1996), and gadolinium-enhanced fat-suppressed images (SHOENUT et al. 1993a), have been shown to perform well in colorectal cancer and have been recommended to determine the depth of invasion into the bowel wall.

Endorectal MR imaging has proved able to demonstrate lymph nodes as small as 2 mm (SCHNALL et al. 1994). Similar to CT, however, MRI is unable to

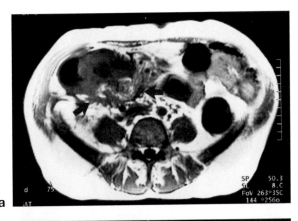

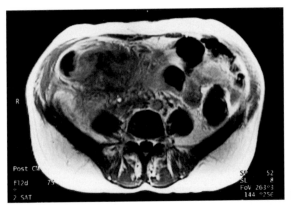

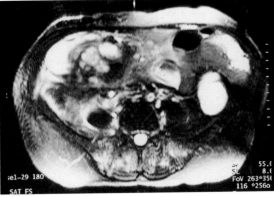

Fig. 15.10 a–c. Carcinoma of the ascending colon. The T1-weighted breath-hold FLASH sequence in the transverse orientation (**a**) shows a low signal intensity inhomogeneous mass filling the entire colonic lumen and penetrating through the dorsal wall into the pericolonic fat tissue (*arrows*). After contrast enhancement (**b**) the tumor shows mild enhancement with delineation of nonenhancing necrotic areas. T2-weighted fat-saturated imaging after retrograde filling with aqueous methylcellulose suspension (**c**) allows delineation of intraluminal tumor from anterior colonic wall. The necrotic areas show high signal intensity

recognize tumor foci in normal-sized nodes (Fig. 15.3f) and is dependent on the same size criteria for the diagnosis of lymph node abnormality (short-axis diameter larger than 1 cm). (VINNICOMBE et al. 1995). MRI readily distinguishes enlarged nodes from vessels without the use of intravenous contrast. Lymph node metastases present with low to intermediate signal internsity on unenhanced T1-weighted images and with intermediate to high signal intensity on T2-weighted sequences.

Invasion of adjacent organs is best demonstrated on the transverse or coronal plane of section; however, for rectal carcinoma additional sagittal imaging is mandatory to evaluate the craniocaudal tumor extent and tumor spread to adjacent organs (Fig. 15.3f). Loss of the separating fat plane and high signal intensity of the vaginal or bladder wall on T2-weighted images is highly suggestive of tumor invasion.

15.5.2.2
Anal Carcinoma

The MR imaging characteristics of anal carcinoma resemble those of colorectal adenocarcinoma, al-

though histologically most anal carcinomas are squamous cell carcinomas. Evaluation of the extent of disease is facilitated by using orthogonal imaging planes and by administration of intravenous gadolinium. Since sphincter-sparing radiochemotherapy is considered preferable to radical surgery for smaller (<4 cm) tumors (GRABENBAUER et al. 1994; SCHLAG and HUNERBEIN 1995), MR imaging may play a significant role in treatment planning in the future.

15.5.2.3
Lymphoma

Primary non-Hodgkin's lymphoma of the colon is a rare disease. Usually lymphoma of the colon represents a manifestation of widespread disease. Colonic lymphoma may develop in patients with long-standing ulcerative colitis and an association with HIV infection has been described. The most common sites of involvement are the cecum and the rectum. MRI features include single or multiple enhancing masses, or diffuse nodularity combined with an enhancing, thickened colonic wall. Central areas of low signal intensity on T1-weighted images and

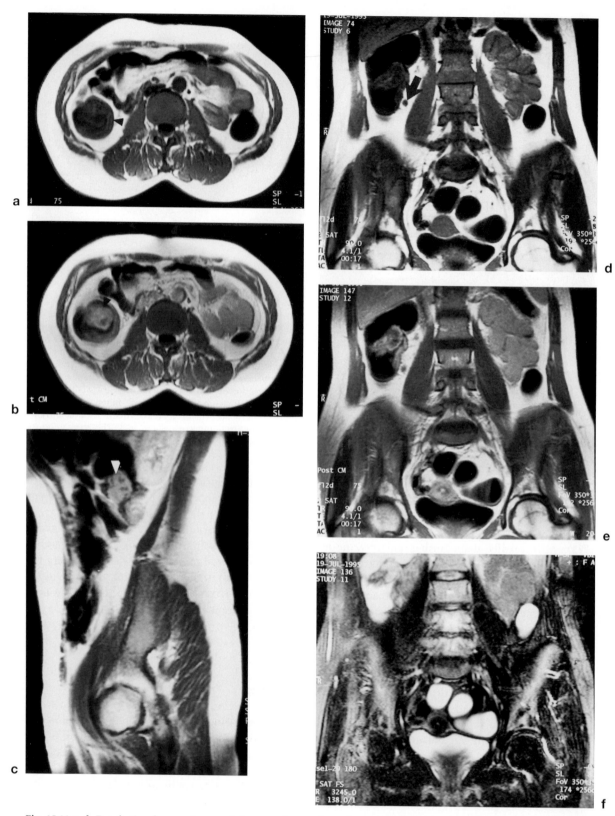

Fig. 15.11 a–f. Exophytic adenocarcinoma of the ascending colon. Axial T1-weighted FLASH images before (**a**) and after i.v. contrast (**b**) and a sagittal contrast-enhanced section (**c**) demonstrate thickening of the medial wall of the ascending colon (*arrowhead* in **a**) containing an exophytic intraluminal enhancing mass (*arrowhead* in **b**). Nonenhancing central areas of the tumor are indicative for necrosis. T1-weighted coronal images before (**d**) and after i.v. contrast administration (**e**) show clear delineation of the thickened colonic wall from mesenteric fat without any signs of tumor invasion into the mesenteric fat. Areas of low signal intensity correspond to locoregional lymph nodes (*arrow* in **d**). T2-weighted fat-suppressed sequence (**f**) after retrograde filling of the colon with aqueous methylcellulose suspension clearly depicts the exophytic tumor mass, but does not allow distinction between bowel wall and mesenteric fat

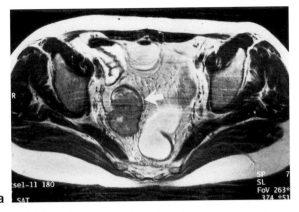

a

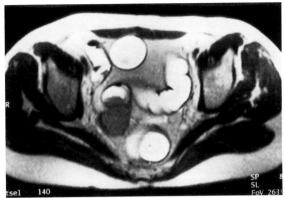

b

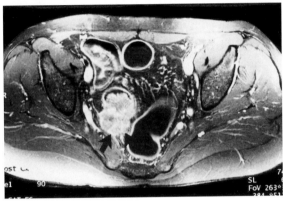

c

Fig. 15.12 a–c. Carcinoma of the sigmoid. T2-weighted axial images obtained with the TSE (a) and HASTE (b) techniques after rectal application of aqueous methylcellulose suspension demonstrate a mass occupying the entire lumen of the sigmoid colon (*arrow* in a). Due to full-thickness tumor infiltration, the normal layers of the bowel wall with their linear pattern of enhancement are destroyed (c). Additionally, tumor invasion of the perisigmoid fat (*arrow*) is present on the T1-weighted contrast-enhanced fat-suppressed sequence (c)

high signal intensity on T2-weighted images reflect the tendency toward necrosis. The combination of these features with bulky retroperitoneal and mesenteric lymphadenopathy and enlargement of the spleen is indicative of the diagnosis.

15.5.2.4
Carcinoid

Carcinoids also occur in the colon although most commonly they are found in the small bowel. The most frequent sites in the colon are the appendix and the rectum. In contrast to appendiceal carcinoids, which are almost invariably benign, rectal carcinoids are usually malignant. Frequently these malignant tumors are too small to be detectable by MR imaging. Large tumors produce asymmetric bowel wall thickening that enhances after intravenous gadolinium. As on CT, stranding in the mesenteric root is characteristic for the desmoplastic response surrounding the tumor. Multiple nodularities are suggestive of lymph node involvement.

15.5.2.5
Metastases

Cervical and ovarian carcinoma are the two most common malignancies to secondarily involve the colon, mostly through direct tumor invasion (cervical carcinoma) or intraperitoneal tumor spread (ovarian carcinoma). The sigmoid colon and the area close to the ileocecal valve are common sites for metastatic seeds. Peritoneal implants of ovarian cancer are best demonstrated on T1-weighted fat-suppressed contrast-enhanced studies (SEMELKA et al. 1993). When peritoneal implants and metastatic tumor masses are present in ovarian cancer, examination of the entire abdomen, including the supramesocolic space, is mandatory to allow for optimal planning of surgical debulking.

15.5.3
Cancer Recurrence

Diagnosis of rectal cancer recurrence is one of the most common applications for MR imaging of the

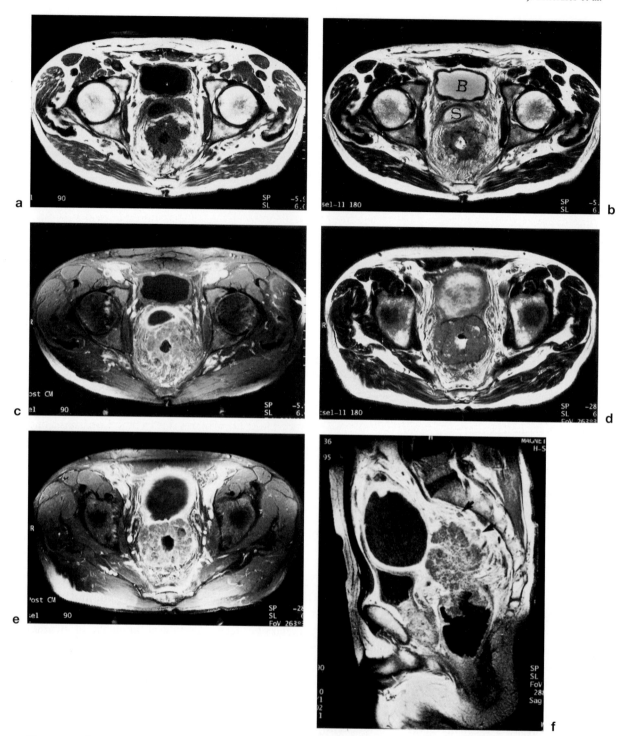

Fig. 15.13 a–f. Carcinoma of the rectum. Axial T1-weighted
SE (**a**) and T2-weighted TSE (**b**) sequences demonstrate
irregular thickening of the rectal bowel wall with streaky
infiltration of the perirectal tissue. Anteriorly the bladder (*B*)
and a contrast filled part of the sigmoid colon (*S*) are identified
(**b**) with strong contrast enhancement of the wall of the
sigmoid colon on the fat-suppressed T1-weighted image (**c**).
Two centimeters above the level of **a–c**, T2-weighted (**d**) and
fat-suppressed images (**e**) demonstrate a large, fluid-filled,
enhancing structure anterior to the tumor which represents
the distended cecum. The craniocaudal extension of the carcinoma and the infiltration of the cecum are best encountered
in the sagittal plane of section (**f**; contrast-enhanced T1-
weighted image). Although there was no significant enlargement, perirectal lymph nodes (*arrows*) were infiltrated by the
tumor

colon and rectum since breath-hold imaging is not necessarily required. Sagittal MR imaging capabilities permit evaluation of the rectum in the best plane and give MR imaging an edge over CT. Recurrence rates vary between 8% and 50% depending on tumor stage at primary presentation (DE LANGE et al. 1989). Recurrences are typically found in the vicinity of the surgical margin, usually at the site of anastomosis. Recurrent tumor masses are often of low signal intensity on T1-weighted images and high signal intensity on T2-weighted sequences (EBNER et al. 1988; KRESTIN et al. 1988). After i.v. administration of gadolinium, tumor recurrences show significant enhancement. On fat-suppressed T1-weighted sequences, however, a moderate degree of enhancement may also be encountered in postoperative scars. Postradiation fibrosis is low in signal intensity on T2-weighted images with negligible enhancement (BUTCH et al. 1986; DE LANGE et al. 1989; THOENI 1991; ITO et al. 1992). Especially in the early postoperative phase (<1 year after surgery) there is considerable overlap in the MR imaging features which precludes reliable differentiation between fibrosis and recurrent tumor. Furthermore, a desmoplastic reaction as a common host response to various benign and malignant conditions can resemble the appearance of benign fibrosis with low signal intensity on T2-weighted images when actually tumor recurrence is present (BUTCH et al. 1986; DE LANGE et al. 1989; THOENI 1991; ITO et al. 1992). Therefore, diagnosis of recurrence should not be based only on signal intensity and contrast enhancement, but also on tissue morphology (platelike appearance of fibrosis vs nodularity of recurrence), the patient's symptomatology, and clinical data.

15.5.4
Role of Endorectal Ultrasound, CT, and MRI in the Diagnosis and Staging of Primary and Recurrent Colorectal Malignancies

The preoperative evaluation of patients diagnosed as having colorectal cancer is influenced by: (a) the anatomic location of the primary tumor; (b) the knowledge that 10%–25% of patients harbor detectable metastases at the time of initial diagnosis; (c) the observation that as many as one-third of patients with isolated metastases may achieve significant survival benefit by aggressive surgery; and (d) the need to accurately stage rectal cancers to permit selection of appropriate surgery. Endorectal ultrasound is an established imaging modality for the evaluation of

rectal cancer (RIFKIN and MARKS 1985). Overstaging seems to be the most frequent error, both in the staging of rectal carcinoma (TIO et al. 1991) and in the determination of the malignant potential of adenomas (HULSMANS et al. 1992). One reason for overstaging is inflammatory peritumoral changes that mimic direct tumor extension. The accuracy of transrectal ultrasound is 77% for demonstration of tumor invasion into the perirectal fat and 50% for perirectal lymph node involvement (RIFKIN et al. 1989). Limitations of endorectal ultrasound are its dependence on the experience of the operator and the fact that the instrument is unable to pass severe luminal stenosis. Ultrasound assessment of colorectal carcinoma above the peritoneal reflection is clinically less important because the findings currently do not alter clinical management. MR imaging with endorectal coils and endorectal ultrasound are equally effective in the staging of colorectal cancer. A range of accuracy of 72%–100% has been reported for endorectal MRI tumor staging (JOOSTEN et al. 1995; MURANO et al. 1995; MEYENBERGER et al. 1996). MRI is superior to endoscopic ultrasound for the assessment of lymphadenopathy (MEYENBERGER et al. 1996). Limitations of endorectal MRI are artifacts due to bowel peristalsis and movement of the endorectal coil, which may lead to nondiagnostic images especially on T2-weighted imaging (MURANO et al. 1995). Although MRI with endorectal coils provides superb resolution and contrast-to-noise, the small field of view of the coil limits its use to tumors located in the rectum and sigmoid colon.

Magnetic resonance imaging has not yet proven its superiority over CT for the staging of colorectal cancer although initial reports found MRI to compare favorably with CT in terms of overall staging accuracy (BUTCH et al. 1986; THOENI 1991). A recently published large multicenter study (ZERHOUNI et al. 1996) found similar accuracy of both modalities for the depiction of transmural tumor extension of colon cancer and for the detection of lymph node (62%–64%) and liver metastases (85% each). CT was more accurate than MR imaging in the detection and characterization of transmural penetration of rectal tumors (74% vs 58%). All of the examinations, however, were performed in the period 1989–1993 and did not include contrast-enhanced sequences. Additionally, modern imaging techniques (fat suppression, fast spin-echo, and breath-hold sequences) as well as endorectal and phased array coils were not available during the study period. These recent technological advances in MR imaging may affect the results.

One of the most widely used applications of MR imaging is the postoperative evaluation of patients for tumor recurrence. The relatively fixed position of the rectum allows for superior image quality without the need for breath-hold imaging. MRI is well suited for detecting recurrent rectal carcinoma because of the ability to acquire images directly in the sagittal plane. MR imaging has been found to be superior to CT and transrectal ultrasound (Gomberg et al. 1986; Krestin et al. 1988; de Lange et al. 1989; Waizer et al. 1991; Pema et al. 1994). MRI detected recurrent rectal cancer in 83% of patients, whereas endorectal ultrasound identified recurrence in only 42% (Waizer et al. 1991). Use of gadolinium-enhanced T1-weighted sequences in addition to standard T1- and T2-weighted imaging increased the accuracy to 93% (Balzarini et al. 1990). Dynamic MR imaging revealed significantly greater and faster enhancement of recurrences compared with postoperative fibrotic changes and therefore may further increase the utility of MRI for the diagnosis of recurrent rectal carcinoma (Mueller-Schimpfle et al. 1993).

15.6
Conclusion

The role of MR imaging for investigating colorectal disease is increasing. Current indications for MR imaging include staging of colorectal cancer, suspicion of rectal cancer recurrence, and the preoperative evaluation of anorectal fistulae. A role of MR imaging is emerging for the determination of the extent and activity of Crohn's disease and ulcerative colitis. Future directions include comprehensive ultrafast scanning of the entire gastrointestinal tract with single-shot fast spin-echo sequences (Beall and Regan 1996) and echo-planar techniques. The development of dedicated interventional MR scanners will allow for therapeutic interventions with real-time MR guidance and monitoring.

References

Anderson CM, Brown JJ, Balfe DM, Heiken JP, Borrello JA, Clouse RE, Pilgram TK (1994) MR imaging of Crohn disease: use of perflubron as a gastrointestinal contrast agent. J Magn Reson Imaging 4:491–496

Balzarini L, Ceglia E, D'Ippolito G, Petrillo R, Tess JD, Musumeci R (1990) Local recurrence of rectosigmoid cancer: what about the choice of MRI for diagnosis? Gastrointest Radiol 15:338–342

Beall DP, Regan F (1996) MRI of bowel obstruction using the HASTE sequence. J Comput Assist Tomogr 20:823–825

Bernardino ME, Weinreb JC, Mitchell DG, Small WC, Morris M (1994) Safety and optimum concentration of a manganese chloride-based oral MR contrast agent. J Magn Reson Imaging 4:872–876

Brown JJ, Duncan JR, Heiken JP, et al. (1991) Perfluoroctyl-bromide as a gastrointestinal contrast agent for MR imaging: use with and without glucagon. Radiology 181:455–460

Butch RJ, Stark DD, Wittenberg J, et al. (1986) Staging rectal cancer by MR and CT. AJR Am J Roentgenol 146:1155–1160

Chou CK, Chen LT, Sheu RS, Wang ML, Jaw TS, Liu GC (1994) MRI manifestations of gastrointestinal wall thickening [see comments]. Abdom Imaging 19:389–394

Davis MA, Mei H, Ritsema GH (1994) Optimization of a negative oral contrast agent for magnetic resonance imaging. Invest Radiol 29 (Suppl 2):S120–S122

de Lange EE, Fechner RE, Wanebo HJ (1989) Suspected recurrent rectosigmoid carcinoma after abdominoperieneal resection: MR imaging and histopathologic findings. Radiology 170:323–328

deSouza NM, Kmiot WA, Puni R, Hall AS, Burl M, Bartram CI, Bydder GM (1995) High resolution magnetic resonance imaging of the anal sphincter using an internal coil. Gut 37:284–287

Ebner F, Kressel HY, Mintz MC, et al. (1988) Tumor recurrence versus fibrosis in the female pelvis: differentiation with MR imaging at 1.5 T. [published erratum appears in Radiology (1988);168:286]. Radiology 166:333–340

Gomberg JS, Friedman AC, Radecki PD, Grumbach K, Caroline DF (1986) MRI differentiation of recurrent colorectal carcinoma from postoperative fibrosis. Gastrointest Radiol 11:361–363

Grabenbauer GG, Panzer M, Hultenschmidt B, et al. (1994) Prognostische Faktoren nach simultaner Radiochemotherapie des Analkanalkarzinoms in einer multizentrischen Serie von 139 Patienten Onkol 170:391–399

Haggett PJ, Moore NR, Shearman JD, Travis SP, Jewell DP, Mortensen NJ (1995) Pelvic and perineal complications of Crohn's disease: assessment using magnetic resonance imaging. Gut 36:407–410

Haldemann-Heusler RC, Wight E, Marincek B (1995) Oral superparamagnetic contrast agent (Ferumoxsil): tolerance and efficacy in MR imaging of gynecologic diseases. J Magn Reson Imaging 4:385–391

Hancock BJ, Vajcner A (1988) Lipomas of the colon: a clinicopathologic review. Can J Surg 31:178–181

Hirohashi S, Uchida H, Yoshikawa K, et al. (1994) Large scale clinical evaluation of bowel contrast agent containing ferric ammonium citrate in MRI. Magn Reson Imaging 12:837–846

Hopper KD, Sherman JL, Luethke JM, Ghaed N (1987) The retrorenal colon in the supine and prone patient. Radiology 162:443–446

Hricak H, Swift PS, Campos Z, Quivey JM, Gildengorin V, Goranson H (1993) Irradiation of the cervix uteri: value of unenhanced and contrast-enhanced MR imaging. Radiology 189:381–388

Huch-Böni RA, Meyenberger C, Pok Lundquist J, Trinkler F, Lutolf U, Krestin GP (1996) Value of endorectal coil versus body coil MRI for diagnosis of recurrent pelvic malignancies. Abdom Imaging 21:345–352

Hulsmans FH, Tio TL, Mathus-Vliegen EM, Bosma A, Tytgat GN (1992) Colorectal villous adenoma: transrectal US in screening for invasive malignancy. Radiology 185:193–196

Hussain SM, Stoker J, Lameris JS (1995) Anal sphincter complex: endoanal MR imaging of normal anatomy. Radiology 197:671–677

Hussain SM, Stoker J, Schouten WR, Hop WC, Lameris JS (1996) Fistula in ano: endoanal sonography versus endoanal MR imaging in classification. Radiology 200:475–481

Ito K, Kato T, Tadokoro M, Ishiguchi T, Oshima M, Ishigaki T, Sakuma S (1992) Recurrent rectal cancer and scar: differentiation with PET and MR imaging. Radiology 182:549–552

Joosten FB, Jansen JB, Joosten HJ, Rosenbusch G (1995) Staging of rectal carcinoma using MR double surface coil, MR endorectal coil, and intrarectal ultrasound: correlation with histopathologic findings. J Compout Assist Tomogr 19:752–758

Kaminsky S, Laniado M, Gogoll M, et al. (1991) Gadopentetate dimeglumine as a bowel contrast agent: safety and efficacy. Radiology 178:503–508

Kettritz U, Isaacs K, Warshauer DM, Semelka RC (1995) Crohn's disease. Pilot study comparing MRI of the abdomen with clinical evaluation. J Clin Gastroenterol 21:249–253

Kier R, Wain S, Troiano R (1993) Fast spin-echo MR images of the pelvis obtained with a phased-array coil: value in laocalizing the staging prostatic carcinoma. AJR Am J Roentgenol 161:601–606

Krestin GP, Steinbrich W, Fiedmann G (1988) Rezidivdiagnostik der Rektumkarzinome: Verg MR. ROFO Fortschr Geb Rontgenstr Nuklearmed 148:28–33

Krestin GP, Steinbrich W, Friedmann G (1988) Recurrent rectal cancer: diagnosis with MR imaging versus CT. Radiology 168:307–311

Langmo L, Ros PR, Torres GM, Erquiaga E (1992) Comparison of MR imaging after barium administration with CT in pelvic disease. J Magn Reson Imaging 2:89–91

Masuko E, Homma H, Mezawa S, Matsuyama T, Watanabe N, Niitsu Y (1996) Determining depth of invasion of advanced colorectal cancer using MRI short inversion time inversion recovery sequences. J Gastroenterol 31:361–365

Meyenberger C, Wildi S, Kulling D, Bertschinger P, Zala GF, Klotz HP, Krestin GP (1996) Tumorstaging und Nachsorge des rektosigmoi Karzinoms: die koloskopische Endosonographie im Vergleich mit der CT, MRT und endorektalen MRT. Schweiz Rundsch Med Prax 85:622–631

Mirowitz SA, Heiken JP, Brown JJ (1994) Evaluation of fat saturation technique for T2-weighted endorectal coil MRI of the prostate. Magn Reson Imaging 12:743–747

Mueller-Schimpfle M, Brix G, Layer G, et al. (1993) Recurrent rectal cancer: diagnosis with dynamic MR imaging. Radiology 189:881–889

Murano A, Sasaki F, Kido C, et al. (1995) Endoscopic MRI using 3D-spoiled GRASS (SPGR) sequence for local staging of rectal carcinoma. J Comput Assist Tomogr 19:586–591

Myhr GE, Myrvold HE, Nilsen G, Thoresen JE, Rinck PA (1994) Perianal fistulas: use of MR imaging for diagnosis. Radiology 191:545–549

Outwater E, Schiebler ML (1993) Pelvic fistulas: findings on MR images. AJR Am J Roentgenol 160:327–330

Panaccione JL, Ros PR, Torres GM, Burton SS (1991) Rectal barium in pelvic MR imaging: initial results. J Magn Reson Imaging 1:605–607

Patten RM, Moss AA, Fenton TA, Elliott S (1992) OMR, a positive bowel contrast agent for abdominal and pelvic MR imaging: safety and imaging characteristics. J Magn Reson Imaging 2:25–34

Patten RM, Lo SK, Phillips JJ, et al. (1993) Positive bowel contrast agent for MR imaging of the abdomen: phase II and III clinical trials. Radiology 189:277–283

Pema PJ, Bennett WF, Bova JG, Warman P (1994) CT vs MRI in diagnosis of recurrent rectosigmoid carcinoma. J Comput Assist Tomogr 18:256–261

Rifkin MD, Marks GJ (1985) Transrectal US as an adjunct in the diagnosis of rectal and extrarectal tumors. Radiology 157:499–502

Rifkin MD, Ehrlich SM, Marks G (1989) Staging of rectal carcinoma: prospective comparison of endorectal US and CT. Radiology 170:319–322

Rogers J, Lewis J, Josephson L (1994) Use of AMI-227 as an oral MR contrast agent. Magn Reson Imaging 12:631–639

Ros PR, Steinman RM, Torres GM, Burton SS, Panaccione JL, Rappaport DC, McGorray SP (1991) The value of barium as a gastrointestinal contrast agent in MR imaging: a comparison study in normal volunteers. AJR Am J Roentgenol 157:761–767

Rubin DL, Muller HH, Sidhu MK, Young SW, Hunke WA, Gorman WG (1993) Liquid oral magnetic particles as a gastrointestinal contrast agent for MR imaging: efficacy in vivo. J Magn Reson Imaging 3:113–118

Rubin DL, Muller HH, Young SW, Hunke WA, Gorman WG (1994) Optimization of an oral magnetic particle formulation as a gastrointestinal contrast agent for magnetic resonance imaging. Invest Radiol 29:81–86

Rubinstein MC, Fisher RL (1996) Pouchitis: pathogenesis, diagnosis, and management. Gastroenterologist 4:129–133

Scheidler J, Heuck AF, Bruening R, Kohz P, Kimmig R, Stehling MK, Reiser MF (1997a) Magnetic resonance imaging of the female pelvis. New circularly polarized body array coil versus standard body coil. Invest Radiol 32:1–6

Scheidler J, Heuck AF, Meier W, Reiser MF (1997b) MR imaging of pelvic masses: efficacy of the rectal superparamagnetic contrast agent ferumoxisil. J Magn Reson Imaging 7:1027–1032

Schlag PM, Hunerbein M (1995) Anal cancer: multimodal therapy. World J Surg 19:282–286

Schnall MD, Furth EE, Rosato EF, Kressel HY (1994) Rectal tumor stage: correlation of endorectal MR imaging and pathologic findings [see comments]. Radiology 190:709–714

Semelka RC, Lawrence PH, Shoenut JP, Heywood M, Kroeker MA, Lotocki R (1993) Primary ovarian cancer: prospective comparison of contrast-enhanced CT and pre- and postcontrast, fat-suppressed MR imaging, with histologic correlation. J Magn Reson Imaging 3:99–106

Shoenut JP, Semelka RC, Silverman R, Yaffe CS, Micflikier AB (1993a) Magnetic resonace imaging evaluation of the local extent of colorectal mass lesions. J Clin Gastroenterol 17:248–253

Shoenut JP, Semelka RC, Silverman R, Yaffe CS, Micflikier AB (1993b) Magnetic resonance imaging in inflammatory bowel disease. J Clin Gastroenterol 17:73–78

Shoenut JP, Semelka RC, Magro CM, Silvernman R, Yaffe CS, Micflikier AB (1994) Comparison of magnetic resonance imaging and endoscopy in distinguishing the type and severity of inflammatory bowel disease. J Clin Gastroenterol 19:31–35

Smith RC, Reinhold C, Lange RC, McCauley TR, Kier R, McCarthy S (1992) Multicoil high-resolution fast spin-echo MR imaging of the female pelvis. Radiology 184:671–675

Spencer JA, Ward J, Beckingham IJ, Adams C, Ambrose NS (1996) Dynamic contrast-enhanced MR imaging of perianal fistulas. AJR Am J Roentgenol 167:735–741

Stahlberg D, Gullberg K, Lijeqvist L, Hellers G, Lofberg R (1996) Pouchitis following pelvic pouch operation for ulcerative colitis. Incidence, cumulative risk, and risk factors. Dis Colon Rectum 39:1012–1018

Stoker J, Hussain SM, van Kempen D, Elevelt AJ, Lameris JS (1996) Endoanal coil in MR imaging of anal fistulas. AJR Am J Roentgeneol 166:360–362

Thoeni RF (1991) Colorectal cancer: cross-sectional imaging for stanging of primary tumor and detection of local recurrence. AJR Am J Roentgenol 156:909–915

Thoeni RF, Rogalla P (1994) Current CT/MRI examination of the lower intestinal tract. Baillieres Clin Gastroenterol 8: 765–796

Tio TL, Coene PP, van Delden OM, Tytgat GN (1991) Colorectal carcinoma: preoperative TNM classificiation with endosonography. Radiology 179:165–170

Vinnicombe SJ, Norman AR, Nicolson V, Husband JE (1995) Normal pelvic lymph nodes: evaluation with CT after bipedal lymphangiography [published erratum appears in Radiology (1995) Sep;196:800]. Radiology 194:349–355

Vlahos L, Gouliamos A, Athanasopoulou A, et al. (1994) A comparative study between Gd-DTPA and oral magnetic particles (OMP) as gastrointestinal (GI) contrast agents for MRI of the abdomen. Magn Reson Imaging 12:719–726

Waizer A, Powsner E, Russo I, et al. (1991) Prospective comparative study of magnetic resonance imaging versus transrectal ultrasound for preoperative staging and follow-up of rectal cancer. Preliminary report. Dis Colon Rectum 34:1068–1072

Wesbey GE, Brasch RC, Engelstad BL, Moss AA, Crooks LE, Brito AC (1983) Nuclear magnetic resonance contrast enhancement study of the gastrointestinal tract of rats and a human volunteer using nontoxic oral iron solutions. Radiology 149:175–180

Younathan CM, Ros PR, Burton SS (1991) MR imaging of colonic lipoma. J Comput Assist Tomogr 15:492–494

Zerhouni EA, Rutter C, Hamilton SR, et al. (1996) CT and MR imaging in the staging of colorectal carcinoma: report of the Radiology Diagnostic Oncology Group II. Radiology 200:443–451

16 Bladder

U.G. Müller-Lisse, A.F. Heuck, and J.O. Barentsz

CONTENTS

16.1
Introduction

Since its early days more than a decade ago, magnetic resonance imaging (MRI) of the pelvis has been advocated as the best noninvasive imaging technique to examine regional pathologies of various organ systems (Hricak et al. 1983). Among the pelvic pathologies studied with MRI, however, diseases of the bladder received relatively little attention until the advent of fast imaging methods. The inclusion of

U.G. Müller-Lisse, MD, Department of Diagnostic Radiology, Klinikum Großhadern, Ludwig-Maximilians University, Marchioninistrasse 15, D-81377 München, Germany
A.F. Heuck, MD, Department of Diagnostic Radiology, Klinikum Großhadern, Ludwig-Maximilians University, Marchioninistrasse 15, D-81377 München, Germany
J.O. Barentsz, MD, Department of Diagnostic Radiology, University Hospital Nijmegen, P.O. Box 9101, 6500 HB Nijmegen, The Netherlands

dynamic imaging sequences in study protocols particularly spurred the development of MRI of the bladder (Tanimoto et al. 1992; Kim et al. 1994; Barentsz et al. 1996a,b).

With few exceptions, MRI examinations of the bladder have been limited to tumor patients. Nonneoplastic bladder pathologies, such as uncomplicated inflammatory bladder disease, often do not require any imaging. Sonography and conventional radiographic techniques, including intravenous urography, retrograde urethrocystography, and various fluoroscopic methods, suffice to depict most malformations, injuries and their sequelae, concrements, fistulas, foreign bodies, and functional disorders. Bladder tumors, however, require thorough staging that goes beyond the confines of the urinary tract lumina. While computed tomography (CT) was the first cross-sectional imaging method among the noninvasive staging tools, MRI has been establishing a role in the evaluation of the more advanced stages of invasive bladder cancer (stages T2 and higher) (Patel and Hricak 1995).

This chapter concentrates on the development and current options of MRI for imaging of the bladder affected with urothelial carcinoma.

16.2
Imaging Techniques and Protocols

16.2.1
Conventional MRI

16.2.1.1
Spin-Echo Imaging

Early imaging protocols were based on T1- and T2-weighted spin-echo (SE) sequences whose typical repetition times and echo times are shown in Table 16.1. Fields of view typically ranged from 28 to 36 cm, and matrix sizes from 128×256 to 256×256. The section thickness was typically ca. 0.8 cm (0.5–1.2 cm), and the intersection gap ca. 0.2 cm

Table 16.1. Examination parameters in conventional MRI of the bladder: SE sequences

Authors	Magnetic field strength	T1-weighted SE sequence	T2-weighted SE sequence
FISHER et al. (1985)	Not reported	TR 0.5 s, TE 28 ms	TR 1.0–2.0 s, TE 28–56 ms
AMENDOLA et al. (1986)	0.35 T, body coil	TR 0.5 s, TE 28 ms	TR 1.0–2.0 s, TE 28–56 ms
KÜPER et al. (1986)	1.5 T, body coil	TR 0.4–0.8 s, TE 30 ms	TR 0.8–3.2 s, TE 90–240 ms
BRYAN et al. (1987)	0.3 T and 1.0 T, body coil	TR 0.5 s, TE 30–35 ms	TR 1.0–2.0 s, TE 60–90 ms
RHOLL et al. (1987)	0.35–0.5 T, body coil	TR 0.5 s, TE 30–35 ms	TR 1.5–2.1 s, TE 90 ms
BARENTSZ et al. (1988)	0.5 T, body coil Double surface coil	TR 0.25–0.5 s, TE 30 ms	TR 2.0 s, TE 30/60–150 ms
BUY et al. (1988)	0.5 T, body coil	TR 0.4 s, TE 28 ms	TR 1.6 s, TE 40/80/120 ms
KOELBEL et al. (1988)	1.5 T, body coil	TR 0.8 s, TE 30 ms	TR 2.0 s, TE 30–90 ms
HUSBAND et al. (1989)	1.5 T, body coil	TR 0.5 s, TE 17 ms	TR 2.1 s, TE 30–70 ms

(0–1.0 cm) (FISHER et al. 1985; AMENDOLA et al. 1986; KÜPER et al. 1986; BRYAN et al. 1987; RHOLL et al. 1987; BARENTSZ et al. 1988; BUY et al. 1988; KOELBEL et al. 1988; HUSBAND et al. 1989).

Based on these parameters, the bladder wall shows an intermediate signal intensity on T1-weighted images, while urine has a low signal and perivesical fat tissue a high signal intensity. The different layers of the bladder wall cannot be differentiated on T1-weighted SE images, and the bladder floor and trigone do not contrast sufficiently with the prostate (FISHER et al. 1985; KÜPER et al. 1986). On T2-weighted images, urine shows a very bright signal that contrasts strongly with the low signal intensity bladder wall. Perivesical fat tissue is moderately bright, and the prostate has a slightly higher signal intensity than the bladder wall. The seminal vesicles are readily distinguished by their bright internal signal and the low signal intensity of their walls (FISHER et al. 1985; KÜPER et al. 1986). T2-weighted images are prone to chemical shift artifact that may produce low signal intensity lines on one side of the bladder and high signal intensity lines on the other, due to differences in the precessional frequencies of water and fat. These lines may be misinterpreted as bladder wall pathology. In case of doubt, the direction of the readout gradient should be swapped and the sequence repeated (HEIKEN and LEE 1988). With any of the unenhanced sequences that have been applied in MRI of the bladder, it is not possible to reliably differentiate between tumor and surrounding inflammatory reaction or edema of the bladder wall (HRICAK et al. 1983; FISHER et al. 1985; KÜPER et al. 1986; RHOLL et al. 1987; HEIKEN and LEE 1988).

Transitional cell (urothelial) carcinoma of the bladder, on the other hand, may present with T1 and T2 relaxation times so similar to uninvolved bladder wall that differentiation of tumor and healthy surrounding tissue becomes very difficult on the basis of

Table 16.2. FSE protocols for T2-weighted MRI of the bladder

Author	KIM et al. (1994)	BARENTSZ et al. (1996b)
Magnetic field strength	1.5 T, body/phased array coil	1.5 T, Helmholtz surface coil
TR	4.0–5.0 s	3.0 s
TE eff.	102 ms	90 ms
Section thickness	0.5 cm	0.8 cm
Intersection gap	0.1 cm	0.2 cm
Slice orientation	Not specified	In plane of best tumor visibility
No. of acquisitions	4	3
Matrix	192 × 256	320 × 512
Field of view	32–40 cm	30 cm

signal intensity on both T1- and T2-weighted SE images (KOELBEL et al. 1988). However, bladder cancers may show a signal intensity higher than that of unaffected bladder wall on T2-weighted images (KIM et al. 1994). If the echo time (TE) does not exceed 100 ms, bladder cancer usually shows a higher signal intensity on T2-weighted images when compared with normal bladder wall. In presence of fibrosis, however, signal intensity of urothelial carcinoma may be as low as signal intensity of bladder wall (BARENTSZ et al. 1990).

16.2.1.2
Fast Spin-Echo Imaging

The introduction of fast spin-echo (FSE) techniques has made T2-weighted MRI considerably faster, particularly at higher magnetic field strengths (KIM et al. 1994; BARENTSZ et al. 1996a). As a result, imaging time can be reduced, or the matrix or number of slices increased and slice section thickness reduced (Table 16.2, Fig. 16.1).

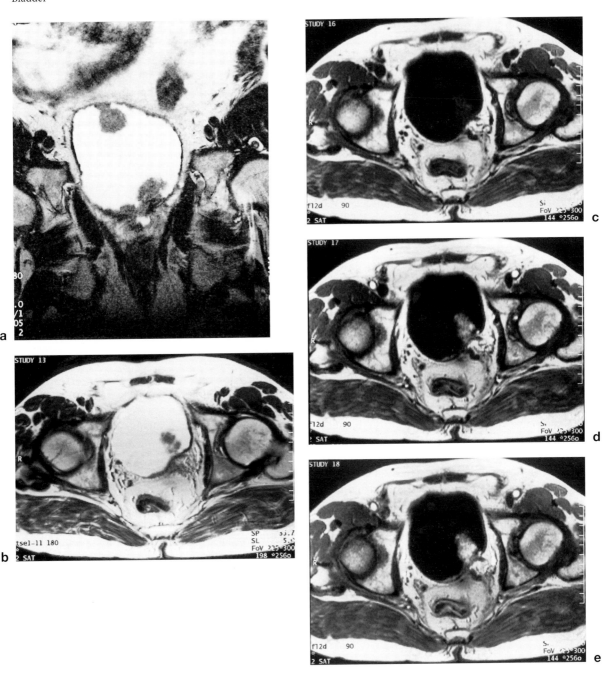

Fig. 16.1 a–e. Multifocal stage Ta papillary urothelial carcinoma of the bladder in a 63-year-old male patient. T2-weighted coronal (**a**) and axial (**b**) FSE images show papillary tumor growth, while depth of invasion cannot be perceived. Dynamic, contrast-enhanced gradient-echo (GRE) images obtained prior to (**c**), 30 s after (**d**), and 60 s after (**e**) intravenous contrast administration show superficial tumor staged T1 or below

16.2.1.3
Other Imaging Techniques

Spin-echo sequences with T1-weighting have been replaced by a three-dimensional magnetization-prepared rapid gradient-echo (MPRAGE) sequence by the group of BARENTSZ et al. (1994, 1996a,b). With a repetition time (TR) of 10 ms, a TE of 4 ms, an inversion time (TI) of 500 ms, a flip angle of 10°, an effective section thickness of 0.12 cm, two acquisitions, a 192 × 256 matrix, and a 30-cm field of view, the MPRAGE sequence allows for multiplanar image reconstruction and improved visualization of both the tumor and perivesical lymph nodes (BARENTSZ et al. 1996b).

16.2.2
Contrast-Enhanced and Dynamic MRI

Since 1989, various authors have included contrast-enhanced T1-weighted sequences in their imaging protocols. The dose of contrast media applied was invariably the standard dose of 0.1 mmol Gd-DTPA per kg body weight (NEUERBURG et al. 1989; SOHN et al. 1990; DORINGER et al. 1991; SPARENBERG et al. 1991; TACHIBANA et al. 1991; TANIMOTO et al. 1992; BARENTSZ et al. 1994; KIM et al. 1994; BARENTSZ et al. 1996b).

More recent reports also include dynamic contrast-enhanced studies with short TR/short TE sequences repetitively acquired after intravenous bolus injection of Gd-DTPA (NEUERBURG et al. 1989; TACHIBANA et al. 1991; TANIMOTO et al. 1992; KIM et al. 1994; BARENTSZ et al. 1996b). The different protocols used are listed in Table 16.3.

The different approaches to rapid dynamic imaging show that this aspect of MRI of the bladder is still in an early phase of development. One of the most severe problems to date is that only a very limited number of slices can be obtained with the high repetition rate that characterizes dynamic imaging. The problem of missing the tumor has been addressed by BARENTSZ et al. (1996b), who reported failure of tumor inclusion in the single slice depicted

by their dynamic sequence in 2 of 49 cases. In fact, successful dynamic imaging with a single- or dual-slice technique requires recognition of tumor location prior to slice selection. It is, therefore, likely to fail in cases of flat, superficial, or superficially invasive tumors, e.g., stages Tis or T1. In prebiopsy MRI examinations, the target is likely to be missed when focal edema or an inflammatory reaction leads to local bladder wall distension. In multifocal bladder cancer, it may be difficult to include all foci recognized in preceding multislice sequences in one or two slices for dynamic evaluation (Fig. 16.1). Also, in recurrent bladder cancer, it may be difficult to select the site of recurrence among focal alterations in the bladder wall brought about by earlier therapeutic measures.

16.3
Staging of Bladder Cancer

16.3.1
Classification and Histologic Characterization of Bladder Tumors

Bladder tumors may be benign or malignant, and derive from epithelial or mesenchymal cells. Primary tumors of the bladder have to be distinguished from secondary tumors that infiltrate the bladder from without or represent metastases of other, distant tumors. Among the latter, tumors infiltrating the bladder include malignancies of the female reproductive organs, the prostate, or the colon and rec-

Table 16.3. Protocols for rapid dynamic MRI of the bladder

Author	NEUERBURG et al. (1989)	TACHIBANA et al. (1991)	TANIMOTO et al. (1992)	KIM et al. (1994)	BARENTSZ et al. (1996b)
Filed strength	1.5 T	1.5 T	1.5 T	1.5 T	1.5 T
Sequence	FLASH	FSE	SE	GRE	TurboFLASH
TR	50 ms	100 ms	100 ms	40–130 ms	7 ms
TE	10 ms	14 ms	12 ms	4.5–12 ms	3 ms
Flip angle	60°			70°–80°	10°
TI					15 ms
No. of Acq.	1–2	1	1	1–2	1–2
No. of slices	1	1	1–2	Not reported	1
Acq. time	13–22 s	14 s	6.7–14 s	20–40 s	1.25–2.50 s
Slice thickness	0.8 cm	1.0 cm	1.0 cm	Not reported	0.8 cm
Interslice gap			Not reported	Not reported	
Orientation	Various[a]	Various[a]	Various[a]	Not reported	Various[a]
Matrix	256 × 256	Not reported	128 × 256	128 × 256	128 × 256
FOV	Not reported	Not reported	28–32 cm	32–40 cm	35 cm

Acq., acquisitions; FOV, field of view; FLASH, fast low-angle shot; FSE, fast spin-echo; GRE, spoiled gradient echo.
[a] Perpendicular to tumor base.

tum. Metastases often derive from carcinoma of the stomach, melanoma, breast cancer, or bronchial cancer. Primary epithelial tumors include papilloma, transitional cell carcinoma (urothelial carcinoma), squamous cell carcinoma, adenocarcinoma, and undifferentiated carcinoma. Mesenchymal primaries include benign fibroma, myxoma, leiomyoma, hemangioma, neurofibroma, neurinoma, pheochromocytoma, and other rare benign tumors as well as malignant leiomyosarcoma, fibrosarcoma, osteochondrosarcoma, rhabdomyosarcoma, and reticuloendothelial tumors.

The majority of bladder tumors are of epithelial (urothelial) origin. Normal urothelium in the bladder consists of three to seven layers of transitional cells, mainly of elongated shape with eccentric nuclei. Most cells are in contact with the basal membrane. Structural and cellular alterations of the urothelium are described as hyperplasia, metaplasia, dysplasia, and carcinoma. Epithelial hyperplasia consists of an increased number of transitional cell layers that are regularly arrayed. Squamous cell metaplasia describes a situation where urothelium is replaced by nonkeratinized squamous cell epithelium. Metaplasia in the presence of keratinization and cellular atypia that may extend into deeper layers of the bladder wall is described as leukoplakia. Leukoplakia is considered to represent a precancerotic state with a 20% chance of developing into bladder cancer (BENSON et al. 1983). Squamous cell epithelial bladder cancer is a rare type of urothelium-derived carcinoma often associated with *Schistosoma haematobium* and squamous cell metaplasia. The differential diagnosis of metaplasia includes von Brunn's cell nests, which represent inclusions of normal-looking urothelium into deeper layers of the bladder wall. A similar lesion is found in cystitis cystica, urothelial inclusions in the bladder wall surrounding a center of amorphic, eosinophilic matter. In cystitis follicularis, lymphatic follicles develop in the submucosa layer as a reaction to chronic inflammatory disorder. In combination with metaplastic changes, urothelial inclusions in the bladder wall are a sign of cystitis glandularis, which is considered to represent a precancerotic alteration. Inverted papilloma, which shows a preference for invasion into the fibromuscular stroma, also represents a precancerotic lesion. Urothelial dysplasia represents various degrees of nuclear alteration in the absence of an increased number of mitoses or cell layers. It is often difficult to distinguish between urothelial dysplasia and transitional cell carcinoma in situ (JOCHAM 1994).

In situ carcinoma (Tis) has been defined as an anaplastic (grade 3) urothelial tumor without exophytic, papillary protrusion into the bladder lumen or infiltration beyond the basal membrane ("flat tumor"). Loss of the usual array of epithelial cell layers distinguishes carcinoma in situ from urothelial dysplasia. While primary Tis is relatively seldom (5% of all superficial bladder tumors), its importance lies in both its extreme aggressiveness (almost 80% risk of progression; 38%–83% risk of developing into a muscle-infiltrating tumor) and the high rate of coincidence of secondary carcinoma in situ with exophytic, papillary or solid urothelial carcinoma (20%–75%) (ALTHAUSEN et al. 1976; JAKSE et al. 1989). Also, Tis is frequently found in recurrent or primary multifocal bladder cancer.

Among the various types of urothelial carcinoma of the bladder, papillary exophytic tumors are most frequent (ca. 70%, Fig. 16.1), while solid, infiltrating or nodular types (10%) or mixed types (20%) are less common. Cell morphology and differentiation within the tumor is generally described as good (G1), intermediate (G2), or poor (G3). With the exception of Tis tumors that are defined by their poor differentiation, tumor size and depth of invasion correlate both with the degree of cell differentiation and with the risk of progression.

Adenocarcinoma of the bladder represents less than 2% of all bladder cancers and may derive from remnants of the urachus, primary adenomatous cells anywhere in the bladder, or secondary metastatic clusters of adenocarcinoma cells in the bladder (JOCHAM 1994).

16.3.2
Staging Systems for Urothelial Carcinoma of the Bladder

The TNM classification of bladder cancers includes only carcinomas, excluding papillomas and other tumors. Local tumor staging (T-staging) is guided by clinical examination, various imaging methods, endoscopy, and biopsy. Lymph node staging (N-staging) includes clinical examination and imaging methods. The earliest staging system was developed in the 1940s (JEWETT and STRONG 1946; MARSHALL 1952) and integrates local tumor extent, lymph node infestation, and metastatic extension under one common staging symbol. The TNM system of the Union Internationale Contre le Cancrum (UICC) stages local tumor extent (T-stage, Fig. 16.2), lymph node invasion (N-stage), and metastasis (M-stage) individually. Table 16.4 lists both staging systems and their staging criteria.

16.4
Accuracy of MRI in the Staging of Bladder Cancer

The accuracy of MRI in the staging of bladder cancer will depend to a considerable extent on the individual experience of the radiologist with bladder cancer as a pathologic and a radiologic entity. However, careful selection among the ever-increasing spectrum of MRI sequences and staging criteria and consideration of the biopsy status of the patient's bladder are likely to determine the clinical value of MRI in the staging of bladder cancer. The classical staging criteria for unenhanced MR images refer to SE sequences with a matrix size of 128 × 256 or 256 × 256 and a field of view of 32 × 32 cm to 36 × 36 cm, acquired with the body coil at various field strengths ranging from 0.35 to 1.5 T (FISHER et al. 1985; KÜPER

et al. 1986). While criteria for the absence of tumor (T0) or the presence of low-grade superficial tumors (Ta) are not included, FISHER et al. (1985) list in situ (Tis) bladder cancers as "too small for current resolution." According to their criteria, invasive tumor is best recognized as a high signal intensity defect in the bladder wall on T2-weighted images that either leaves an undisrupted layer of low signal intensity, representing the outer bladder wall and indicating stage T1 or T2 bladder cancer, or involves most of its width, indicating T3a bladder cancer. Complete disruption of the low signal intensity line of the bladder wall and abnormal tissue external to the bladder wall in perivesical fat are indicative of stage T3b bladder cancer. Extension of abnormal tissue to contiguous pelvic organs (e.g., seminal vesicles, prostate, vagina, and rectum) are suggestive of T4a disease. Stage T4b bladder cancer is characterized by the extension of abnormal tissue to distant organs or to the pelvic sidewalls (FISHER et al. 1985). While the criteria indicating stage T3b and above are based on findings on both T1- and T2-weighted

a) histological layers of the bladder wall

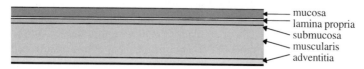

— mucosa
— lamina propria
— submucosa
— muscularis
— adventitia

b) stage Ta carcinoma of the bladder (papillary growth pattern)

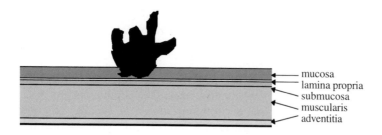

— mucosa
— lamina propria
— submucosa
— muscularis
— adventitia

c) stage Tis carcinoma of the bladder (flat tumor)

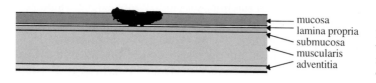

— mucosa
— lamina propria
— submucosa
— muscularis
— adventitia

Fig. 16.2. Histologic layers of the bladder wall and different stages of urothelial carcinoma of the bladder according to the TNM classification

Table 16.4. Comparison of the Jewett-Strong-Marshall system and the TNM system of bladder cancer staging according to histopathologic criteria

Jewett-Strong-Marshall stages	TNM stages	Staging criteria
No stage	T0	No tumor
0	Tis	Carcinoma in situ
0	Ta	Superficial tumor, confined to mucosal epithelium
A	T1	Invasive tumor, confined to lamina propria
B1	T2	Invasive tumor, confined to inner half of muscle layer
B2	T3a	Invasive tumor, confined to outer half of muscle layer
C	T3b	Extravesical tumor growth, confined to perivesical fat
D1	T4a	Extravesical tumor growth, invading other pelvic organs
D1	T4b	Extravesical tumor growth, invading pelvic or abdominal wall
D1	N1	Solitary homolateral internal or external iliac lymph node metastasis
D1	N2	Contralateral or bilateral or multiple internal or external iliac lymph node metastases
D1	N3	Fixed regional lymph node metastases
D2	N4	Juxtaregional (common iliac, inguinal, or aortic) lymph node metastases
D2	M1	Distant organ metastases

d) stage T1 carcinoma of the bladder with submucosal invasion

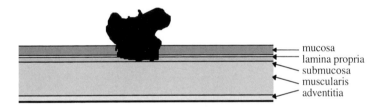

mucosa
lamina propria
submucosa
muscularis
adventitia

e) stage T2 carcinoma of the bladder invading inner half of muscle layer

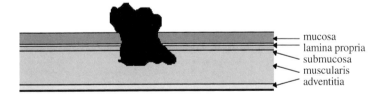

mucosa
lamina propria
submucosa
muscularis
adventitia

f) Stage T3a carcinoma of the bladder invading outer half of muscle layer

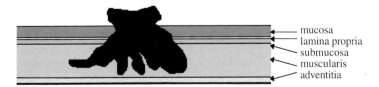

mucosa
lamina propria
submucosa
muscularis
adventitia

Fig. 16.2. (*Continued*)

g) stage T3b carcinoma of the bladder invading perivesical fat tissue   Fig. 16.2. (*Continued*)

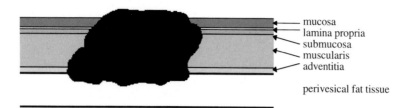

mucosa
lamina propria
submucosa
muscularis
adventitia

perivesical fat tissue

h) stage T4a (left) and T4b (right) carcinoma of the bladder

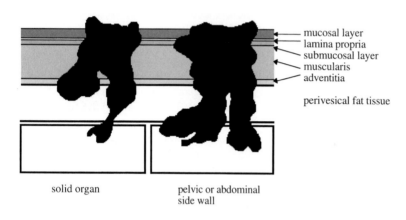

mucosal layer
lamina propria
submucosal layer
muscularis
adventitia

perivesical fat tissue

solid organ   pelvic or abdominal
                     side wall

Table 16.5. Accuracy of MRI in the T-staging of pT0 carcinoma of the bladder

Author	MRI technique	No. correct T-staging	% correct T-staging	Comment
Sohn et al. (1990)	Contrast-enhanced	6/7	86%	MRI prebiopsy
Barentsz et al. (1994)	Dynamic + MPRAGE	5/7	71%	MRI postbiopsy
Barentsz et al. (1996b)	Unenhanced	4/12	33%	MRI postbiopsy
Barentsz et al. (1996b)	Unenhanced + dynamic	11/12	92%	MRI postbiopsy

images, recognition of tumor confined to the bladder relies greatly on the presence of a high signal intensity defect on a T2-weighted image. Possible reasons for staging error in the lower stages include generation of a high signal intensity lesion by entities other than tumor, e.g., inflammation and edema alone, in the presence of tumor, or after tumor biopsy, or by motion artifact or chemical shift artifact, and erroneous assumption of another depth of infiltration due to the high or low filling state of the bladder and corresponding variation in wall thickness.

16.4.1
Absence of Bladder Cancer

Magnetic resonance imaging-assisted staging in cases of tumor absence, either primary or secondary to tumor resection at cystoscopy, has received relatively little attention. Among the studies listed in Table 16.5, less than 30 urothelial carcinoma patients without bladder cancer have undergone MRI of the bladder. One early study (Sohn et al. 1990) included seven patients without evidence of bladder cancer who underwent contrast-enhanced MRI of the bladder. While MRI staging of T0 carcinoma was correct in six of the cases, the authors did not list the criteria they used to rule out cancer on MR images. The other studies (BARENTSZ et al. 1994, 1996b) included only postbiopsy patients. Their staging criteria included presence of a biopsy defect in the bladder wall and absence of tumor signs. Without contrast enhancement, absence of tumor was correctly diagnosed in only four of 12 patients, the other eight being overstaged (in six cases stages Ta–T2; in two cases stage T3a). Adding dynamic, contrast-enhanced imaging, 11 of 12 cases were correctly staged as being free from tumor, the criterion being absence of bladder wall enhancement in the suspicious area within 10 s of arterial peak enhancement (BARENTSZ et al. 1996b). The results illustrate that, without contrast enhancement, and particularly in patients who have undergone cystoscopy and biopsy prior to MRI, staging carcinoma as T0 or absent is virtually impossible (Fig. 16.3).

16.4.2
Superficial Bladder Cancers

Bladder cancers whose most deeply growing parts (i.e., those parts penetrating furthest in a centrifugal direction from the urothelial surface) do not infiltrate the muscle layer of the bladder wall are called superficial. The superficial bladder cancers include stages Ta, Tis, and T1. Together, they comprise about 80% of all bladder cancers (JEWETT 1973; JOCHAM 1994). In these stages, carcinoma of the bladder in principle can be cured with local therapy and the bladder maintained. Therapy regimens include electrocoagulation, laser therapy, thermal or photodynamic tumor destruction, topical chemotherapy or immunotherapy, and radiation therapy, either alone or in combination with the most frequently applied diagnostic and therapeutic modality, transurethral electroresection of the bladder (TUR-B). However, 5-year survival, rate of metastasis, and rate of progression differ among the stages. In stage Ta tumors, about 95% of patients survive over a follow-

up period of 5 years. Metastases occur in 0.7%, and tumor progression is found in 4.4% of these patients. Five-year survival is equal among patients with and without Ta tumor recurrence (JOCHAM 1994). It is therefore important for an imaging method applied in the staging of bladder cancer to distinguish between superficial and muscle-infiltrating urothelial carcinoma, and to be as accurate as possible in the differentiation of the three stages of superficial tumor.

16.4.2.1
Superficial Cancers of Stages Ta and Tis

As a group of their own, stage Ta and Tis tumors have received little attention in the MRI literature (Table 16.6). Their staging is difficult, because the tumors may be small and flat and also may differ little from metaplastic or dysplastic urothelium (Figs. 16.1, 16.3). Thus, particularly flat tumors may escape detection by MRI, which is currently based on focal bladder wall thickening or thinning and altered contrast enhancement behavior. The only MRI series to include more than ten Ta/Tis tumors understaged seven of 12 tumors as T0 and overstaged two tumors, while only three were correctly identified (SOHN et al. 1990). However, the criteria applied to stage the tumors were not cited (SOHN et al. 1990). FISHER et al. (1985), in their initial study, suggested that Ta/Tis bladder cancer is too small for the spatial resolution MRI could achieve at that time. However, there is as yet no study to show that even current MRI methods are capable of correctly staging Ta/Tis bladder cancer.

16.4.2.2
Superficially Invasive Bladder Cancer of Stage pT1

Stage T1 bladder cancer may represent the most difficult stage for surgical decision-making. One reason is the vast prognostic difference between highly dif-

Table 16.6. Accuracy of MRI in the T-staging of pTa and pTis carcinoma of the bladder

Author	MRI technique	No. correct T-staging	% correct T-staging	Comment
FISHER et al. (1985)	Unenhanced	0/1	0%	Biopsy status not specified
BRYAN et al. (1987)	Unenhanced	0/1	0%	Biopsy status not specified
SOHN et al. (1990)	Contrast-enhanced	3/12	25%	MRI prebiopsy
KIM et al. (1994)	Dynamic	0/2	0%	MRI postbiopsy

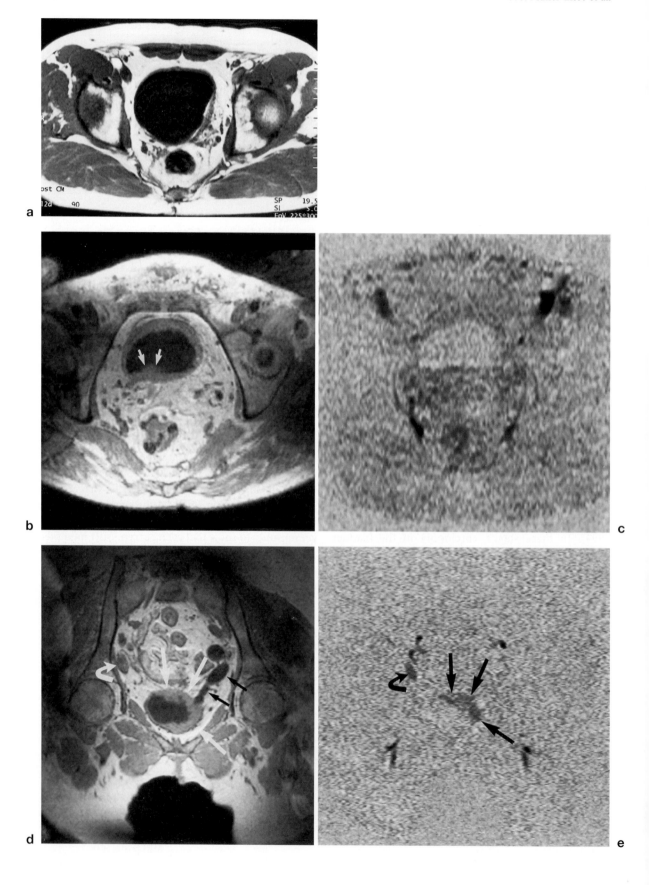

Table 16.7. Accuracy of MRI in the cumulative T-staging of pTa to pT1 carcinoma of the bladder

Author	MRI technique	No. correct T-staging	% correct T-staging	Comment
TAVARES et al. (1990)	Unenhanced	3/4	75%	MRI prebiopsy
SPARENBERG et al. (1991)	Unenhanced	4/12	33%	MRI postbiopsy
SPARENBERG et al. (1991)	Contrast-enhanced	10/14	71%	MRI postbiopsy

ferentiated (histologic grades G1 and G2; 5-year survival rate 81%, rate of metastasis 13.9%, progression rate 18.8% after transurethral electroresection) and poorly differentiated or anaplastic (histologic grades G3 and G4; 5-year survival rate 64%, rate of metastasis 22.1%, progression rate 31.4% after transurethral electroresection) stage T1 tumors (JOCHAM 1994). While TUR-B is likely to be adequate to treat the better-differentiated T1 bladder cancers, cystectomy will in many instances be recommended for poorly differentiated T1 tumors. The importance of differentiating between superficial Ta/Tis tumor, superficially invasive T1 tumor, and muscle-infiltrating tumor that is unlikely to be cured by electroresection alone has not yet been addressed by many MRI studies. Only one series has included more than ten patients with stage T1 bladder cancers. In this series, unenhanced MRI alone failed to contribute significantly to the correct staging of Ta–T1 carcinoma of the bladder. With contrast enhancement, about 70% of Ta–T1 tumors were correctly staged by MRI (SPARENBERG et al. 1991; Table 16.7).

16.4.3
Muscle-Infiltrating Bladder Cancers Confined to the Bladder Wall (Stages pT2 and pT3a)

The treatment of choice for muscle-infiltrating bladder cancers that do not invade extravesical tissues is radical cystectomy. Cystectomy shows a high local efficacy; local tumor recurrence occurs at a rate of 10%–20% (JOCHAM 1994). In principle, invasive tumors of stages pT2 and pT3a can also be cured by transurethral electroresection. Up to 45% of solitary stage pT2 tumors can be transurethrally resected with tumor-free margins, while another 30% can be fully resected in up to three follow-up operations. However, more than 60% of stage pT3 tumors cannot be entirely resected by TUR-B (O'FLYNN et al. 1975; BARNES et al. 1977; HERR 1987; HENRY et al. 1988; SOLSONA et al. 1992). Partial resection of the bladder in open surgery is restricted to tumors in bladder diverticula, tumors at the vertex of the bladder (carcinoma of the urachus), circumscribed lesions in the vicinity of an ureteral orifice, and patients with superficial tumors who cannot undergo transurethral resection, e.g., due to severe coxarthritis (JOCHAM 1994). Five-year survival among patients with pT2 tumors averages 58% after TUR-B, and 59% after radical cystectomy. In patients with pT3a tumors, the respective rates are 30% and 30% (RAGHAVAN et al. 1990).

The different therapy options and prognoses for muscle-infiltrating bladder cancers make it desirable to locate exactly the cancerous lesion and to distinguish tumor stages pT2 and pT3a from both superficial and extravesically growing tumors. Also, exact differentiation of stages pT2 and pT3a can be crucial for prognosis and, therefore, for decisions on additional follow-up examinations

◄
Fig. 16.3. a Superficial scar tissue in the left lateral bladder wall with contrast enhancement 30 s after intravenous contrast administration in a patient with recurrent Ta urothelial carcinoma who had undergone superficial transurethral electroresection 3 months prior to MRI. Stage Ta or Tis flat tumor within the scar cannot be ruled out with certainty. **b,c** Granulation tissue after transurethral electroresection. The T1-weighted image shows a mass (*arrows* in **b**), while rapid dynamic contrast-enhanced MRI does not show enhancement in the subtraction image obtained with a turboFLASH sequence 15 s after first arterial enhancement (**c**). Findings at pathologic examination confirmed granulation tissue. **d,e** Urothelial carcinoma of the bladder that appears as a mass along the left lateral bladder wall, bladder floor, and bladder roof (*large arrows* in **d**) with dilatation of the left ureter (*small arrows* in **d**) and an enlarged contralateral lymph node (*curved arrow* in **d**) demonstrates more rapid enhancement than surrounding tissues on dynamic contrast-enhanced MRI. The subtraction image obtained with a turboFLASH sequence 6.25 s after first arterial enhancement (**e**) shows contrast uptake both in the tumor (*large arrows*) and in the enlarged lymph node (*curved arrow*). (**b–e** from BARENTSZ et al. 1996b)

and therapies (chemotherapy, radiation therapy) (Fig. 16.4).

In the largest series published, eight of nine patients (89%) with stage T2 bladder cancer were correctly staged with MRI, when dynamic contrast-enhanced images obtained prior to biopsy were evaluated (TANIMOTO et al. 1992). In the same series, CT, with an accuracy of 55%, was superior to unenhanced MRI and delayed contrast-enhanced MRI (TANIMOTO et al. 1992; Table 16.8).

Various authors have published series of eight or more patients with stage T3a bladder cancers (Table 16.9). Independent of both the MRI technique applied (unenhanced, contrast-enhanced, or dynamic, contrast-enhanced imaging) and the biopsy status of the bladder, the staging accuracy varied between 64% and 100%. Two of the studies (TANIMOTO et al. 1992; KIM et al. 1994) included comparison with CT staging results. In these studies, the accuracy of CT in the staging of T3a bladder cancer was 43%–50%. Similar accuracies were achieved with unenhanced or delayed postcontrast MRI sequences (TANIMOTO et al. 1992; KIM et al. 1994).

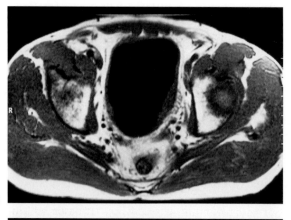

a

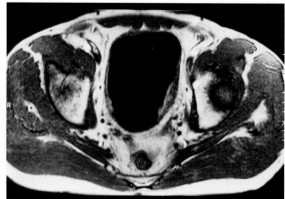

b

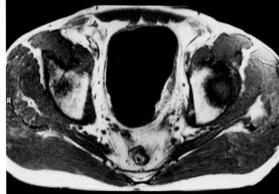

c

Fig. 16.4 a–c. Stage T2 urothelial carcinoma of the right and left bladder wall (postbiopsy) in a 66-year-old male patient who subsequently underwent radical cystoprostatovesiculectomy. Dynamic, contrast-enhanced GRE images at 0 (**a**), 30 (**b**), and 60 (**c**) s after intravenous contrast administration show tumor invading the inner half of the muscle layer

Table 16.8. Accuracy of MRI in the T-staging of pT2 carcinoma of the bladder

Author	MRI technique	No. correct T-staging	% correct T-staging	Comment
AMENDOLA et al. (1986)	Unenhanced	0/3	0%	MRI prebiopsy
TAVARES et al. (1990)	Unenhanced	1/2	50%	MRI prebiopsy
TANIMOTO et al. (1992)	Unenhanced	2/9	22%	MRI prebiopsy
TANIMOTO et al. (1992)	Contrast-enhanced	4/9	45%	MRI prebiopsy
TANIMOTO et al. (1992)	Dynamic	8/9	89%	MRI prebiopsy

Table 16.9. Accuracy of MRI in the T-staging of pT3a carcinoma of the bladder

Author	MRI technique	No. correct T-staging	% correct T-staging	Comment
FISHER et al. (1985)	Unenhanced	2/2	100%	Biopsy status not specified
AMENDOLA et al. (1986)	Unenhanced	2/2	100%	MRI prebiopsy
TAVARES et al. (1990)	Unenhanced	9/9	100%	MRI prebiopsy
DORINGER et al. (1991)	Unenhanced	2/3	67%	MRI prebiopsy
DORINGER et al. (1991)	Contrast-enhanced	2/3	67%	MRI prebiopsy
TACHIBANA et al. (1991)	Dynamic	7/11	64%	MRI prebiopsy
TANIMOTO et al. (1992)	Unenhanced	3/6	50%	MRI prebiopsy
TANIMOTO et al. (1992)	Dynamic	4/6	67%	MRI prebiopsy
TANIMOTO et al. (1992)	Contrast-enhanced	3/6	67%	MRI prebiopsy
BARENTSZ et al. (1994)	Dynamic + 3D	8/8	100%	MRI postbiopsy
KIM et al. (1994)	Dynamic	3/6	50%	MRI postbiopsy
BARENTSZ et al. (1996b)	Unenhanced	7/10	70%	MRI postbiopsy
BARENTSZ et al. (1996b)	Unenhanced + dynamic	9/10	90%	MRI postbiopsy

16.4.4
Cumulative Evaluation of Tumors of Stages pT1 to pT3a

Urologic centers tending to a more aggressive surgical approach even for superficially infiltrating (T1) tumors may benefit from cumulative evaluation of imaging results for stages T1 to T3a that in theory can be cured by cystectomy alone. With the exception of one particularly small group of patients whose bladder cancers were all incorrectly staged by MRI (BRYAN et al. 1987), results in groups of more than ten patients show an average 90% staging accuracy of MRI (Table 16.10). RHOLL et al. (1987) examined 10 of 14 patients with bladder cancer of stages T1 to T3a with both MRI and CT. In their study, CT correctly staged nine of these ten tumors.

16.4.5
Bladder Cancers Infiltrating Neighboring Tissues

In view of the morbidity of locally progressive, infiltrating bladder cancers, which includes recurrent hematuria, decreased bladder capacity, intestinovesical fistula, and formation of a cloaca, palliative cystectomy is now more frequently applied. Since higher tumor stages bear a higher risk of local and distant metastasis, chemotherapy with schemes including methotrexate and cisplatin is frequently used following radical cystectomy as an adjuvant therapy for stage T3b and T4a tumors, particularly when lymph node metastases have been found at surgery. Sometimes, inductive or neoadjuvant chemotherapy is used for tumor reduction (downstaging) or to sterilize occult micrometastases prior to radical cystectomy or TUR-B (SCHER 1988; SPLINTER 1990; DEBRUYNE 1991). The combination of cystectomy with radiation therapy has also been discussed (WHITMORE et al. 1977).

16.4.5.1
Tumor Extension into Perivesical Fat Tissue (Stage pT3b)

Correct recognition of perivesical fat tissue infiltration with MRI is possible in 74%–100% of patients with pT3b bladder cancer when bigger patient groups are examined. Although stage T3b bladder cancer is often correctly diagnosed with unenhanced MRI, contrast enhancement and dynamic imaging tend to improve accuracy (Table 16.11). The accuracy of CT in the staging of T3b bladder cancer in studies also reporting MRI results varies between 0% (0/2 patients, KIM et al. 1994) and 100% (5/5 patients, RHOLL et al. 1987; 10/10 patients, HUSBAND et al. 1989).

16.4.5.2
Tumor Extension into Neighboring Organs or into the Pelvic or Abdominal Wall (Stages pT4a and pT4b)

Infiltration into neighboring organs (T4a) and into the pelvic or abdominal wall (T4b) represents tumor stages that mostly cannot be treated with a curative intention. The 5-year survival rate of patients with stage T4 tumors lies between 0% and 29% with cystectomy, and is greater than 10% with definitive

Table 16.10. Accuracy of MRI in the cumulative T-staging of pT1 to pT3a carcinoma of the bladder

Author	MRI technique	No. correct T-staging	% correct T-staging	Comment
Bryan et al. (1987)	Unenhanced	0/3	0%	Biopsy status not specified
Rholl et al. (1987)	Unenhanced	14/14	100%	Biopsy status not specified
Barentsz et al. (1988)	Unenhanced	13/15	87%	Biopsy status not specified
Sohn et al. (1990)	Contrast-enhanced	9/10	90%	MRI prebiopsy

Table 16.11. Accuracy of MRI in the T-staging of pT3b carcinoma of the bladder

Author	MRI technique	No. correct T-staging	% correct T-staging	Comment
Fisher et al. (1985)	Unenhanced	6/7	86%	Biopsy status not specified
Amendola et al. (1986)	Unenhanced	4/4	100%	MRI prebiopsy
Küper et al. (1986)	Unenhanced	1/2	50%	MRI postbiopsy
Rholl et al. (1987)	Unenhanced	5/5	100%	Biopsy status not specified
Barentsz et al. (1988)	Unenhanced	5/5	100%	Biopsy status not specified
Nicolas et al. (1988)	Unenhanced	4/4	100%	MRI postbiopsy
Husband et al. (1989)	Unenhanced	8/10	80%	MRI postbiopsy
Sohn et al. (1990)	Contrast-enhanced	14/19	74%	MRI prebiopsy
Tavares et al. (1990)	Unenhanced	10/10	100%	MRI prebiopsy
Sparenberg et al. (1991)	Unenhanced	3/5	60%	MRI postbiopsy
Sparenberg et al. (1991)	Contrast-enhanced	3/5	60%	MRI postbiopsy
Tachibana et al. (1991)	Dynamic	4/6	67%	MRI prebiopsy
Tanimoto et al. (1992)	Unenhanced	7/11	64%	MRI prebiopsy
Tanimoto et al. (1992)	Dynamic	10/11	91%	MRI prebiopsy
Tanimoto et al. (1992)	Contrast-enhanced	9/11	82%	MRI prebiopsy
Barentsz et al. (1994)	Dynamic + 3D	5/5	100%	MRI prebiopsy
Kim et al. (1994)	Dynamic	1/2	50%	MRI postbiopsy
Barentsz et al. (1996b)	Unenhanced	11/14	79%	MRI postbiopsy
Barentsz et al. (1996b)	Unenhanced + dynamic	12/14	86%	MRI postbiopsy

radiation therapy (60 Gy) (Raghavan et al. 1990). On the one hand, survival is linked with the radicality of treatment possible in each individual case. Tumors extending into the prostate in men can be fully excised with radical cystovesiculoprostatectomy as long as they are organ-confined. Partial or complete exenteration of the small pelvis is another surgical means to treat locally extensive disease that does not infiltrate the pelvic sidewalls (Fig. 16.5). In stage T4b tumors, surgery often is not radical, since tumor tissue can remain after sharp tumor detachment from the pelvic or abdominal wall. On the other hand, the likelihood of occult metastasis via lymphatic or blood vessels increases with increasing tumor stage. Five-year survival data are thus a reflection of both local and distant tumor control.

Correct MRI staging of T4a tumors requires contrast-enhanced imaging. One recent study (Barentsz et al. 1996b) shows that the addition of a dynamic contrast-enhanced study to the protocol improves accuracy in the staging of T4 tumors by more than 25% (Table 16.12). The accuracy of CT in studies reporting both MRI and CT staging results is similar to the accuracy of MRI (ca. 60%–80%; Husband et al. 1989; Tachibana et al. 1991; Kim et al. 1994).

Although the numbers of patients examined in the individual studies listed in Table 16.13 are rather small, there remains little doubt that, independently of both the MRI technique used and the biopsy status of the patients, almost all patients with T4b tumors are correctly T-staged by MRI. Results of CT staging of T4b tumors in studies also including MRI examinations are very similar (Husband et al. 1989; Tachibana et al. 1991; Kim et al. 1994).

When stages T4a and T4b are looked at together (Table 16.14), the staging accuracy of MRI is 75%–100% using unenhanced images (with the exception of the data published by Sparenberg et al. 1991), and approaches 100% using contrast-enhanced sequences.

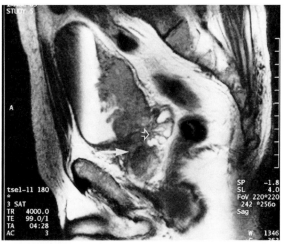

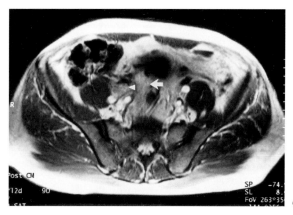

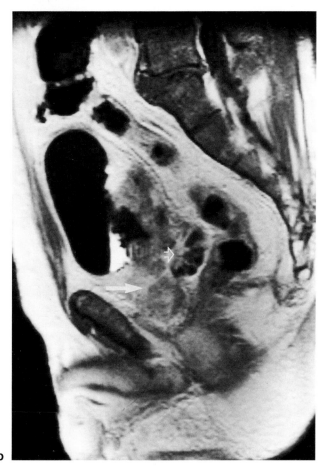

Fig. 16.5 a–c. Stage T4aN2 urothelial carcinoma of the bladder invading the prostate and seminal vesicles and metastasizing to lymph nodes along the external iliac artery on the right in a 67-year-old patient. Prostate (*arrow*) and seminal vesicle (*open arrow*) invasion is more easily recognized on the sagittal T2-weighted FSE image (**a**) than on the contrast-enhanced GRE image (**b**). Tumor (*arrow*) and lymph node (*arrowhead*) enhancement is recognized on the axial contrast-enhanced GRE image (**c**)

16.5
Regional Lymph Node Staging

The prevalence of lymph node metastases of bladder cancer correlates with the T-stage. While pT1 tumors present with positive lymph nodes in about 5% of cases, the likelihood of nodal metastasis increases to about 30% in stages pT2/pT3a and is higher than 60% in stage pT3b bladder cancer (JOCHAM 1994).

Bladder cancer cells prefer certain routes of lymph node infiltration over others. Metastases are most frequently found in lymph nodes of the obturatorius group (75%) and along the external

Table 16.12. Accuracy of MRI in the T-staging of pT4a carcinoma of the bladder

Author	MRI technique	No. correct T-staging	% correct T-staging	Comment
Amendola et al. (1986)	Unenhanced	2/2	100%	MRI prebiopsy
Küper et al. (1986)	Unenhanced	3/4	75%	MRI postbiopsy
Barentsz et al. (1988)	Unenhanced	1/1	100%	Biopsy status not specified
Nicolas et al. (1988)	Unenhanced	3/3	100%	MRI postbiopsy
Husband et al. (1989)	Unenhanced	4/5	80%	MRI postbiopsy
Sohn et al. (1990)	Contrast-enhanced	7/7	100%	MRI prebiopsy
Tavares et al. (1990)	Unenhanced	0/3	0%	MRI prebiopsy
Tachibana et al. (1991)	Dynamic	4/7	57%	MRI prebiopsy
Barentsz et al. (1994)	Dynamic + 3D	4/4	100%	MRI postbiopsy
Kim et al. (1994)	Dynamic	9/10	90%	MRI postbiopsy
Barentsz et al. (1996b)	Unenhanced	7/11	64%	MRI postbiopsy
Barentsz et al. (1996b)	Unenhanced + dynamic	10/11	91%	MRI postbiopsy

Table 16.13. Accuracy of MRI in the T-staging of pT4b carcinoma of the bladder

Author	MRI technique	No. correct T-staging	% correct T-staging	Comment
Küper et al. (1986)	Unenhanced	1/1	100%	MRI postbiopsy
Barentsz et al. (1988)	Unenhanced	3/3	100%	Biopsy status not specified
Husband et al. (1989)	Unenhanced	2/2	100%	MRI postbiopsy
Sohn et al. (1990)	Contrast-enhanced	4/5	80%	MRI prebiopsy
Tavares et al. (1990)	Unenhanced	5/7	71%	MRI prebiopsy
Tachibana et al. (1991)	Dynamic	2/2	100%	MRI prebiopsy
Barentsz et al. (1994)	Dynamic + 3D	2/2	100%	MRI postbiopsy
Kim et al. (1994)	Dynamic	4/4	100%	MRI postbiopsy
Barentsz et al. (1996b)	Unenhanced	4/4	100%	MRI postbiopsy
Barentsz et al. (1996b)	Unenhanced + dynamic	4/4	100%	MRI postbiopsy

Table 16.14. Accuracy of MRI in the cumulative T-staging of pT4a and pT4b carcinoma of the bladder

Author	MRI technique	No. correct T-staging	% correct T-staging	Comment
Fisher et al. (1985)	Unenhanced	3/4	75%	Biopsy status not specified
Rholl et al. (1987)	Unenhanced	3/4	75%	Biopsy status not specified
Nicolas et al. (1988)	Unenhanced	3/3	100%	MRI postbiopsy
Sparenberg et al. (1991)	Unenhanced	4/7	57%	MRI postbiopsy
Sparenberg et al. (1991)	Contrast-enhanced	7/7	100%	MRI postbiopsy
Tanimoto et al. (1992)	Unenhanced	5/6	83%	MRI prebiopsy
Tanimoto et al. (1992)	Dynamic	6/6	100%	MRI prebiopsy
Tanimoto et al. (1992)	Contrast-enhanced	6/6	100%	MRI prebiopsy

iliac artery (65%). Common iliac artery nodes are infiltrated in 19%, and internal iliac artery nodes in 15% of patients. Lymph nodes along the hypogastric artery and the perivesical vessels are infiltrated in 15% (Jocham 1994).

In a study of 57 patients, Barentsz et al. (1996b) detected 12/14 cases of pelvic lymph node metastasis with combined unenhanced and contrast-enhanced, dynamic MRI. Criteria were rapid contrast uptake

(less than 10 s after peak arterial enhancement at a sequence repetition rate of one in 1.25–2.50 s) and a shortest axial size/long axis ratio of more than 0.8 in nodes of more than 8 mm in diameter. Other pathologic signs were a nodal diameter of more than 10 mm and an asymmetric cluster of small nodes. Barentsz et al. reported an accuracy of 93%, a sensitivity of 86%, a specificity of 95%, a positive predictive value of 86%, and a negative predictive value of

95%. Without contrast enhancement, they recognized lymph node metastasis in 10/14 cases. JAGER et al. (1996) reported an accuracy of 92%, a sensitivity of 83%, a specificity of 98%, a positive predictive value of 96%, and a negative predictive value of 89% in 71 patients with bladder cancer who underwent MRI for nodal staging.

16.6
Distant Metastasis

Blood-borne metastasis is found in more than 60% of patients with bladder cancer of stage T3b or higher. About 40% of distant metastases are exclusively skeletal. Other locations of predilection include the liver, the lung, the central nervous system, and endocrine organs like the thyroid gland and the adrenal glands (JOCHAM 1994). Due to the spatial restriction of MRI examinations, most of these locations cannot be covered during an MRI examination of the bladder.

16.7
MRI of Other Neoplastic Bladder Lesions

Neurofibromatosis (von Recklinghausen disease) is a congenital, hereditary dysplasia that affects all three germ cell layers and may involve any organ system in the body. Involvement of the urogenital system is rare. However, in these cases, the bladder is often affected. Neurofibromas usually show signal intensities similar to that of skeletal muscle on T1-weighted images, but present with a markedly increased signal on T2-weighted images, and with strong enhancement following intravenous administration of gadolinium-containing contrast agents. Bladder wall involvement may be nodular or diffuse, and is accompanied by pelvic sidewall and adjacent soft tissue alterations (SHONNARD et al. 1992).

Non-Hodgkin's lymphoma rarely presents as primary extranodal disease of the urinary bladder wall. Bladder lymphoma may appear as a large, lobulated submucosal mass. On the basis of MRI signal characteristics or contrast enhancement patterns, however, lymphoma of the bladder wall cannot be differentiated from transitional cell carcinoma (YEOMAN et al. 1991).

Leiomyomas are seldom found in the retrovesical pouch. Leiomyomas may indent the posterior bladder wall as an extravesical tumorous lesion. They are characterized by their low signal intensity on both T1- and T2-weighted MR images, although they may be inhomogeneous on T2-weighted images when hyaline, myxomatous, or fatty degeneration has occurred (THURNHER et al. 1992).

Tumorous invasion of the bladder wall by other pelvic malignancies lends itself to diagnostic MRI investigation due to the high soft tissue contrast and free choice of imaging plane that MRI offers over other modalities. Various recent studies have shown the value of MRI in staging extensive gynecologic cancers (SEMELKA et al. 1993; HOUVENAEGHEL et al. 1993; KAJI et al. 1994; IWAMOTO et al. 1994). However, while MRI staging is correct in more than 80% of the cases, some authors prefer MRI over CT but find endoscopic ultrasound a reliable alternative (HOUVENAEGHEL et al. 1993; IWAMOTO et al. 1994).

16.8
Conclusion

In contrast to its frequency of application in the staging and follow-up of other pelvic malignancies, MRI of the bladder in patients with transitional cell carcinoma is still in its early development. The wide variety of MRI sequences applied in the 20 studies published between 1985 and 1996 that are cited in this chapter shows that there is as yet no basic rule on how to shape an examination protocol. The general direction, however, is towards rapid, contrast-enhanced, repetitive ("dynamic") imaging with the same sequence. While various authors (NEUERBURG et al. 1989; TACHIBANA et al. 1991; TANIMOTO et al. 1992; KIM et al. 1994; BARENTSZ et al. 1996b) obtained higher staging accuracies when they included dynamic imaging sequences in their MRI protocols, BARENTSZ et al. (1996b) took the concept furthest when they reported that dynamic MRI with sequence repetition frequencies of one in 1.25–2.50 s allows the differentiation of inflammatory reaction from active bladder cancer in patients who have undergone bladder biopsy. The drawback of rapid dynamic imaging to date has been the limitation to one or two slices, which requires careful preselection of the area of the bladder wall and its surrounding tissues to be included in the dynamic imaging process. Preselection necessitates the recognition of the tumor-infiltrated area by multislice imaging prior to the dynamic sequence. Sources of error include flat tumor, multifocality, and previous therapies or biopsies that have left focal bladder wall irregularities. Integration of the advantages of multislice acquisition and rapid imaging will be necessary if such sources of error are to be excluded; this will be a demanding task.

The small overall number of patients with bladder cancer in the studies cited here who have undergone MRI staging examinations, along with their varying biopsy status and the different MRI protocols applied, makes it difficult to reach conclusions on the value of MRI in the staging of carcinoma of the bladder at this juncture. While most studies include rather small patient populations, there is at least a strong trend towards superiority of MRI over CT in locoregional staging efforts, particularly since MRI demonstrates a high capability to detect regional lymph node metastasis.

The basic advantage of CT lies in the ability to perform whole-body imaging within one examination. However, the superior locoregional performance of combined cystocopy and MRI (differentiation of stages Ta–T2 by cystoscopy and biopsy; differentiation of stages T2–T4b by MRI), as compared with combined cystoscopy and CT, seems to constitute a good reason to omit CT, at least in those institutions that can offer rapid, dynamic, contrast-enhanced MRI examinations.

References

Althausen AFG, Prout GR Jr, Daly JJ (1976) Noninvasive papillary carcinoma of the bladder associated with carcinoma in situ. J Urol 116:575

Amendola MA, Glazer GM, Grossman HB, Aisen AM, Francis IR (1986) Staging of bladder carcinoma: MRI-CT-surgical correlation. Am J Roentgenol 146:1179–1183

Barentsz JO, Lemmens JAM, Ruijs SHJ, et al. (1988) Carcinoma of the urinary bladder: MR imaging with a double surface coil. Am J Roentgenol 151:107–112

Barentsz JO, Debruyne FMJ, Ruijs SHJ (1990) MR imaging of carcinoma of the urinary bladder. Kluiver Academic Publishers, Dordrecht

Barentsz JO, Jager G, Mugler JP III, Oosterdorf G, Peters H, van Erning LTJO, Ruijs SHJ (1994) Staging urinary bladder cancer: value of T1-weighted three-dimensional magnetization prepared-rapid gradient-echo and two-dimensional spin-echo sequences. Am J Roentgenol 164:109–115

Barentsz JO, Jager GJ, Witjes JA, Ruijs SHJ (1996a) Primary staging of urinary bladder carcinoma: the role of MRI and a comparison with CT. Eur Radiol 6:129–133

Barentsz JO, Jager GJ, van Vierzen PBJ, et al. (1996b) Staging urinary bladder cancer after transurethral biopsy: value of dynamic contrast-enhanced MR imaging. Radiology 201:185–193

Barnes RW, Dick AL, Hadley HL, Johnston OL (1977) Survival following transurethral resection of bladder carcinoma. Cancer Res 37:2895

Benson RC Jr, Tomera KM, Kelalis PP (1983) Transitional cell carcinoma of the bladder in children and adolescents. J Urol 130:54

Bryan PJ, Butler HE, LiPuma JP, Resnick MI, Kursh ED (1987) CT and MR imaging in staging bladder neoplasms. J Comput Assist Tomogr 11:96–101

Buy JN, Moss AA, Guinet C, Ghossain MA, Malbec L, Arrive L, Vadrot D (1988) MR staging of bladder carcinoma: correlation with pathologic findings. Radiology 169:695–700

Debruyne FMJ (1991) Induktive Chemotherapie des Blasenkarzinoms. Eine kritische Beurteilung. Urologe [A] 30:81–84

Doringer E, Joos H, Forstner R, Schmoller HJ (1991) MRT des Harnblasenkarzinoms: Tumorstaging und Gadoliniumkontrastverhalten. Fortschr Röntgenstr 154:357–363

Fisher MR, Hricak H, Tanagho EA (1985) Urinary bladder MR imaging. II. Neoplasm. Radiology 157:471–477

Heiken JP, Lee JKT (1988) MR imaging of the pelvis. Radiology 166:11–16

Henry K, Miller J, Mori M (1988) Comparison of transurethral resection to radical therapies for stage B bladder tumors. J Urol 140:964

Herr HW (1987) Conservative management of muscle-infiltrating bladder cancer: prospective experience. J Urol 138:1162

Houvenaeghel G, Delpero JR, Rosello R, et al. (1993) Results of a prospective study with comparison of clinical, endosonographic, computed tomography, magnetic resonance imaging and pathologic staging of advanced gynecologic carcinoma and recurrence. Surg Gynecol Obstet 177:231–236

Hricak H, Williams RD, Spring DB, Moon KL Jr, Hedgcock MW, Watson RA, Crooks LE (1983) Anatomy and pathology of the male pelvis by magnetic resonance imaging. Am J Roentgenol 141:1101–1110

Husband JES, Olliff JFC, Williams MP, Heron CW, Cherryman GR (1989) Bladder cancer: staging with CT and MR imaging. Radiology 173:435–440

Iwamoto K, Kigawa J, Minagawa Y, Miura H, Terakawa N (1994) Transvaginal ultrasonographic diagnosis of bladder-wall invasion in patients with cervical cancer. Obstet Gynecol 83:217–219

Jager GJ, Barentsz JO, Oosterhof G, Ruijs JHJ (1996) 3D MR imaging in nodal staging of bladder and prostate cancer. AJR 167:1503–1507

Jakse G, Putz A, Feichtinger J (1989) Cystectomy: the treatment of choice in patients with carcinoma in situ of the urinary bladder? Eur J Surg Oncol 15:211–216

Jewett HJ (1973) Cancer of the bladder. Cancer 32:1072–1074

Jewett HJ, Strong GH (1946) Infiltrating carcinoma of the bladder. Relation of depth of penetration of the bladder wall to incidence of local extension and metastases. J Urol 55:366–372

Jocham D (1994) Maligne Tumoren der Harnblase. In: Jocham D, Miller K (eds) Praxis der Urologie, Band II, Teil 2. Thieme, Stuttgart, pp 49–115

Kaji Y, Sugimura K, Kitao M, Ishida T (1994) Histopathology of uterine cervical carcinoma: diagnostic comparison of endorectal surface coil and standard body coil MRI. J Comput Assist Tomogr 18:785–792

Kawakami S, Togashi K, Kojima N, Morikawa K, Mori T, Konishi J (1995) MR appearance of malignant lymphoma of the uterus. J Comput Assist Tomogr 19:238–242

Kim B, Semelka RC, Ascher SM, Chalpin DB, Carroll PR, Hricak H (1994) Bladder tumor staging: comparison of contrast-enhanced CT, T1- and T2-weighted MR imaging, dynamic gadolinium-enhanced imaging, and late gadolinium-enhanced imaging. Radiology 193:239–245

Koelbel G, Schmiedl U, Griebel J, Hess CF, Kueper K (1988) MR imaging of urinary bladder neoplasms. J Comput Assist Tomogr 12:98–103

Küper K, Kölbel G, Schmiedl U (1986) Kernspintomographische Untersuchungen von Harnblasenkarzinomen bei 1,5 T. Fortschr Röntgenstr 144:674–680

Marshall VF (1952) The relation of the preoperative estimate to the pathologic demonstration of the extent of vesical neoplasms. J Urol 68:714–723

Neuerburg JM, Bohndorf K, Sohn M, Teufl F, Guenther RW, Daus HJ (1989) Urinary bladder neoplasms: evaluation with contrast-enhanced MR imaging. Radiology 172:739–743

Nicolas V, Harder T, Steudel A, Krahe T, Schindler G, van Ahlen H, Jaeger N (1988) Die Wertigkeit bildgebender Verfahren bei der Diagnostik und dem Staging von Harnblasentumoren. Fortschr Röntgenstr 148:234–239

O'Flynn JD, Smith JD, Hanson JS (1975) Transurethral resection for the assessment and treatment of vesical neoplasm. A review of 800 consecutive cases. Eur Urol 1:38

Patel MD, Hricak H (1995) Current role of magnetic resonance imaging in urology. Curr Opin Urol 5:67–74

Raghavan D, Shipley WU, Garnick MB (1990) Biology in management of bladder cancer. N Engl J Med 322:1129

Rholl KS, Lee JKT, Heiken JP, Ling D, Glazer HS (1987) Primary bladder carcinoma: evaluation with MR imaging. Radiology 163:117–121

Scher HI, Yagoda A, Herr HW, et al. (1988) Neoadjuvant M-VAC (methotrexate, vinblastine, adriamycin and cisplatin) effect on the primary bladder lesion. J Urol 139:470–474

Semelka RC, Lawrence PH, Shoenut JP, Heywood M, Kroeker MA, Lotocki R (1993) Primary ovarian cancer: prospective comparison of contrast-enhanced CT and pre- and postcontrast, fat-suppressed MR imaging, with histologic correlation. J Magn Reson Imaging 3:99–106

Shonnard KM, Jelinek JS, Benedikt RA, Kransdorf MJ (1992) CT and MR of neurofibromatosis of the bladder. J Comput Assist Tomogr 16:433–438

Sohn M, Neuerburg J, Teufl F, Bohndorf K (1990) Gadolinium-enhanced magnetic resonance imaging in the staging of urinary bladder neoplasms. Urol Int 45:142–147

Solsona E, Iborra I, Ricos JV, Monros JL, Dumont R (1992) Feasibility of transurethral resection for muscle-infiltrating carcinoma of the bladder: prospective study. J Urol 147:1513–1515

Sparenberg A, Hamm B, Hammerer P, Samberger V, Wolf KJ (1991) Diagnostik von Harnblasenkarzinomen in der Kernspintomographie: Verbesserung mit Gd-DTPA? Fortschr Röntgenstr 155:117–122

Splinter TAW (1990) Neoadjuvante Chemotherapie des invasiven Blasenkarzinoms. Akt Urol 21:173–174

Tachibana M, Baba S, Deguchi N, et al. (1991) Efficacy of gadolinium-diethylenetriamninepentaacetic acid-enhanced magnetic resonance imaging for differentiation between superficial and muscle-invasive tumor of the bladder: a comparative study with computerized tomography and transurethral ultrasonography. J Urol 145:1169–1173

Tanimoto A, Yuasa Y, Imai Y, Izutsu M, Hiramatsu K, Tachibana M, Tazaki H (1992) Bladder tumor staging: comparison of conventional and gadolinium-enhanced dynamic MR imaging and CT. Radiology 185:741–747

Tavares NJ, Demas BE, Hricak H (1990) MR imaging of bladder neoplasms: correlation with pathologic staging. Urol Radiol 12:27–33

Thurnher S, Marincek B, Hauri D (1992) Retrovesical leiomyoma: CT and contrast-enhanced MR imaging findings. Urol Radiol 13:190–193

Whitmore WF, Batata MA, Ghoneim MA, Grabstald H, Unal A (1977) Radical cystectomy with or without prior irradiation in the treatment of bladder cancer. J Urol 118:184–187

Yeoman LJ, Mason MD, Olliff JFC (1991) Non-Hodgkin's lymphoma of the bladder – CT and MRI appearances. Clin Radiol 44:389–392

17 Prostate and Seminal Vesicles

J. Scheidler and H. Hricak

CONTENTS

17.1 Introduction

The diagnosis and management of prostate cancer are developing into a major health care issue. The annual incidence of prostate cancer in the United States has increased from 86 000 (1985) to approximately 244 000 (1995) with the number of deaths due to prostate cancer estimated to be 40 400 each year (Silverberg 1985; Wingo et al. 1995). In light of these statistics, accurate diagnosis and staging of prostate cancer to ascertain effective therapy is essential.

The use of magnetic resonance imaging (MRI) in the evaluation of the prostate has engendered both enthusiasm and controversy. Its high contrast resolution allows excellent depiction of the prostate anatomy and pathology. MRI combines the best features of transrectal ultrasonography (TRUS), including high soft tissue contrast and multiplanar imaging, with the volumetric imaging characteristic of computed tomography (CT). Absence of ionizing radiation and lack of need for intravenous contrast media are additional advantages of MRI over CT. However, MRI findings are not tissue specific, MR image quality varies greatly, and experience plays a significant role in image interpretation (Tempany et al. 1994; Yu et al. 1997). In this chapter the normal and pathologic appearance of the prostate on MRI will be discussed, with special emphasis on the evaluation of prostate cancer.

17.2 Technical Considerations

17.2.1 Pulse Sequences

Adequate evaluation of the prostate and seminal vesicles requires both T1- and T2-weighted images. T1-weighted images provide tissue characterization (postbiopsy hemorrhage, fluid, fat) and are essential for the detection of lymph node metastasis. Therefore, T1-weighted sequences have to cover the anatomic region between the aortic bifurcation and the symphysis pubis. Since T1-weighted fast spin-echo (FSE) imaging does not provide coverage from the symphysis pubis to the aortic bifurcation, spin-echo (SE) methods are used for T1-weighted imaging. T2-weighted images, obtained either with the SE or, more efficiently, with the FSE technique (Kier et al. 1993), best demonstrate the zonal anatomy and intrinsic pathology of the prostate and seminal

J. Scheidler, MD, Department of Diagnostic Radiology, Klinikum Großhadern, Ludwig-Maximilians University, Marchioninistrasse 15, D-81377 München, Germany
H. Hricak, MD, Department of Radiology, Abdominal Imaging Section, University of California, San Francisco, 505 Parnassus Avenue, San Francisco, CA 94143-0628, USA

vesicles. Although T2-weighted fat-suppressed sequences might be helpful to improve image quality, significant advantages over conventional T2-weighted images have not as yet been shown (MIROWITZ et al. 1994). MRI with gradient-recalled echo (GRE) sequences plays a minor role in the pelvis. Such sequences are sometimes used for differentiation between lymph nodes and vascular structures and are also indicated where the patency of a vessel is questioned.

The use of contrast-enhanced sequences (gadolinium chelates) is not supported by the literature (MIROWITZ et al. 1993; SOMMER et al. 1993). Contrast-enhanced imaging with an endorectal coil also revealed no improvement in the accuracy of MR staging of prostate cancer over T2-weighted FSE sequences (HUCH-BÖNI et al. 1995a). However, a recent study showed that dynamic contrast-enhanced MRI may be helpful for the diagnosis of extracapsular extension (BROWN et al. 1995), and specifically seminal vesicle invasion.

17.2.2
Transmitter and Receiver Coils

When using endorectal and/or multicoil array systems as receiver coils, radiofrequency pulses are generally transmitted by the body coil. Endorectal and multicoil array systems, either alone or in combination, significantly improve image resolution over that obtained with body coils (mainly by increasing the signal-to-noise level and permitting the use of a smaller field of view), and thus improve the accuracy of staging of prostate cancer (SCHNALL et al. 1991; HRICAK et al. 1994). Prior to placement of an endorectal coil, the patient should be properly screened. The endorectal coil should not be used in the following conditions: previous rectal surgery, recent radiation therapy to the pelvis, inflammatory bowel disease (ulcerative colitis or Crohn's disease), bleeding diathesis, and obstruction of the rectum or colon, including large hemorrhoids. Patient preparation (use of laxatives), coil placement, and maximum balloon distention are all important factors in assuring optimal quality with endorectal coil MR images.

17.2.3
Suggested Imaging Protocol

Imaging of the prostate is typically performed in two or three orthogonal planes, preferably with contiguous, 3- to 5-mm-thick sections. In general, T1- and T2-weighted images in the transaxial plane, supplemented with T2-weighted images in the coronal plane, provide adequate evaluation of most abnormalities of the prostate and seminal vesicles. The transaxial plane of imaging optimizes differentiation of the transition and peripheral zones. Delineation of the central zone at the base of the prostate on axial sections is difficult. Differentiation between the central and the peripheral zone is assessed in the coronal plane of section.

The relationship between the prostate and adjacent organs is well depicted on multiplanar images. Axial images show the prostate in relation to the seminal vesicles, periprostatic veins, and rectum, as well as the levator ani and obturator internus muscles. Sagittal images depict the relationship of the prostate to the bladder base, seminal vesicles, and rectum. The coronal plane is most useful for evaluation of the seminal vesicles, the base and apex of the prostate, and its relation to the levator ani muscles.

Respiratory compensation techniques diminish artifacts caused by respiratory motion and their routine use is recommended when available. Glucagon (1 mg IM) or butylscopolamine (20 mg IV) reduce motion artifacts, as does fat suppression (KIER et al. 1993; MIROWITZ et al. 1994). Anterior and posterior saturation bands are helpful to avoid ghosting artifacts due to abdominal wall movement and also reduce image nonuniformity when multicoil array systems are used.

17.3
Normal MRI Appearance

17.3.1
Prostate

The prostate shows a homogeneous intermediate signal intensity without zonal differentiation on T1-weighted images (Fig. 17.1). Detailed zonal anatomy with differentiation between the glandular and the nonglandular portion of the prostate can be delineated on T2-weighted images (Fig. 17.2; SOMMER et al. 1986; SCHNALL and POLLACK 1990). On T2-weighted images, the peripheral zone (PZ), the largest portion of the prostate, demonstrates a homogeneously high signal intensity that is equal to or higher than that of the surrounding fat (SCHNALL and POLLACK 1990). The central zone (CZ) is an inverted cone-shaped structure, with its broad surface

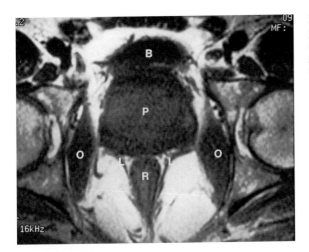

Fig. 17.1. Normal anatomy of the prostate. T1-weighted axial plane of section (1.5 T, SE, TR/TE 550/16) at the midgland level shows normal intermediate signal intensity of the entire gland without zonal differentiation. *B*, Bladder; *L*, levator ani muscle; *O*, obdurator internus muscle; *P*, prostate; *R*, rectum

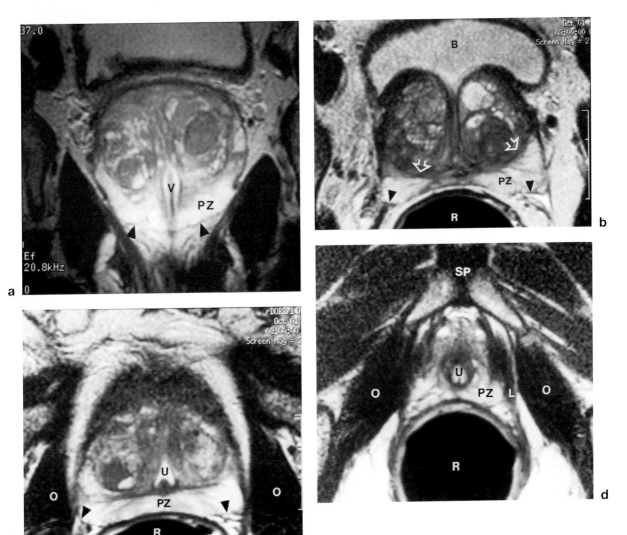

Fig. 17.2 a–d. Normal anatomy of the prostate. Coronal T2-weighted (**a**) and axial T2-weighted images (1.5 T, FSE, TR/eff. TE 3500–5000/102) at the base (**b**), midgland (**c**), and apex (**d**). The normal peripheral zone (*PZ*) demonstrates high signal intensity. Heterogeneous signal intensity of the transitional zone (*TZ*) is due to benign prostatic hypertrophy with mixed stromal and glandular proliferation. A low signal intensity surgical pseudocapsule is seen in **b** (*arrow*). The true prostatic capsule can be identified as a thin layer with low signal intensity separating the PZ from the surrounding periprostatic fat

(*arrowheads*). At the level of the verumontanum (**c**), the urethra (*U*) has an inverted Y configuration. At the apex (**d**), the distal prostatic urethra (*U*) demonstrates a "doughnut"-like appearance with the outer muscle layer showing low signal intensity. As seen on the coronal plane of section, the central zone is conical in shape with its apex at the verumontanum (*V*). The ejaculatory ducts open into the prostatic urethra at the level of the verumontanum. *L*, Levator ani muscle; *O*, obturator internus muscle; *B*, bladder; *R*, rectum; *SP*, symphysis pubis

lying at the prostatic base and its apex extending to the level of the verumontanum. It demonstrates homogeneous low signal intensity on T2-weighted images. The signal intensity of the CZ and the transition zone (TZ), two small paraurethral lobes along the proximal segment of the prostatic urethra, is similar at all imaging parameters. The CZ and TZ can be differentiated only by knowledge of their respective anatomic locations (HRICAK et al. 1987a). The CZ and TZ are often referred to as the central gland.

The nonglandular parts of the prostate include the fibromuscular stroma, urethra, and prostatic capsule. The fibromuscular stroma forms the anterolateral surface of the prostate. It demonstrates low signal intensity on both T1- and T2-weighted images (HRICAK et al. 1987a). The distal prostatic urethra can be identified on T2-weighted images. It demonstrates a "doughnut"-like appearance with the outer muscular layer demonstrating a low signal intensity. The prostatic capsule surrounds the outer margin of the prostate, except in the region of the anterior fibromuscular stroma and the apex (STAMEY et al. 1990). The prostatic capsule is composed of fibromuscular tissue about 1 mm thick. On T2-weighted images the capsule can be depicted as a low signal intensity stripe at the periphery of the gland. The surgical pseudocapsule is present at the interface between the TZ and the PZ (SCHNALL and POLLACK 1990). It also demonstrates low signal intensity on T2-weighted images.

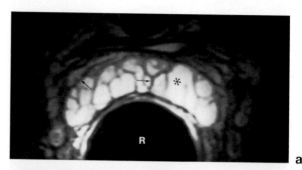

a

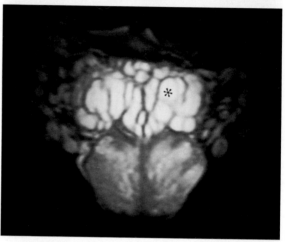

b

Fig. 17.3 a,b. Normal anatomy of the seminal vesicles. Axial (a) and coronal (b) T2-weighted images (1.5 T, FSE, TR/eff. TE 3000–5000/102). Typical graplike configuration of the seminal vesicles, with differentiation between high signal intensity seminal fluid (*asterisk*) and low signal intensity septa and wall (*arrow*). *R*, Rectum

17.3.2
Seminal Vesicles

T2-weighted images demonstrate best the characteristic, grape-like configuration of the seminal vesicles, with the high signal intensity fluid differentiated from the low signal intensity of the inner convolutions and outer wall (Fig. 17.3). Symmetry of signal intensity should be maintained in normal seminal vesicles. On T1-weighted images, normal seminal vesicles are homogeneous and symmetric, with intermediate signal intensity similar to that of the adjacent pelvic muscles. Intravenously administered gadolinium (Gd-DTPA) enhanced T1-weighted images permit demonstration of the internal architecture of the seminal vesicles, enhancing the walls of convolutions while the seminal fluid remains of low signal intensity (SECAF et al. 1991). The seminal vesicles reveal androgen-dependent changes in size and signal intensity. Although great variations in the

size of normal seminal vesicles can occur in adult men of the same age group, the seminal vesicles tend to be largest during the fifth and sixth decades of life, subsequently regressing slowly (SECAF et al. 1991). Prior to puberty, little or no seminal vesicle fluid is present; thus they are small and of low signal intensity on T2-weighted images.

17.4
Pathology of the Prostate

17.4.1
Congenital and Acquired Abnormalities

17.4.1.1
Agenesis

Agenesis of the prostate is recognized when no tissue is interposed between the rectum and urethra. Congenital prostatic hypoplasia is often found in conjunction with the Eagle-Barrett (prune belly) syndrome (GEVENOIS et al. 1990). An adult prostate of less than 4g is considered hypoplastic (GRESKOICH and NYBERG 1988). A hypoplastic prostate furthermore demonstrates diffuse low signal intensity, and the zonal anatomy on T2-weighted MR images is not differentiated.

17.4.1.2
Prostatic Cysts

Congenital cysts of the prostate are rare. Two types of congenital cyst may be diagnosed: utricle and müllerian duct cysts. A utricle cyst is a midline lesion, located posteriorly to the verumontanum and confined within the prostate. Since there is an association with unilateral renal agenesis, undescended testicle, and hypospadia (HRICAK 1991), they are usually discovered in childhood.

Müllerian duct cysts (Fig. 17.4) are usually found in middle-aged adults. the clinical symptoms most commonly mimic those of benign prostatic hyperplasia. They can be distinguished from utricle cysts by their paramedian location and large size. The cysts usually extend toward the prostatic base along the embryonal course of the müllerian duct.

Other prostatic cysts are acquired as the result of inflammation, trauma, or retention. Retention cysts are formed by ductal obstruction in the glandular

acini of the prostate. Benign hyperplastic nodules can also undergo cystic degeneration. Their MRI appearance is similar to that of retention cysts, presenting as small cysts with high signal intensity on T2-weighted images.

All types of cyst are well depicted on MR images and their location can be precisely displayed using multiplanar techniques. The signal intensity of a cyst is variable, depending on its fluid content (THURNER et al. 1988). Cysts filled with serous fluid usually show low signal intensity on T1-weighted images and high signal intensity on T2-weighted images. Complicated cysts manifest a range of signal intensity on both T1- and T2-weighted images. An infected or hemorrhagic cyst may demonstrate high signal intensity on T1-weighted images (THURNER et al. 1988).

17.4.2
Infectious Disease

Acute prostatitis is most commonly caused by gram-negative organisms (especially *E. coli*), usually by direct extension from the posterior urethra or urinary bladder, and often following surgical manipulation of these structures (LIPSKY 1989). The most common MRI appearance is diffuse enlargement of the prostate. The inflammatory focus demonstrates high signal intensity on T2-weighted images. It can be seen in the PZ or in the periurethral region (if it is secondary to a long-term indwelling catheter), or there can be widespread involvement of the PZ and central gland (Fig. 17.5). Gd-chelate enhanced T1-weighted images depict the area of inflammation with an increasing signal intensity (HRICAK 1991).

Chronic prostatitis is more common than the acute form, is frequently recurrent, and is often clinically silent (LIPSKY 1989). It frequently demonstrates low signal intensity on T2-weighted images. When chronic infection involves the PZ, its appearance is indistinguishable from prostate cancer (SCHNALL and POLLACK 1990).

A prostatic abscess usually develops as a sequela of prostatitis, although it may occur rarely as a result of hematogenous dissemination of a distant infection. On MRI, it may be seen as focal glandular enlargement with obliteration of periprostatic fat on T1-weighted images. The abscess is usually depicted as a high intensity signal area with indistinct margins on T2-weighted images (STAMEY et al. 1988).

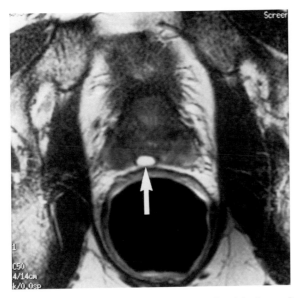

Fig. 17.4. Müllerian duct cyst. T2-weighted axial plane of section (1.5T, FSE, TR/eff. TE 4000/102). The paramedian location of the cyst (*arrow*) led to the diagnosis

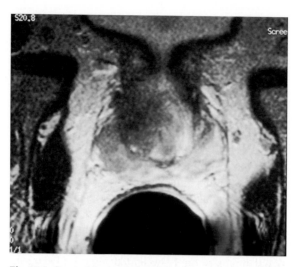

Fig. 17.5. Prostatitis. Axial T2-weighted image (1.5 T, FSE, TR/ eff. TE 4000/102). There is a diffuse inhomogeneous signal pattern predominantly on the right side and ill-defined delineation of the TZ and PZ indicative for prostatitis. However, differentiation between prostatitis and carcinoma is impossible based on MRI alone

17.4.3
Benign Prostatic Hyperplasia

Benign prostatic hypertrophy (BPH) occurs predominantly in the TZ and periurethral glandular tissue. The progressive prostate enlargement causes compression and narrowing of the urethra and the bladder neck, leading to bladder outlet obstruction. Preferential proliferation of the periurethral glands, if present, causes enlargement of the "median portion" of the prostate, leading to focal protrusion of the subvesicular part of the gland into the bladder base (McNeal 1983). Only 5% of cases of BPH can be found in the PZ (Oyen et al. 1993). Histologically, BPH can be predominantly glandular, stromal, or of mixed type (McNeal 1983). The histologic type will influence its MRI appearance (Lovett et al. 1992; Ishida et al. 1994). On T1-weighted images, BPH exhibits a medium signal intensity and is indistinguishable from the remainder of the prostate. On T2-weighted images, all types of BPH demonstrate heterogeneous signal intensity (Fig. 17.2). In addition, the glandular type of BPH demonstrates high signal intensity, while stromal hyperplasia has an intermediate to low signal intensity. BPH adenoma can manifest as a single, centrally located, round or oval nodule with a distinct margin. Bilobed or multiple variably sized nodules can also be demonstrated. The changes can be distributed symmetrically or asymmetrically throughout the central

gland. The central gland with enlarged hyperplastic nodules can be separated from the compressed PZ by a surgical pseudocapsule (Schnall and Pollack 1990), which demonstrates low signal intensity on T2-weighted images. MRI allows not only a more accurate measurement of the total gland volume than ultrasound, but also direct volumetric measurement of BPH. This provides the opportunity to assess temporal changes of BPH volume during medical treatment. The volume measurement can be obtained either by planimetry or by the prolate ellipse formula (length × width × anteroposterior diameter × 0.52) (Hricak et al. 1987b). The difference between the two methods is less than 10%, and the more practical ellipse method is generally accepted.

17.4.4
Prostatic Carcinoma

17.4.4.1
Tumor Detection

Carcinoma of the prostate usually originates in the PZ (68%), although tumors can occur in the TZ (24%) and CZ (8%) (Stamey et al. 1988). The location of the tumor and the imaging sequences applied determine the MRI appearance and influence the detectability of the cancer (Kier et al. 1993; Rifkin et al. 1990; Schnall et al. 1991). On T1-weighted images, prostate cancer is often poorly delineated. Prostate cancer is best depicted on T2-weighted images, where most tumors are shown as foci of low signal intensity located within the high signal area of the normal PZ (Carrol et al. 1987; Schnall and Pollack 1990). A normal MRI appearance of the PZ, however, does not exclude the presence of carcinoma. Rarely, mucin-producing prostatic carcinoma can be similar or higher in signal intensity than the peripheral zone on T2-weighted images. Tumors arising outside the PZ are not detectable on MRI, since the inhomogeneous, low intensity signal pattern of the TZ or CZ prevents differentiation of tumor from BPH (Rifkin et al. 1990; Schnall et al. 1991).

Hemorrhage, prostatitis, postradiation, or dystrophic changes can be misdiagnosed as cancer. Bleeding within the prostate and the seminal vesicles commonly occurs after transrectal biopsy and presents the primary diagnostic problem hampering tumor detection and staging on MRI (Bezzi et al. 1988; Carrol et al. 1992; White et al. 1995). The MRI appearance is dependent on the time interval between biopsy and MR study. During the first 2 weeks following biopsy, high signal intensity on T1-weighted images and low signal intensity on T2-weighted images may be noted at the biopsy site. After approximately 2 weeks, high signal intensity is demonstrated at the biopsy site on both T1- and T2-weighted images due to the presence of extracellular methemoglobin (Figs. 17.6, 17.7). It has been shown that at least a 3-week delay after biopsy is required to avoid diagnostic difficulties on MRI (WHITE et al. 1995).

With the introduction of combined endorectal-multicoil array systems, high-resolution MR spectroscopy (MRS) of the prostate has been developed and is currently under investigation as an adjunct to MRI in prostate cancer. A promising technique uses three-dimensional proton MRS imaging, allowing simultaneous MRS data acquisition of multiple regions within the prostate with a spatial resolution of $0.24\,cm^3$ voxel size (KURHANEWICZ et al. 1996a). An elevated choline + creatine-to-citrate ratio has been shown to be indicative for prostate cancer

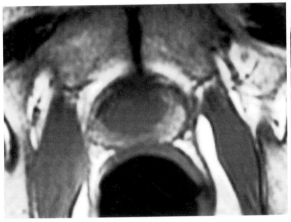
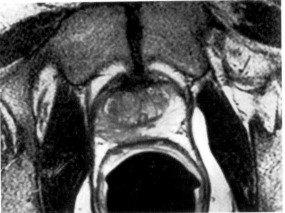

Fig. 17.6 a,b. Subacute postbiopsy hemorrhage and prostate cancer stage pT2b (Jewett B). **a** Axial T1-weighted image (1.5 T, SE, TR/TE 700/8). **b** Axial T2-weighted image (1.5 T, FSE, TR/eff. TE 6350/96). The T1-weighted image demon-strates diffuse increased signal intensity within the entire PZ, representing hemorrhage due to multiple biopsies. Low signal intensity stage T2b carcinoma in the right PZ is seen on the T2-weighted image

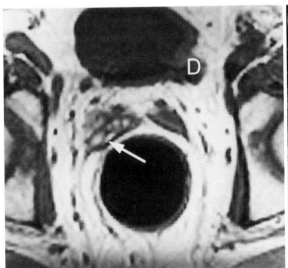
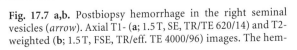
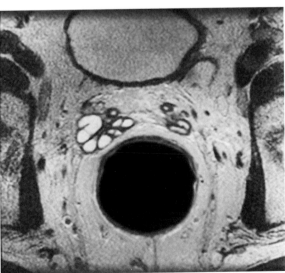

Fig. 17.7 a,b. Postbiopsy hemorrhage in the right seminal vesicles (*arrow*). Axial T1- (**a**; 1.5 T, SE, TR/TE 620/14) and T2-weighted (**b**; 1.5 T, FSE, TR/eff. TE 4000/96) images. The hem-orrhage presents with high signal intensity on both T1- and T2-weighted images. *D*, Bladder diverticula

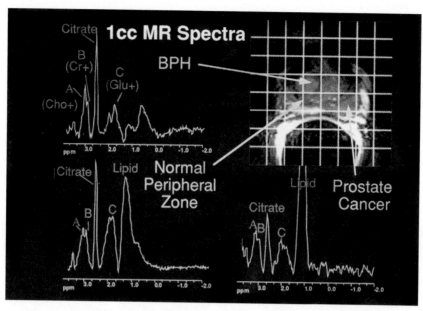

Fig. 17.8. MR spectroscopy. Typical specta of the PZ, BPH, and prostate cancer. Note the lower peaks of citrate and higher peaks of choline in cancer compared with BPH and normal PZ tissue. (Courtesy of Dr. Kurhanewicz, San Francisco)

(KURHANEWICZ et al. 1993), whether primary or recurrent. Preliminary results show the ability of MRS imaging to differentiate between tumor, PZ tissue, and BPH (Fig. 17.8) based on choline + creatine-to-citrate ratio (KURHANEWICZ et al. 1995).

17.4.4.2
Tumor Staging

Appropriate choice of therapeutic modalities in prostate cancer is dependent on accurate staging. If the tumor is entirely intracapsular, radical prostatectomy offers an excellent chance of cure. If extracapsular extension (ECE) of tumor is present, however, surgical methods are less successful, and the disease is usually treated by radiation and/or hormonal therapy. MRI of prostatic carcinoma allows both evaluation of local tumor extent and detection of nodal and distant metastasis. Staging of prostatic carcinoma can be based on either the modified JEWETT (1975) or the TNM (PIESSL et al. 1989) classification (Table 17.1).

Stage A (T1) cancers are clinically silent nonpalpable lesions (Fig. 17.9). Most of them arise from the TZ. They are often found incidentally during surgery for benign disease. Stage B (T2) disease indicates organ-confined cancer. On MRI, the tumor area with abnormal low signal intensity on T2-weighted images is limited to the prostate. A smooth

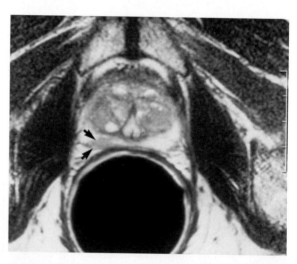

Fig. 17.9. Prostate cancer, stage pT1b (Jewett stage A). T2-weighted axial image (1.5 T, FSE, TR/eff. TE 4000/102). A small focus of low signal intensity (arrows) on the right side indicates prostate cancer. There is no evidence of ECE

tumor bulge may be demonstrated (Fig. 17.10). The prostatic capsule should be intact. Stage C (T3) disease indicates extracapsular cancer extension (stage T3a, T3b; Fig. 17.11) and/or seminal vesicle invasion (stage T3c; Figs. 17.12, 17.13). The following parameters may be suggestive of ECE: contour deformity with step-off or an angulated margin, broad area of cancer–capsule contact, obliteration of the rectoprostatic angle, asymmetry of the neurovascular bundle,

Table 17.1. MRI staging criteria following the Jewett and the TNM classifications of prostate cancer (modified according to SCHROEDER et al. (1992)

Jewett	TNM	System description
A	T1	Tumor is incidental histologic finding
	T1a/b	<5%[a]/>5% of gland involved with cancer
B	T2	Tumor present clinically, but grossly limited to the gland
	T2a	<50% of lobe involved with cancer
	T2b	>50% of lobe involved with cancer
	T2c	Both lobes involved with cancer
C	T3	Tumor invades into the prostatic apex or into or beyond the prostatic capsule, bladder neck, or seminal vesicle but is not fixed
	T3a	Unilateral extracapsular extension
	T3b	Bilateral extracapsular extension
	T3c	Seminal vesicle invasion
D	T (any)	Any size of local tumor plus lymph nodes and systemic metastases
	N (any)	
	M (any)	
D1	T (any)	Metastasis in a single pelvic lymph node, 2 cm or less in greatest dimension
	N1	
	M0	
D2	T (any)	Distant metastases
	N (any)	
	M1	

[a] Cannot be detected on MRI.

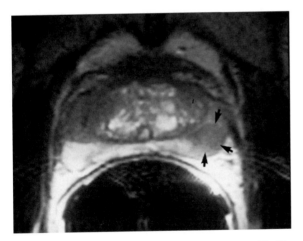

Fig. 17.10. Prostate cancer, stage pT2a (Jewett stage B). T2-weighted axial image (1.5 T, FSE, TR/eff. TE 4000/102). A well-defined focus of low signal intensity (prostate cancer) is demonstrated in the left PZ (*arrows*), presenting as a smooth bulge of the gland. There is no evidence of ECE

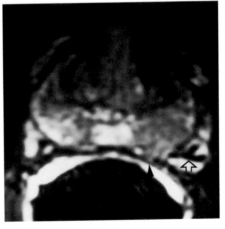

Fig. 17.11. Bilateral prostate cancer, stage pT3b (Jewett stage C). T2-weighted axial image (1.5 T, FSE, TR/eff. TE 4000/102). Cancer in the left PZ demonstrating breach of the capsule (*arrow*) with direct tumor extension into the periprostatic tissue and asymmetry of the neurovascular bundles (*open arrow*), indicating extracapsular tumor extension

irregular capsule bulge, and a direct tumor extension with breach of the capsule. Among these, obliteration of the rectoprostatic angle and asymmetry of the neurovascular bundle are the most valid predictive findings of ECE (OUTWATER et al. 1994; YU et al. 1997). Tumor length, broad contact, and smooth and irregular tumor bulge are unreliable criteria (SCHIEBLER et al. 1992; CHELSKY et al. 1993;

OUTWATER et al. 1994). Stringent diagnosis of ECE on MRI is necessary to ensure that as few patients as possible will be unnecessarily deprived of potentially curative therapy on the basis of false-positive MRI results (LANGLOTZ et al. 1995).

Tumor infiltration of the seminal vesicles (Figs. 17.12, 17.13) follows three distinct pathways (WHEELER 1989):

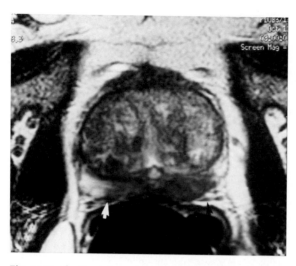 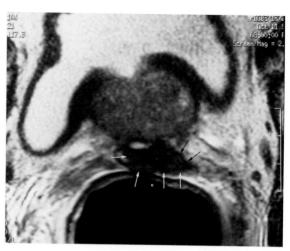

Fig. 17.12 a,b. Prostate cancer, stage pT3c (Jewett stage C). T2-weighted axial sections (1.5 T, FSE, TR/eff. TE 4000/102) at the midgland (**a**) and base (**b**). **a** Diffuse low signal intensity tumor is present bilaterally. Note the obliteration of the rectoprostatic angle with retraction of the neurovascular bundles (*arrows*) on both sides, indicative for ECE. **b** There is tumor involvement (*arrows*) of both sides (left > right) of the seminal vesicles

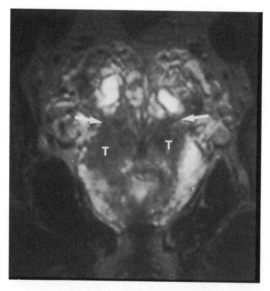

Fig. 17.13. Stage pT3c (Jewett stage C) prostate cancer. T2-weighted coronal plane of section (1.5 T, FSE, TR/eff. TE 3500/108). Tumor (*T*) at the base of the prostate shows direct seminal vesicle invasion, resulting in obliteration of the angle (*arrow*) between the base of the gland and the seminal vesicles. Both seminal vesicles demonstrate low signal intensity. Findings indicate bilateral seminal vesicle invasion

1. Via the ejaculatory duct complex (40%), resulting in nonvisualization of the ejaculatory duct and decreased signal intensity of the seminal vesicles on T2-weighted sequences, chiefly in the central portion

2. Via direct transcapsular extension (30%), shown by the contiguous extension of the low signal intensity cancer into and/or around the seminal vesicles

3. By hematogenous metastasis (30%), seen as an area of low signal intensity, either localized or diffuse in the seminal vesicles

Hemorrhage, chronic inflammation, diabetes mellitus, alcoholism, previous pelvic irradiation, and amyloidosis can also cause low signal intensities within the seminal vesicles on T2-weighted sequences (KALI et al. 1992). In addition to changes in signal intensity, prostatic cancer invasion can also result in changes in the size and configuration of the seminal vesicles. Identification of tumor invasion into the urinary bladder can be evaluated on T2-weighted images, when the continuity of the normal low signal intensity of the bladder wall is interrupted, and the perivesical fat stripe at the bladder base is obliterated. The same imaging criteria can be applied for the diagnosis of direct tumor invasion into the rectum.

Stage D prostate cancer can be subdivided into D1 and D2 disease. Stage D1 prostate cancer denotes the presence of pelvic lymphadenopathy, with a size greater than 1 cm in the short axis. The diagnostic criteria and accuracy of MRI and CT in the evaluation of lymphadenopathy are similar (BEZZI et al. 1988). Both modalities suffer from low sensitivity of nodal detection and the routine use of cross-sectional imaging is not endorsed. When distant metastases in bone or other organs are found, the cancer is staged as D2. The most common form of osseous metastases is osteoblastic. In contrast to most metastases from other primary tumors, these osteoblastic metastases are of low signal intensity on T1- as well as on T2-weighted images.

17.4.5
Role of TRUS and MRI in the Diagnosis and Staging of Prostate Cancer

The combination of prostate-specific antigen (PSA) screening, digital rectal examination, and TRUS-guided biopsy offers the best approach for the detection of prostate cancer. The selection of treatment for prostate cancer, however, remains controversial, and ranges from watchful waiting to radiation therapy, cryosurgery, chemotherapy, hormonal therapy, radical prostatectomy, or a combination there of (BORING et al. 1995; CHODAK et al. 1994; FAIR et al. 1993). The choice of treatment is an important yet often empirical decision, guided by the patient's age and general condition, serum PSA level, and Gleason score, as well as the physician and patient preference. Cancer staging, including both its locoregional extent and the presence of metastasis, should play an important role in treatment decisions. It is generally agreed that radical prostatectomy is the method of choice for gland-confined cancer, while nonsurgical therapy should be prescribed for stage C and D cancers (Table 17.1). Cancers with seminal vesicle involvement (SVI) or extracapsular extension (ECE) have high recurrence rates after radical prostatectomy (EPSTEIN et al. 1993a). In addition, the extent of ECE (focal versus gross) and surgical margin status will influence the disease-free survival (EPSTEIN et al. 1993b).

Clinical staging of prostate cancer is inaccurate, with reported understaging occurring in as many as 30%–72% of patients (MUKAMEL et al. 1987; CARTER and COFFEY 1988; RITCHIE 1994; D'AMICO et al. 1995). Diagnostic imaging is a helpful adjunct to clinical staging. Endorectal ultrasound is the most widely use imaging modality for local staging of prostate cancer. However, controversy remains regarding its diagnostic efficacy, with reported accuracies of TRUS ranging from 58% to 90% and sensitivities for ECE and SVI of 49% and 25%, respectively (SALO et al. 1987; RIFKIN et al. 1990).

The development of surface coils (endorectal, phased-array multicoil, or a combination, improved the staging accuracy of MRI. Endorectal MRI surpasses TRUS in the local staging of prostate cancer (HUCH-BÖNI et al. 1995b; PRESTI et al. 1996). In particular, endorectal coil MRI is superior to TRUS in both the localization of tumor (97% vs 70%) and sensitivity for ECE (90% vs 48%) (PRESTI et al. 1996). Furthermore, MRI, with its multiplanar capability, is superior to TRUS in the evaluation of cancers located at the prostatic base and apex.

The overall staging accuracy of MRI, however, varies widely and has been reported to range from as low as 54% (TEMPANY et al. 1994) to as high as 82%–88% in two recent studies (HUCH-BÖNI et al. 1995a; BARTOLOZZI et al. 1996). Differences in MR technique (TEMPANY et al. 1994), image quality (LANGLOTZ et al. 1995; YU et al. 1997), and reader experience (TEMPANY et al. 1994; QUINN et al. 1994; HARRIS et al. 1995; YU et al. 1997) are responsible for the wide variability in the reported accuracy of prostate MRI. Furthermore, the use of different imaging features may have affected the accuracy in detecting ECE on MRI. Multivariate analysis has shown that obliteration of the rectoprostatic angle and asymmetry of the neurovascular bundle are reliable signs of ECE (OUTWATER et al. 1994; YU et al. 1997) and should be used to ensure high specificity of prostate MRI in the diagnosis of gross extracapsular tumor extension.

If the nodal status needs to be evaluated, either CT or MRI can provide the information. Due to the low probability of lymph node metastasis in early stage prostate cancer, cross-sectional lymph node staging has not been advocated unless the PSA level is higher than 20 ng/ml (HUNCHAREK and MUSCAT 1996).

In conclusion, TRUS combined with biopsy plays a pivotal role in the diagnosis of prostatic cancer. In patients with a small tumor volume, a low PSA, and a low Gleason score, whose cancer is very likely confined to the gland, no further imaging is needed. In patients with large, multifocal high-grade tumors (seen by a combination of TRUS and needle biopsy) and obvious TRUS findings of ECE, further imaging is also not needed. There is, however, a group of patients in whom clinical parameters of PSA, Gleason score, and number of positive biopsies, as well as TRUS staging findings, remain indeterminate in differentiating intraprostatic cancer from ECE. This group of patients will benefit from MR staging, as MRI is superior to TRUS for the evaluation of ECE and SVI.

17.5
Pathology of the Seminal Vesicles

17.5.1
Congenital Abnormalities

Congenital agenesis of the seminal vesicles can be unilateral or bilateral. Unilateral agenesis is frequently associated with ipsilateral agenesis of the ductus deferens and the kidney. The contralateral seminal vesicle is often hypoplastic. A seminal vesicle is considered hypoplastic when it is less than 2 cm in length, less than 5 mm in width, and lacks normal convolutions. Bilateral agenesis of the seminal vesicles is rare. On MRI seminal vesicle agenesis is indicated by the absence of any structures typical for seminal vesicles within the fibroadipose tissue between the bladder base and the rectum (THURNER et al. 1988). Agenesis of the seminal vesicles can be best depicted on axial T1-weighted images, but for complete evaluation both T1- and T2-weighted images are needed.

Seminal vesicle cysts can be either congenital or acquired. Ipsilateral renal agenesis and infertility are commonly associated with the latter (NAZLI et al. 1994; HELLERSTEIN 1995). Congenital cysts are usually unilateral and can be either unilocular or multilocular. Whereas small cysts are usually found incidentally during cross-sectional imaging of the pelvis for other reasons, large cysts are often symptomatic. MRI provides precise anatomic localization of these cysts, allowing differentiation of the laterally located seminal vesicle cysts from the midline congenital prostatic cysts. The signal intensity of a seminal vesicle cyst depends on its fluid composition. Hemorrhage is often present within the cysts. The signal intensity depends on the age of the bleeding, being either high on both T1- and T2-weighted studies or high on T1-weighted images and low on T2-weighted sequences.

17.5.2
Infectious Disease

Inflammation of the seminal vesicles is usually secondary to prostatitis or epididymitis. In acute inflammation, the seminal vesicles may be normal in size or enlarged. The signal intensity varies from hypointense to normal on T1- and T2-weighted (SECAF et al. 1991). A common finding in subacute infection is hemorrhage within the seminal vesicles (Fig. 17.14). The MR appearance depends on

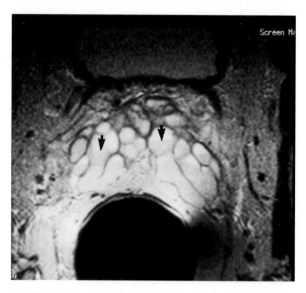

Fig. 17.14. Inflammatory disease of the seminal vesicles secondary to prostatitis. T2-weighted axial images (1.5 T, FSE, TR/eff. TE 5500/96). Note the diffuse enlargement of the seminal vesicles with multiple fluid–fluid levels (*arrows*) that represent hemorrhage

the age of the hemorrhage. Chronic inflammation causes atrophy of the seminal vesicles which con-tain a reduced amount of fluid, resulting in lower than normal signal intensity on T2-weighted images. Abscesses within the seminal vesicles are developed as sequelae of acute infection. MRI demonstrates a focal, low signal intensity lesion with poorly defined margins and infiltrative strands into the adjacent perivesicular fat on T1-weighted images that enhances after contrast administration.

17.5.3
Tumors

The vast majority of malignant tumors of the seminal vesicles are secondary to prostatic carcinoma (see Sect. 17.4.4.2). Occasionally, secondary tumor involvement of the seminal vesicles can occur by direct extension from tumors of the bladder or rectum. Primary neoplasms of the seminal vesicles are rare. The most frequent benign tumors are leiomyomas, whereas primary malignant neoplasms are most commonly adenocarcinomas (MURPHY and GEATA 1986). Benign tumors of the seminal vesicles typically appear as a smooth, well-marginated mass with intermediate signal intensity on T1-weighted and moderately increased signal intensity on T2-weighted images (McClure and Hricak 1986; Secaf et al. 1991).

17.6
Posttherapeutic MRI

17.6.1
MRI After Surgery

The MRI appearance following prostate surgery depends on the type of surgical procedure performed. After transurethral resection of the prostate (TURP; Fig. 17.15), the proximal prostatic urethra from the base of the bladder to the verumontanum is dilated, and no scar tissue is identified in the suprapubic region. After suprapubic or retropubic prostatectomy for BPH, scar tissue in the suprapubic region, the subcutaneous tissues, and the lower anterior abdominal wall muscles can be found in addition to a widened proximal prostatic urethra. There may also be some irregularity in the bladder wall in patients who have had suprapubic surgery. After either type of simple prostatectomy, a diffuse, homogeneously decreased signal intensity can be seen in the peripheral zone on T2-weighted images (Carroll et al. 1992).

Surgical treatments for prostate cancer include radical retropubic prostatectomy, radical transperineal prostatectomy, and cryosurgery. Radical retropubic or transperineal prostatectomy is the treatment of choice when the tumor is confined within the gland (stages T1 and T2, or if the Jewitt classification is used, stages A2, B1, and B2). The

procedures include the removal of the prostate, the seminal vesicles, and the prostatic urethra. Depending on the extent of tumor involvement, some portion of the bladder base may also be excised. During the procedure, the vesicoprostatic plexus are ligated, the puboprostatic ligament is transected, and Denonvillier's fascia is used as the plane of dissection between the prostate and rectum (Walsh 1992). The residual bladder base is anastomosed to the membranous urethra, and the patient relies on the external sphincter mechanism of the urogenital membrane for continence. In addition, in retropubic radical prostatectomy, the obturator nodes and both internal and external iliac lymph nodes are dissected and removed to the level of the common iliac bifurcation.

On MRI there is absence of prostate and seminal vesicles and the site of anastomosis can be identified by a signal void effect due to surgical metallic clips and by a low signal intensity region on both T1- and T2-weighted images representing fibrous scar tissue. After lymph node dissection, additional surgical clips are usually present adjacent to the iliac vessels, extending to the common iliac bifurcation.

17.6.2
Cancer Recurrence

Local tumor recurrence following radical prostatectomy is reported in 4%–22% of patients, varying with stage, volume, and grade of the primary tumor (Walsh 1987; Robey and Schellhammer 1987). Obtaining serial PSA levels is the method of

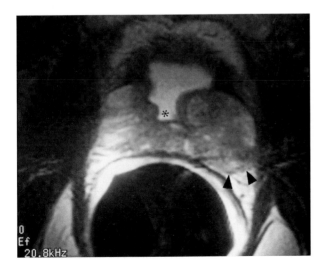

Fig. 17.15. Prostate cancer, stage pT3c (Jewett stage C) and status post-TURP. T2-weighted axial plane of section (1.5 T, FSE, TR/eff. TE 4000/102). There is diffuse low signal intensity tumor infiltration of the left and right base. ECE is demonstrated on the left side (*arrowheads*) with obliteration of the rectoprostatic angle and breach through the capsule. A post-TRUP defect is present in the central gland (*asterisk*)

choice for following postprostatectomy patients. MRI using an endorectal coil is recommended in patients with elevated PSA levels in whom metastatic spread has been ruled out (Huch-Böni et al. 1996) and TRUS of the postoperative bed has rendered equivocal results.

Recurrent tumor is most commonly found in the vicinity of the surgical margin, usually at the site of anastomosis (Fig. 17.16). It is diagnosed as a mass lesion with heterogeneous, often low signal intensity on T2-weighted images and medium signal intensity on T1-weighted images (Ebner et al. 1988; Carrington and Hricak 1991). The imaging differentiation between recurrent cancer and scar tissue can pose problems. Both recurrent tumor and postoperative fibrosis may demonstrate contrast enhancement. MR spectroscopic imaging has been explored for noninvasive improvement of tissue specificity. An elevated choline/citrate ratio has been shown not only in primary, but also in recurrent cancers (Kurhanewicz et al. 1995).

17.6.3
MRI After Cryosurgery

Improved cryotechnology and expertise in TRUS has focused attention on cryoablation for patients with organ-confined prostate cancer not eligible for radical prostatectomy as well as patients with stage

T3 disease or with local recurrence after radiation. Although cryosurgical ablation is considered to be a low morbidity treatment, early and late post-therapy complications can be seen in up to 50% of patients and include impotence, outflow obstruction, incontinence, osteitis pubis, and development of rectourethral fistula (Shinohara et al. 1996). MRI (Kalbhen et al. 1996) and MR spectroscopy (Kurhanewicz et al. 1996b) have been used for monitoring the effects and complications of cryosurgery.

As demonstrated on MRI, the prostate often enlarges immediately after cryosurgery, and loses its zonal anatomy with heterogenous signal intensity on T2-weighted images. Approximately 2 weeks after the procedure the prostate volume decreases by 30%–50%, but the zonal anatomy remains indistinct (Kalbhen et al. 1996). Areas of necrosis can be seen in about half of the patients, involving the urethra, the TZ, and the PZ (Fig. 17.17). A thick capsule involving the prostate and the neurovascular bundles on T2-weighted images develops in most patients (Fig. 17.18). Its appearance correlates with the impotency rate (Kalbhen et al. 1996). Other findings in the periprostatic tissue include abnormal high signal intensity on T2-weighted sequences in the levator ani muscles and/or obturator internus muscles as well as high signal intensity foci in the symphysis pubis representing osteonecrosis (Kalbhen et al. 1996).

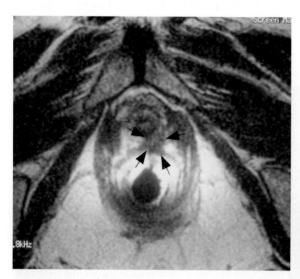

Fig. 17.16. Local tumor recurrence after radical prostatectomy. T2-weighted axial section (1.5 T, FSE, TR/eff. TE 4000/102) demonstrates a well-defined low signal intensity focus of recurrent cancer (*arrows*) at the apex

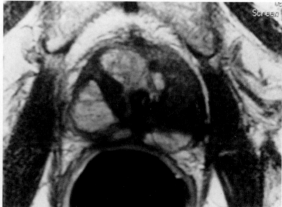

Fig. 17.17. Partial cryotherapy (3 weeks postreatment). T2-weighted axial image (1.5 T, FSE, TR/eff. TE 5000/108). Large high signal areas of necrosis are present in the PZ bilaterally and in the central gland predominantly on the right side

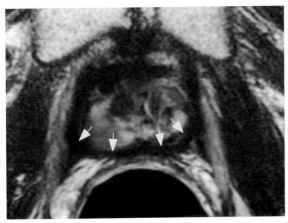

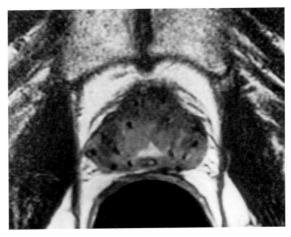

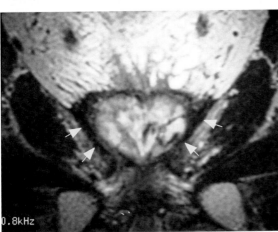

Fig. 17.19. Status following brachytherapy. T2-weighted axial image (1.5 T, FSE, TR/eff. TE 5000/96). Note the multiple scattered signal voids throughout the gland due to radiation seeds. The prostate demonstrates diffuse low signal intensity and differentiation between PZ and TZ is no longer feasible

Fig. 17.18 a,b. Status following cryotherapy (1 year after treatment). T2-weighted axial (**a**) and coronal (**b**) planes of section (1.5 T, FSE, TR/eff. TE 3500–5000/102). Zonal anatomy is no longer seen. There is a thick scar (*arrows*) around the gland encasing the neurovascular bundle and thus causing the patient's impotence

17.6.4
MRI of the Prostate in Radiation Therapy

Magnetic resonance imaging is helpful in the determination of the prostatic volume before radiotherapy. 3D MR therapy simulation is more accurate than 3D CT therapy planning since CT overestimates the tumor volume by approximately 32% (ROACH et al. 1996).

After radiotherapy, the volume of the prostate decreases. The prostate reveals low signal intensity and a loss of zonal anatomy (Fig. 17.19) on T2-weighted images (SUGIMURA et al. 1990; CHAN and KRESSEL 1991). Occasionally, the signal intensity of the PZ can be lower than that of the central gland. Postradiation changes of the seminal vesicles are demonstrated as a reduction in their size and signal

intensity (SUGIMURA et al. 1990; CHAN and KRESSEL 1991), probably due to glandular atrophy and stromal fibrosis.

17.6.5
MRI After Hormonal Therapy

Hormonal ablation of prostate cancer is preferred for patients with metastatic disease, but in selected patients it is also used in conjunction with radical prostatectomy, cryosurgery, and radiation therapy. As a new approach, neoadjuvant hormonal treatment prior to radical prostatectomy has proven to result in significant reductions in PSA, prostate volume, and tumor volume, and a lower rate of tumor-positive surgical margins (SOLOWAY et al. 1995; PEDERSEN et al. 1995).

Hormonal therapy causes a reduction in the volume of the prostate that is more pronounced in the PZ than in the TZ. More than 50% of patients exhibit diffuse low signal intensity in the PZ on T2-weighted images (CHEN et al. 1996). Therefore, detection of residual cancer or cancer recurrence in these patients is often very difficult or even impossible (Fig. 17.20). Furthermore, ECE is overestimated (CHEN et al. 1996), which is especially bothersome when ECE was present before treatment. Hormonal therapy also affects the appearance of the seminal vesicles on MRI. A symmetrical decrease in size and signal intensity on T2-weighted images has been reported (SECAF et al. 1991; CHEN et al. 1996).

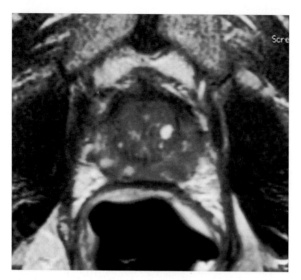

Fig. 17.20. Status following hormonal therapy. T2-weighted axial image (1.5 T, FSE, TR/eff. TE 6000/96) demonstrates low signal intensity of the PZ and the TZ, precluding reliable tumor detection

17.6.6
MRI After Laser-Induced Thermotherapy

Laser-induced thermotherapy (LITT), as a minimal invasive modality, has been used for just over 3 years to treat BPH. Laser applicators are placed in the hyperplastic central gland either transurethrally under endoscopic control or transperineally with sonographic guidance. The interstitially by applied neodymium: yttrium-aluminum garnet (Nd:YAG) laser radiation (DIXON 1995) induces coagulation necrosis of BPH that subsequently results in a decrease in hyperplastic tissue and decompression of the intraprostatic urethra. Advantages of LITT include reduced blood loss and shorter hospitalization compared with TURP.

The MRI appearance of the prostate after LITT varies depending on the time interval between LITT and MRI. Immediately after laser application, ill-defined areas of high signal intensity can be visualized on T2-weighted images (DE SOUZA et al. 1995). MRI studies obtained 48 h after LITT show an increase in total gland volume varying between 18% and 108% (MÜLLER-LISSE et al. 1996) due to intraprostatic edema. The laser-induced lesions now reveal low intensity cores surrounded by hyperintense rims on T2-weighted sequences representing perifocal edema (HEUCK et al. 1995; MÜLLER-LISSE et al. 1996). Moderate to severe edema in the periprostatic tissue marked by large areas of hyperintensity on T2-weighted images develops within 24–48 h fol-

lowing LITT. Periprostatic edema resolves 3–6 weeks after LITT; however, prostatic swelling can remain for up to 6 months after LITT (MÜLLER-LISSE et al. 1996). Alterations in prostatic tissue after microwave hyperthermia appear similar to those of LITT on MRI.

References

Bartolozzi C, Menchi I, Lencioni R, et al. (1996) Local staging of prostate carcinoma with endorectal coil MRI: correlation with whole-mount radical prostatectomy specimens. Eur Radiol 6:339–345

Bezzi M, Kressel HY, Allen KS, et al. (1988) Prostatic carcinoma: staging with MR at 1.5 T. Radiology 169:339–346

Boring CC, Squires TS, Tong T, Montgomery S (1995) Cancer statistics, 1995. CA Cancer J Clin 45:11–30

Brown G, Macvicar DA, Ayton V, Husband JE (1995) The role of intravenous contrast enhancement in magnetic resonance imaging of prostatic carcinoma. Clin Radiol 50:601–606

Carrington BM, Hricak H (1991) Postoperation and postradiation pelvis. In: Hricak H, Carrington BM (eds) MRI of the pelvis. Martin Dunitz, London, pp 519–527

Carroll CL, Sommer GF, McNeal JE, Stamey TA (1987) The abnormal prostate: MR imaging at 1.5 T with histopathologic correlation. Radiology 163:521–525

Carrol P, Sugimura K, Cohen MB, Hricak H (1992) Detection and staging of prostate carcinoma after transurethral resection or open enucleation of the prostate: accuracy of magnetic resonance imaging. J Urol 147:402–406

Carter HB, Coffey DS (1988) Prostate cancer: the magnitude of the problem in the United States. In: Coffey DS, Resnick MI, Dorr FA, Karr JP (eds) A multidisciplinary analysis of controversies in the management of prostate cancer. Plenum Press, New Youk, pp 1–7

Chan TW, Kressel HY (1991) Prostate and seminal vesicles after irradiation: MR appearance. J Magn Reson Imaging 1:503–511

Chelsky MJ, Schnall MD, Seidmon EJ, Pollack HM (1993) Use of endorectal surface coil magnetic resonance imaging for local staging of prostate cancer. J Urol 150:391–395

Chen M, Hricak H, Kalbhen CL, et al. (1996) Hormonal ablation of prostatic cancer: effects on prostate morphology, tumor detection, and staging by endorectal coil MR imaging. Am J Radiol 166:1157–1163

Chodak GW, Thisted RA, Gerber GS, et al. (1994) Results of conservative management of clinically localized prostate cancer. N Engl J Med 330:242–248

Cox RL, Crawford ED (1995) Complications of cryosurgical ablation of the prostate to treat localized adenocarcinoma of the prostate. Urology 45:932–935

D'Amico AV, Whittington R, Schnall M, et al. (1995) The impact of the inclusion of endorectal coil magnetic resonance imaging in a multivariate analysis to predict clinically unsuspected extraprostatic cancer. Cancer 75:2368–2372

de Souza NM, Flynn RJ, Coutts GA, et al. (1995) Endoscopic laser ablation of the prostate: MR appearances during and after treatment and their relation to clinical outcome. Am J Radiol 164:1429–1434

Dixon CM (1995) Lasers for the treatment of benign prostatic hyperplasia. Urol Clin North Am 22:413–422

Ebner F, Kressel HY, Mintz MC, et al. (1988) Tumor recurrence versus fibrosis in the female pelvis: differentiation with MR imaging at 1.5 T. Radiology 166:333–340

Epstein J, Carmichael M, Walsh PC (1993a) Adenocarcinoma of the prostate invading the seminal vesicles: definition and relation to tumor volume, grade and margins of resection to prognosis. J Urol 149:1040–1045

Epstein J, Carmichael M, Pizov G, Walsh PC (1993b) Influence of capsular penetration on progression following radical prostatectomy: a study of 196 cases with long term follow-up. J Urol 150:135–141

Fair WR, Aprikian A, Sogani P, et al. (1993) The role of neoadjuvant hormonal manipulation in localized prostatic cancer. Cancer 71:1031–1038

Gevenois PA, Van Sinoy ML, Stintzoff SA Jr, et al. (1990) Cysts of the prostate and seminal vesicles: MR imaging findings in 11 cases. Am J Radiol 155:1021–1024

Greskoich FJ III, Nyberg LM Jr (1988) The prune-belly syndrome: a review of its etiology, defects, treatment and prognosis. J Urol 140:707–712

Harris RD, Schned AR, Heaney JA (1995) Staging of prostate cancer with endorectal MR imaging: lessons from a learning curve. Radiographics 15:813–829

Hellerstein DK (1995) Seminal vesicle cyst, renal agenesis and infertility (letter). Br J Urol 75:113–114

Heuck A, Müller-Lisse U, Muschter R, Schneede P, Scheidler J, Hofstetter A, Reiser M (1995) Magnetic resonance imaging in interstitial laser coagulation of benign prostatic hyperplasia: first experience. Lasermedizin 11:27–33

Hricak H (1991) The prostate gland. In: Hricak H, Carrington BM (eds) MRI of the Pelvis. Martin Dunitz, London, pp 249–260

Hricak H, Dooms GC, McNeal JE, et al. (1987a) MR imaging of the prostate gland: normal anatomy. Am J Radiol 148:51–58

Hricak H, Jeffrey RB, Dooms GS, et al. (1987b) Evaluation of prostate size: a comparison of ultrasound and magnetic resonance imaging. Urol Radiol 9:1–8

Hricak H, White S, Vigneron D, et al. (1994) Carcinoma of the prostate gland: MR imaging with pelvic phased-array coils versus integrated endorectal-pelvic phased-array coils. Radiology 193:703–709

Huch-Böni RA, Boner JA, Lutolf UM, et al. (1995a) Contrast-enhanced endorectal coil MRI in local staging of prostate carcinoma. J Comput Assist Tomogr 19:232–237

Huch-Böni RA, Boner JA, Debatin JF, et al. (1995b) Optimization of prostate carcinoma staging: comparison of imaging and clinical methods. Clin Radiol 50:593–600

Huch-Böni RA, Meyenberger C, Pok Lundquist J, Trinkler F, Lutolf U, Krestin GP (1996) Value of endorectal coil versus body coil MRI for diagnosis of recurrent pelvic malignancies. Abdom Imaging 21:345–352

Huncharek M, Muscat J (1996) Serum prostate-specific antigen as a predictor of staging abdominal/pelvic computed tomography in newly diagnsosed prostate cancer. Abdom Imaging 21:364–367

Ishida J, Sugimura K, Okizuka H, et al. (1994) Benign prostatic hyperplasia: value of MR imaging for determining histologic type. Radiology 190:329–331

Jewett HJ (1975) The present status of radical prostatectomy for stages A and B prostatic cancer. Urol Clin North Am 2:105–124

Kalbhen CL, Hricak H, Shinohara K, et al. (1996) Prostate carcinoma: MR imaging findings after cryosurgery. Radiology 198:807–811

Kali Y, Sugimura K, Nagaoka S, Ishida T (1992) Amyloid deposition in seminal vesicles mimicking tumor invasion from bladder cancer: MR findings. J Comput Assist Tomogr 16:989–991

Kier R, Wain S, Troiano R (1993) Fast spin-echo MR images of the pelvis obtained with a phase-array coil: value in localizing and staging prostatic carcinoma. Am J Radiol 161:601–606

Kurhanewicz J, Dahiya R, Macdonald JM, et al. (1993) Citrate alterations in primary and metastatic human prostatic adenocarcinomas: 1H magnetic resonance spectroscopy and biochemical study. Magn Reson Med 29:149–157

Kurhanewicz, J, Vigneron DB, Nelson SJ, et al. (1995) Citrate as an in vivo marker to discriminate prostate cancer from benign prostatic hyperplasia and normal prostate peripheral zone: detection via localized proton spectroscopy. Urology 45:459–466

Kurhanewicz J, Vigneron DB, Hricak H, et al. (1996a) Three-dimensional H-1 MR spectroscopic imaging of the in situ human prostate with high (0.24–0.7 cm^3) spatial resolution. Radiology 198:795–805

Kurhanewicz J, Vigneron DB, Hricak H, et al. (1996b) Prostate cancer: metabolic response to cryosurgery as detected with 3D H-1 MR spectroscopic imaging. Radiology 200:489–496

Langlotz CP, Schnall MD, Pollack H (1995) Staging of prostate cancer: accuracy of MR imaging. Radiology 194:645–646

Lipsky BA (1989) Urinary tract infections in men. Epidemiology, pathophysiology, diagnosis, and treatment. Ann Intern Med 110:138–150

Lovett K, Rifkin MD, McCue PA, Choi H (1992) MR imaging characteristics of noncancerous lesions of the prostate. J Magn Reson Imaging 2:35–39

McClure RD, Hricak H (1986) Magnetic resonance imaging: its application to male infertility. Urology 27:91–98

McNeal JE (1983) The prostate gland: morphology and pathobiology. Monogr Urol 4:5–13

Mirowitz SA, Brown JJ, Heiken JP (1993) Evaluation of the prostate and prostatic carcinoma with gadolinium-enhanced endorectal coil MR imaging. Radiology 186:153–157

Mirowitz SA, Heiken JP, Brown JJ (1994) Evaluation of fat saturation technique for T2-weighted endorectal coil MR of the prostate. Magn Reson Imaging 12:743–747

Mukamel E, Hanna J, de Kernoin JB (1987) Pitfalls in preoperative staging in prostate cancer. Urology 30:318–321

Müller-Lisse UG, Heuck AF, Schneede P, et al. (1996) Postoperative MRI in patients undergoing interstitial laser coagulation thermtherapy of benign prostatic hyperplasia. J Comput Assist Tomogr 20:273–278

Murphy GP, Geata JF (1986) Tumors of testicular adnexal structures and seminal vesicles. In: Walsh PC, Gittes RF, Perlmutter AD, et al. (eds) Campbell's urology. Saunders, Philadelphia, pp 1607–1614

Nazli O, Apaydin E, Killi R, Ozbek E, Mulazimoglu N (1994) Seminal vesicle cyst, renal agenesis and infertility in a 32-year-old man. Br J Urol 73:467

Outwater EK, Petersen RO, Siegelman ES, Gomella LG, Chernesky CE, Mitchell DG (1994) Prostate carcinoma: assessment of diagnostic criteria for capsular penetration on endorectal coil MR images. Radiology 193:333–339

Oyen RH, Van de Voorde WM, Van Poppel HP, et al. (1993) Benign hyperplastic nodules that originate in the peripheral zone of the prostate gland. Radiology 189:707–711

Pedersen KV, Lundberg S, Ahlgren G, et al. (1995) Neoadjuvant hormonal treatment with triptorelin versus no treatment prior to radical prostatectomy: a prospective randomized multicenter study. J Urol 153:391A

Piessl B, Beahrs O, Hermanek P, et al. (1989) TNM atlas:

illustrated guide to the TNM/pTNM-classification of malignant tumors, 3rd edn. Springer, Berlin Heidelberg New York

Presti JC Jr, Hricak H, Narayan PA, Shinohara K, White S, Carroll PR (1996) Endorectal magnetic resonance imaging and transrectal ultrasound in the local staging of prostatic carcinoma. Am J Radiol 166:103–108

Quinn SF, Franzini DA, Demlow TA, et al. (1994) MR imaging of prostate cancer with an endorectal surface coil technique: correlation with whole-mount specimens. Radiology 190:323–327

Rifkin MD, Zerhouni EA, Gatsonis CA, et al. (1990) Comparison of magnetic resonance imaging and ultrasonography in staging early prostate cancer. Results of a multi-institutional cooperative trial. N Engl J Med 323:621–626

Ritchie JP (1994) Management of patients with positive surgical margins following radical prostatectomy. Urol Clin North Am 21:717–723

Roach M, Faillace-Akazawa P, Malfatti C, Holland J, Hricak H (1996) Prostate volumes defined by magnetic resonance imaging and computerized tomographic scans for three-dimensional conformal radiotherapy. Int J Radiat Oncol Biol Phys 35:1011–1018

Robey EL, Schellhammer PF (1987) Local failure after definitive therapy for prostatic cancer. J Urol 137:613–619

Salo JO, Kivisaari L, Ranniko S, Lehtonen T (1987) Computerized tomography and transrectal ultrasound in the assessment of local extension of prostatic cancer before retropubic prostatectomy. J Urol 137:435–438

Schiebler ML, Yankaskas BC, Tempany C, Holtz P, Zerhouni E (1992) Efficacy of prostate-specific antigen and magnetic resonance imaging in staging stage C adenocarcinoma of the prostate. Invest Radiol 27:575–577

Schnall MD, Pollack HM (1990) Magnetic resonance imaging of the prostate gland. Urol Radiol 12:109–114

Schnall MD, Imai Y, Toaszewski J, et al. (1991) Prostate cancer: local staging with endorectal surface coil MR imaging. Radiology 178:797–801

Schroeder FH, Hermanke P, Denis L, et al. (1992) The TNM classification of prostate cancer. Prostate 4:129–138

Secaf E, Nuruddin RN, Hricak H, et al. (1991) MR imaging of the seminal vesicles. Am J Radiol 156:989–994

Shinohara K, Connolly JA, Presti JC Jr, Carroll PR (1996) Cryo-surgical treatment of localized prostate cancer (stages T1 to T4): preliminary results. J Urol 156:115–121

Silverberg E (1985) Cancer statistics, 1985. CA Cancer J Clin 35:19–35

Soloway MS, Sharifi R, Wood D, et al. (1995) Randomized comparison of medical prostatectomy alone or preceded by androgen deprivation for cT2b prostate cancer. J Urol 154:424–428

Sommer FG, Nghiem HV, Herfkens R, McNeal J (1993) Gadolinium-enhanced MRI of the abnormal prostate. Magn Reson Imaging 11:941–948

Stamey TA, McNeal JE, Freiha FS, Redwine EA (1988) Morphometic and clinical studies on 68 consecutive radical prostatectomies. J Urol 139:1235–1241

Stamey TA, Villers AA, McNeal JE, et al. (1990) Positive surgical margins at radical prostatectomy: importance of the apical dissection. J Urol 143:66–73

Sugimura K, Carrington BM, Quivey JM, Hricak H (1990) Postirradiation changes in the pelvis: assessment with MR imaging. Radiology 175:805–813

Tempany CM, Zhou X, Zerhouni EA, et al. (1994) Staging of prostate cancer: results of radiology diagnostic oncology group project comparison of three MR imaging techniques. Radiology 192:47–54

Tempany CM, Banson ML, D'Amico AV, Propert K, Loughlin KR (1995) Evaluation of endorectal coil MR imaging for the prediction of surgical margin status after radical prostatectomy. Radiology 197(Suppl):253

Thurner S, Hricak H, Tanagho EA (1988) Mullerian duct cysts: diagnosis with MR imaging. Radiology 167:631–636

Walsh PC (1987) Radical prostatectomy. Preservation of sexual function, cancer control: the controversy. Urol Clin North Am 14:663–673

Walsh PC (1992) Radical retropubic prostatectomy. In: Walsh PC, Ratik AB, Stamey TA, Vaughan ED Jr (eds) Campbell's urology. Saunders, Philadelphia, pp 2865–2886

Wheeler TM (1989) Anatomic considerations in carcinoma of the prostate. Urol Clin North Am 16:623–624

White S, Hricak H, Forstner R, et al. (1995) Prostate cancer: effects of postbiopsy hemorrhage on interpretation of MR imaging. Radiology 195:385–390

Wingo PA, Tong T, Bolden S (1995) Cancer statistics, 1995. CA Cancer J Clin 45:8–30

Yu K, Hricak H, Alagappan R, Chernoff D, Bacchetti P, Zaloudek CJ (1997) Detection of extracapsular extension of prostate carcinoma with endorectal and phased-array coil MR imaging: multivariate feature analysis. Radiology 202:697–702

18 Ovaries and Fallopian Tubes

R. Forstner and P. Sattlegger

CONTENTS

18.1
Introduction

Adnexal diseases present a frequent problem in clinical routine as they present a broad spectrum of findings. Cross-sectional imaging modalities are valuable adjuncts in the differential diagnosis. Ultrasonography (US), including endovaginal ultra-

R. Forstner, MD, Zentralroentgeninstitut LKA Salzburg, Müllnerhauptstrasse 48, A-5020 Salzburg, Austria
P. Sattlegger, MD, Zentralroentgeninstitut LKA Salzburg, Müllnerhauptstrasse 48, A-5020 Salzburg, Austria

sonography and color Doppler sonography, has been well established as the primary imaging modality for evaluation of the ovaries. When US findings are equivocal, computed tomography (CT) has been widely used; however, it is often of limited value owing to its poor soft tissue contrast. Recently, especially with the development of new techniques, magnetic resonance imaging (MRI) has emerged as a new imaging modality for the ovaries and may replace CT for many purposes.

18.2
Imaging Technique

The combination of phased-array multicoil systems and fast imaging techniques plays a pivotal role in successful imaging of the ovaries (Fig. 18.1). Phased-array coils should be preferred to body coil imaging because they yield a 2–3 times superior signal-to-noise level (Hayes et al. 1992). Furthermore, they allow high-resolution imaging with a small field of view and high matrix. Saturation bands reduce high signal intensity artifacts in the near field and help to equalize the signal intensity throughout the image (Outwater and Mitchell 1994). The use of phased-array coils, however, is limited in patients with extreme obesity, abdominal protuberances, ostomies, recent surgical incisions, or pelvic pain, because of the limitation in depth penetration and the resulting poor signal-to-noise ratio (Hricak 1993).

To reduce bowel motion artifacts, patients should fast for 4–6 h prior to the MRI study. In addition, administration of glucagon (1 mg) or butylscopolamine bromide, (Buscopan, 40 mg) intramuscularly or both intramuscularly and intravenously is recommended, unless contraindicated.

The use of a negative oral and/or rectal contrast medium improves the differentiation of ovarian lesions and bowel loops and increases the conspicuity of enhancing peritoneal tumors, which is especially important in ovarian cancer staging (Low 1996; Scheidler et al. 1997). Furthermore, rectal air

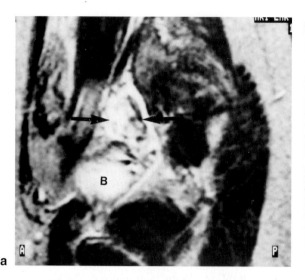

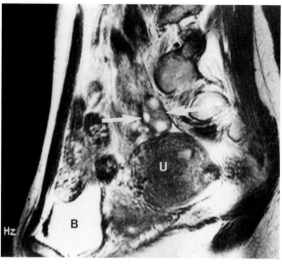

Fig. 18.1 a,b. Normal ovary in two different women of reproductive age. Sagittal T2-weighted image with a body coil (**a**) and sagittal FSE T2-weighted image with a phased-array coil system (**b**). The combination of FSE and a phased-array coil system (**b**) renders superior image quality for the evaluation of the ovary (*arrows*). *B*, Bladder; *U*, uterus

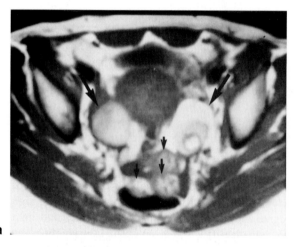

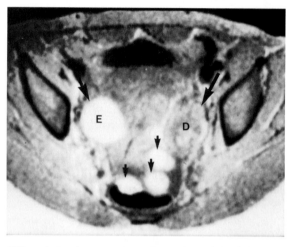

Fig. 18.2 a,b. Fat saturation technique for the differentiation between endometriomas and a dermoid. Transaxial T1-weighted image (**a**) and transaxial T1-weighted image with fat saturation (**b**). Bilateral ovarian lesions (*arrows*) displaying high signal intensity on the T1-weighted image are demonstrated (**a**). The fat saturation technique, however, allows the differentiation between the endometrioma (*E*) of the right ovary and the dermoid (*D*) of the left ovary. Loss of signal on the fat saturation images proves the fatty contents of the dermoid. Endometrial deposits (*small arrows*) can also be identified in the cul-de-sac

insufflation may be used, particularly for improved distension of the rectosigmoid.

Axial T1-weighted spin-echo (SE) imaging (TR/TE 350–700/10–20) and fast spin-echo (FSE) T2-weighted imaging (TR/TE 3000–8000/108–136) are routinely performed with a slice thickness of 4–7 mm. The field of view (FOV) ranges from 18 to 28 cm. Additional planes, e.g., sagittal or coronal FSE with the same imaging parameters, aid in the identification of complex ovarian and uterine disorders and/or pathologies of the fallopian tubes.

Further imaging techniques may be tailored depending on the clinical problem. In patients with a sonographically suspected dermoid, a limited study consisting only of T1-weighted images with and without fat saturation will be diagnostic (STEVENS et al. 1993). Fat-saturated T1-weighted images will allow differentiation between a dermoid and hemorrhagic lesions, e.g., endometrioma (KIER et al. 1992) (Fig. 18.2). Alternatively, chemical shift gradient-echo imaging can be applied (ISHIJIMA et al. 1996).

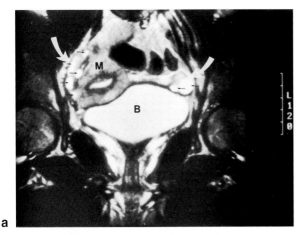

a

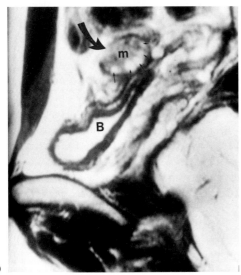

b

Fig. 18.4 a,b. Normal zonal anatomy in a 26-year-old woman. Coronal T2-weighted (a) and sagittal T2-weighted (b) images. Normal ovaries (*curved arrows*) can be identified in both planes of section. The sagittal view (b) shows the left ovary adjacent to the dome of the urinary bladder (*B*). Multiple follicles (*small arrows*) are seen in a subcortical location. The low signal intensity cortex can be differentiated from the central medulla (*m*), the signal intensity of which resembles the myometrium (*M*)

tect more than 90% of ovarian lesions, endovaginal US combined with Duplex or power Doppler, CT, and MRI are all unable to predict malignancy reliably.

High-resolution MRI allows visualization of normal ovaries in both pre- and postmenopausal women. In the latter, MRI is, however, of limited value in depicting small ovaries (1 cm) without follicles (OUTWATER and MITCHELL 1996). Tumor detection in ovaries of normal size is not possible (FORSTNER et al. 1995c). Furthermore, particularly on T1 contrast-enhanced images, normal follicular

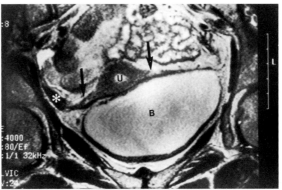

Fig. 18.5. Normal ovary in a postmenopausal woman. Coronal T2-weighted image. The fallopian tubes (*arrows*) and the right ovary (*asterisk*) can be identified lateral to the uterus (*U*). The right ovary measures less than 2 cm and displays homogeneously low signal intensity. Due to a lack of follicles it may easily be missed, especially in the transaxial plane of section. *B*, Urinary bladder

remnants in normal size ovaries may mimic malignancy. Adnexal masses tend to displace the filled bladder inferiorly or inferolaterally, in contrast to the purely lateral displacement which is caused by extraperitoneal lesions (GAMBINO et al. 1993) (Fig. 18.6).

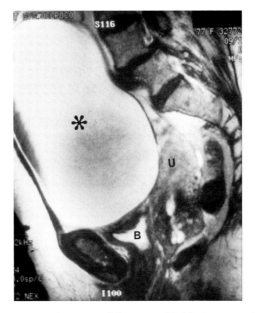

Fig. 18.6. Displacement of the urinary bladder by an ovarian cystadenoma. Sagittal T2-weighted image. The pattern of inferior displacement of the urinary bladder (*B*) by the cystadenoma (*asterisk*) is typical for an intraperitoneal lesion. The uterus (*U*) is displaced posteriorly and is clearly separated from the cystadenoma. Signal loss at the anterior aspect of the bladder is due to a saturation band

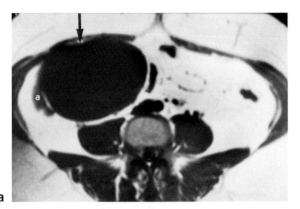

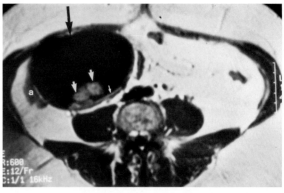

a

b

Fig. 18.7 a,b. Value of contrast-enhanced imaging for tumor characterization: papillary projections in a borderline ovarian cancer. Transaxial T1-weighted image (**a**) and contrast-enhanced T1-weighted image (**b**) at the level of the umbilicus. The contrast-enhanced image (**b**) clearly displays papillary projections (*arrowheads*) and focal wall enhancement (*small arrow*) of an otherwise cystic lesion of the right ovary (*arrow*). Papillary projections rarely can be found in a cystadenoma but should arouse suspicion of an ovarian cancer. *a*, Ascending colon

Tumor size, wall thickness, and internal architecture, including the presence of septations, calcifications, papillary projections, and cystic, necrotic, and solid internal structures, have frequently been used for tumor characterization. The probability of malignancy is related to tumor size. GOLDSTEIN et al. (1989) did not find cancers in cystic lesions less than 5 cm in size, and RULIN and PRESTON (1987) found cancers in only 3% of lesions less than 5 cm and in 11% of lesions measuring 5–10 cm. Sixty-three percent of lesions larger than 10 cm in diameter were malignant in one study (RULIN and PRESTON 1987).

Calcifications are difficult to appreciate on MRI. The internal architecture of ovarian lesions has been shown to be best visualized on contrast-enhanced T1-weighted images with and without fat suppression (THURNHER et al. 1990; STEVENS et al. 1991; THURNHER 1992; SEMELKA et al. 1993; SCOUTT et al. 1994; YAMASHITA et al. 1995; KOMATSU et al. 1996).

Using lesion size >4 cm, wall thickness >3 mm, and presence of solid structures and vegetations in combination with secondary signs (pelvic organ and sidewall invasion, peritoneal, omental or mesenteric involvement, and lymphadenopathy) as criteria of malignancy, STEVENS et al. (1991) reported an accuracy of 95% for differentiation between benign and malignant ovarian lesions. Particularly the presence of papillary projections within an ovarian lesion should raise the suspicion of malignancy and requires surgical evaluation (OUTWATER and MITCHELL 1994; BUY et al. 1991) (Fig. 18.7). Similarly, necrosis within a solid ovarian lesion is highly suggestive of malignancy (Fig. 18.8). Particularly in cases of bilateral necrotic masses (and no clinical evidence of inflammation), metastases should be included in the differential diagnosis. Septations and a wall thickness of >3 mm, however, are less reliable signs of malignancy (STEVENS et al. 1991; SICA et al. 1992). Ascites alone is nonspecific. Absence of ascites in the cul-de-sac in cases of ascites throughout the pelvis or abdomen has been described as a sign of malignancy (WALKEY et al. 1988).

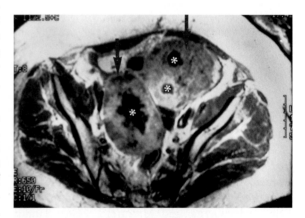

Fig. 18.8. Value of contrast-enhanced imaging for tumor characterization: ovarian metastases from gastric cancer. Transaxial contrast-enhanced T1-weighted image. Bilateral solid ovarian lesions (*arrows*) with central necrosis (*asterisks*) favor the differential diagnosis of metastases

18.5
Nonneoplastic Lesions of the Ovaries

18.5.1
Functional Ovarian Cysts

Functional ovarian cysts constitute the vast majority of completely cystic adnexal lesions. They are frequently found in women of reproductive age but may be seen in the postmenopausal period as well. Follicular or corpus luteum cysts result from failure of ovulation or involution of a mature follicle. Unless several centimeters in size, they cannot be differentiated from normal follicles. *Follicular cysts* are extremely common. They are thin-walled unilocular cysts typically ranging from 1 to 5 cm in size, although rarely they attain a size of 10–12 cm. *Corpus luteum cysts* are also unilocular cysts which tend to be larger than follicular cysts and are often complicated by hemorrhage.

In most cases functional cysts are asymptomatic and not hormonally active. Progesterone production may, however, persist in corpus luteum cysts, resulting in delayed menstruation or bleeding abnormalities. Large cysts often cause abdominal pressure and pain or low back pain. Complications are due to rupture, hemorrhage, or torsion.

Theca lutein cysts are bilateral and, in contrast to follicular and corpus luteum cysts, multilocular cystic lesions. They develop from ovarian hyperstimulation probably secondary to elevation of human chorionic gonadotropin (hCG) levels (COLEMAN 1992). In 25%–50% of cases they are associated with gestational trophoblastic syndrome. Theca lutein cysts are also reported in multiple gestations, molar pregnancies, and pregnancies complicated by hydrops fetalis. Furthermore, they occur in ovarian hyperstimulation syndrome caused by treatment for infertility. Rarely, they can be associated with a normal pregnancy (SUTTON et al. 1992).

MRI Findings. Most functional cysts display intermediate to low signal on T1-weighted images and very high signal on T2-weighted images. Their thin walls can be demonstrated on T2-weighted images and on contrast-enhanced T1-weighted images. *Follicular cysts* cannot be differentiated from normal follicles unless they reach several centimeters in size (Fig. 18.9). *Corpus luteum cysts* tend to show more prominently enhancing walls than follicular cysts and, when complicated by hemorrhage, display high or intermediate signal on

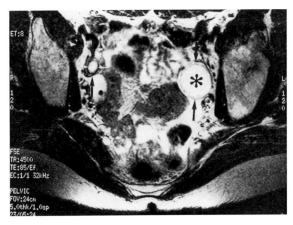

Fig. 18.9. Ovarian cysts. Transaxial T2-weighted image. Bilateral cysts are identified in both ovaries (*arrows*). The left ovary contains a thin-walled cyst of 3.5 cm in diameter (*asterisk*). The right ovary shows a cyst with irregular walls (*small white arrows*) corresponding to an involuted follicular cyst

T1- and intermediate signal on T2-weighted images (OUTWATER and MITCHELL 1996). Layering blood or debris is also often demonstrated within these cysts. Lack of contrast media enhancement aids in the differentiation of clots from papillary projections. After rupture, fluid or blood is found in the cul-de-sac.

Bilateral multilocular cystic enlargement of the ovaries in combination with elevated beta-hCG suggests the diagnosis of *theca lutein cysts*.

Differential Diagnosis. Functional cysts smaller than 2.5–3 cm cannot be differentiated from normal mature follicles. Unilocular cystadenoma may mimic functional cysts. Both corpus luteum cysts and endometrioma show intracystic hemorrhage; however, the prominent T2 shortening of endometrioma is usually not found in hemorrhagic corpus luteum cysts (OUTWATER and DUNTON 1995). Theca lutein cysts may resemble bilateral cystadenoma; however, the clinical background is different.

18.5.2
Parovarian Cysts

Parovarian (paratubal) cysts originate from the mesothelial epithelium of peritoneal inclusions or from paramesonephric remnants within the broad ligaments. Surgical data suggest that they account for 10%–20% of adnexal masses (KIER 1992). They con-

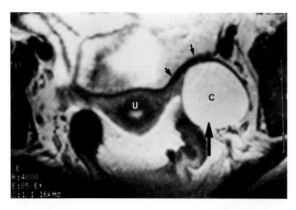

Fig. 18.10. Parovarian cyst. Transaxial T2-weighted image. A thin-walled cyst (*C*) 4 cm in diameter is identified (*arrow*) with displacement of the left adnexa (*small arrows*). Not histologically verified. *U*, Uterus

sist of thin-walled unilocular lesions filled with watery fluid. Their size varies; however, they tend to be large, with an overall size exceeding 6 cm (ALPERN et al. 1984). Although found throughout life, they are encountered most commonly in middle-aged women. They can cause differential diagnostic problems as they do not regress after hormonal therapy or on follow-up, nor are they hormonally active. As with ovarian cysts, complications include torsion, hemorrhage, infection, and rupture. Benign and malignant tumors arising within parovarian cysts are extremely rare. They present as small foci of papillary serous cystadenoma or cystadenocarcinoma (HONORÉ and O'HARA 1980).

MRI Findings. Typically parovarian cysts are seen as large, round or oval, thin-walled cystic lesions within the broad ligaments demonstrating low signal on T1-weighted images and very high signal on T2-weighted images (Fig. 18.10).

Differential Diagnosis. A parovarian cyst can only be differentiated from an ovarian cyst when it is seen distinct from the ipsilateral ovary (KIM et al. 1995). Peritoneal pseudocysts, which occur after surgery, are often not round, their shape instead being defined by the surrounding peritoneal structures. Hydrosalpinx may resemble a parovarian cyst, but it may be differentiated on the basis of its typical tubular form and interdigitating septa. Complicated paratubal cysts cannot be differentiated from abscesses, endometrioma, cystadenoma, or cancer.

18.5.3
Disorders Associated with Ovarian Cysts

18.5.3.1
Polycystic Ovary Syndrome

Polycystic ovary syndrome is a complex endocrine disorder afflicting women in the second or third decade of life. It is believed to result from a complex imbalance in the normal menstrual cycle, resulting in chronic anovulation. Although most notable in Stein-Leventhal syndrome with the classical triad of obesity, hirsutism, and infertility, a wide range of clinical presentations exist (SUTTON et al. 1992). Furthermore, full development of all signs in one patient is rare. In infertile women with polycystic ovaries, serum biochemical analysis demonstrates excessive luteinizing hormone levels, hyperinsulinemia, and increased androgen levels (JACOBS 1995). However, sonographically polycystic ovaries have also been found in normal volunteers, including children and teenagers (FARQUHAR et al. 1994; JACOBS 1995). An increased risk of endometrial cancer in women with polycystic ovary syndrome younger than 40 years of age has been reported (GINBURG and HAVARD 1976).

At pathology, both ovaries are typically involved in polycystic ovary disease. They display hypertrophy of the central ovarian stroma and a thickened, fibrotic capsule. The most striking finding is numerous subcapsular follicular cysts, ranging between 5 and 8 mm in diameter, which represent immature follicles. Mature follicles of 1.5–2.9 cm in size are rare (SUTTON et al. 1992).

MRI Findings. Bilaterally, moderately (up to 5 cm) enlarged, spherical ovaries, or, less commonly, normal size (30%) ovaries with numerous (more than ten) small ringlike, subcapsular cysts are found (SUTTON et al. 1992). Occasionally multiple small follicles may be found randomly distributed throughout the ovary (TOGASHI 1993a). Follicles surround the abundant central ovarian tissue, which typically displays low signal on both T1- and T2-weighted images (MITCHELL et al. 1986) (Fig. 18.11).

Differential Diagnosis. The diagnosis of polycystic ovaries should only be made on the basis of the combination of imaging, clinical, and laboratory findings, as there is an overlap between polycystic and normal ovaries (FARQUHAR et al. 1994; JACOBS 1995; OUTWATER and MITCHELL 1996).

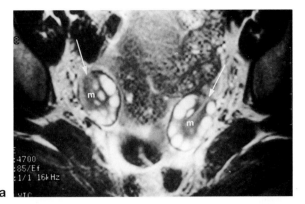

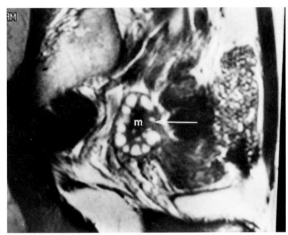

Fig. 18.11 a,b. Polycystic ovaries. Transaxial (**a**) and sagittal (**b**) T2-weighted images. In this infertile woman bilateral moderately enlarged ovaries (*long arrows*) contain numerous ringlike subcapsular follicles of less than 1 cm. The central ovarian medulla (*m*) displays low signal intensity. Note the entrance of the hilar vessels (*long arrows*)

18.5.3.2
Ovarian Hyperstimulation Syndrome

Ovarian hyperstimulation syndrome occurs in various degrees of severity in the majority of women undergoing ovulation induction. Typically, patients complain of symptoms starting from day 5 to day 8 after therapy. They can vary from mild abdominal discomfort, probably due to distension of the ovarian capsule, to severe circulatory and electrolyte imbalance with ascites and/or pleural effusions (FLEISCHER et al. 1992). Furthermore, massive stromal edema can also be associated with ovarian hyperstimulation syndrome. Extremely high levels of estrogen provide proof of the diagnosis.

MRI Findings. In patients with a history of ovulation induction, bilateral markedly enlarged ovaries

(>10 cm in size) can be found. Multiple follicles vary in size, most measuring less than 1.5 cm, and may contain hemorrhage (FLEISCHER et al. 1992; TOGASHI 1993a). Due to stromal edema, in severe cases the ovaries will display a very bright signal on T2-weighted images. Ascites and pleural effusions are associated findings.

18.5.4
Endometriosis

Endometriosis is characterized by functioning endometrial tissue outside the uterus. These ectopic endometriotic lesions are often hormone dependent and undergo cyclic bleeding similar to normal endometrium. In 18% of all laparotomies foci of endometriosis can be identified microscopically. Their prevalence increases to as high as 33% when laparotomy is performed for infertility (FILLY 1993). Although a different clinical entity, endometriosis is associated with adenomyosis of the uterus in 12%–36% of cases (WALSH et al. 1979). Women aged 25–35 years are most commonly affected (incidence 15%).

Although sometimes an incidental finding, endometriosis can become clinically evident as an adnexal mass, or cause infertility, dysmenorrhea, and dyspareunia. No correlation has been found between the extent of the disease and symptoms. Most commonly affected (80% of cases) are the ovaries, which show bilateral lesions in one-third to one-half of all cases. Further endometrial manifestations occur primarily within the pelvis. They are located on the surface of the uterus, the uterosacral ligament, the cul-de-sac, the fallopian tubes, the broad ligament, the urinary bladder, the rectosigmoid, or the pelvic floor. Sites remote from the pelvis, such as the umbilicus, colon, or spleen, are rarely involved.

The originally small endometriotic deposits grow by blood accumulation and show a high tendency to rupture, resulting in subsequent new implants. Endometriomas (endometriotic cysts or chocolate cysts) consist of focal collections of blood caused by recurrent hemorrhage during menses. Typically they display thick irregular walls due to fibrosis and adhesions to surrounding organs. They contain altered blood and display a broad spectrum of findings ranging from cystic to complex lesions with nodules due to clot, fluid debris levels, and solid structure. In 51 patients FRIED et al. (1993) described the internal architecture of endometrioma as complex in 62% of cases, predominantly cystic in 30%, and solid in 8%.

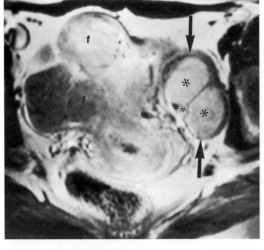

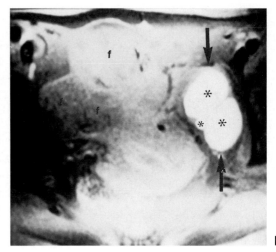

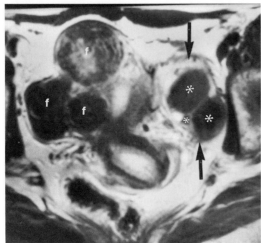

Fig. 18.12 a–c. Endometrioma of the left ovary. Transaxial T1-weighted images without (**a**) and with fat saturation (**b**) and transaxial T2-weighted image (**c**). A septate lesion of the left ovary (*arrows*) displays high signal on the T1-weighted image and following fat saturation (*asterisks*) (**a, b**). On the T2-weighted image (**c**), low signal (*asterisks*) due to concentrated blood products can be identified. This so-called shading is characteristic of an endometrioma. *f,* Uterus with multiple fibroids

Furthermore, multiple lesions in different stages can occur concurrently in the same patient. Although unusual, septations may be found (COLEMAN 1992).

Endometrial cancer originates from endometrial implants with a frequency of 0.3%–0.8%, often as polypoid masses from the lining of an endometrial cyst (KOMATSU et al. 1996). Furthermore, ovarian endometriosis in postmenopausal women seems to be at risk of undergoing malignant transformation (DEPRIEST et al. 1992).

MRI Findings. Endometrioma can form uni- or bilateral ovarian single cysts containing blood products or consist of numerous cysts containing blood of different ages. Such lesions, displaying high signal intensity on T1-weighted images and shading with low signal intensity on T2-weighted images (Figs. 18.12, 18.13), are highly characteristic of endometrioma (sensitivity: 90%–92%; specificity:

91%–98%) (OUTWATER and DUNTON 1995). Furthermore, high signal on both T1- and T2-weighted images can be found; this sign, however, is less specific and may occur with both endometrioma and malignant ovarian lesions (TOGASHI et al. 1991). Small hypointense foci on T1- and T2-weighted images are frequently observed at the periphery of endometrial cysts and are considered signs of fresh rebleeding (TOGASHI et al. 1991; ZAWIN et al. 1989). Endometriomas have a thick low signal intensity wall due to fibrosis and hemorrhage which enhances after gadolinium administration (THURNHER 1992; STEVENS et al. 1991; TOGASHI et al. 1991; SCOUTT et al. 1994). Adhesions are an invariable finding in cases of endometrioma. However, they may be difficult to diagnose, and are nonspecific. Imaging findings may vary from low signal intensity soft tissue strands to severe forms with tethering of pelvic organs (TOGASHI 1993b) (Fig. 18.13).

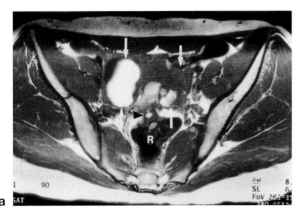
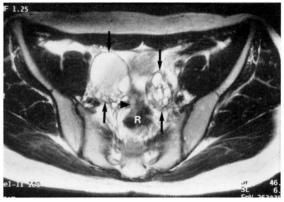

Fig. 18.13 a,b. Pelvic endometrioma. Transaxial T1-weighted image (**a**) and T2-weighted image (**b**). Bilateral adnexal masses (*arrows*) containing some blood-filled loculi are demonstrated in the ovarian fossae. The T2-weighted image displays numerous septations and various signal intensities indicating different ages of the hemorrhage. Tethering of the rectum (*R*) due to implants at the anterior aspect of the rectum (*arrowhead*) can be seen. (Courtesy of A. Heuck, Munich)

Gadolinium is not routinely used in endometrioma; however, it aids in the differentiation between nonenhancing clots in endometrioma and solid lesions, e.g., in endometrial cancer.

Differential Diagnosis. Dermoids display high signal intensity on T1-weighted images, similar to endometrioma (Fig. 18.2), but in contrast to endometriosis they become dark when the fat suppression technique is used. Functional hemorrhagic (corpus luteum cyst) cysts may have similar imaging characteristics to endometrioma; however, typically they do not show profound T2 shortening with low signal on T2-weighted images, which is considered a characteristic finding of endometrioma. In addition, the wall of functional cysts tends to be thinner than in endometrioma. Mucinous cystadenoma may display high signal on T1-weighted images; however, it is usually of lower signal intensity than blood. Hemorrhagic ovarian neoplasms may display high signal intensity on T1-weighted images. Other findings, e.g., large size, multiple septations, and gadolinium enhancement of mural nodules or necrosis, aid in the differential diagnosis. Small solid endometrial implants with low signal intensity on T2-weighted images and enhancement after gadolinium administration cannot be differentiated from scars, especially in cases of previous surgery, nor can they be differentiated from peritoneal implants in carcinosis peritonei (Low and SIGETI 1994).

Endometriomas lacking the typical very high signal on T1-weighted images cannot be differentiated from inflammatory adnexal lesions with high proteinaceous contents, e.g., abscess and hydrosalpinx.

Value of MRI. MRI is the best imaging modality for the detection of endometriomas. Due to the typical signal characteristics of endometriomas, other adnexal lesions can be excluded and high signal intensity on T1- and low signal intensity on T2-weighted images provides excellent sensitivity (90%–92%) and specificity (91%–98%) (TOGASHI et al. 1991; SUGIMURA et al. 1993; SCOUTT et al. 1994). MRI can also be used for prediction of response to and monitoring of hormone therapy. Persistent shading under therapy is likely to be found in nonresponders (SUGIMURA et al. 1996). Due to its limitations regarding small implants and adhesions, MRI cannot replace laparoscopy.

18.6
Benign Neoplastic Lesions of the Ovaries

Benign ovarian neoplasms account for 80% of all tumors involving the ovaries. Although there is a large spectrum of benign ovarian neoplasms, the vast majority are encompassed by only a few different histologic types. It is a matter of debate whether cystadenomas or teratomas are most frequent. In a large series, cystic teratomas accounted for the majority of benign lesions (58%), followed by serous cystadenomas (25%) and mucinous cystadenomas (12%), benign stromal tumors (fibromas/thecomas)

(4%), and Brenner tumors (1%) (KOONINGS et al. 1989).

18.6.1
Dermoid Cysts

Mature teratomas or dermoid cysts account for 25%–58% of all benign ovarian tumors in the reproductive period and for up to 70% of ovarian tumors in females less than 19 years of age. They consist most commonly of unilocular unilateral lesions. In only 10%–15% of cases are bilateral dermoids found.

Dermoid cysts contain mesodermal, endodermal, and ectodermal structures with the last-mentioned as the predominant element. They typically consist of an epithelial lined cyst filled with sebaceous fluid, debris, and hair. An intralesional solid mural nodule, the dermoid plug or Rockitansky nodule, is identified in up to 90% of dermoids (GUINET et al. 1995). It contains a variety of tissues, often including fat, calcifications (18%), or teeth (7%) (SHETH et al. 1988) and is one of the hallmarks of dermoids. The most common complication of dermoids is torsion (16%), which has its peak incidence within the first three decades of life (WARNER et al. 1985). Rare complications include rupture (1%), infection (1%), autoimmunehemolytic anemia (1%), and malignant transformation (1%–2%) (CARRINGTON 1991). Malignant transformation usually arises from the dermoid plug. The risk of malignancy is associated with large size (>10 cm) and postmenopausal age (CARRINGTON 1991).

MRI Findings. Identification of fat within an ovarian lesion allows the diagnosis of a dermoid. The typical findings include a round or oval, sharply delineated lesion with high signal on T1-weighted images and loss of signal on fat-saturated T1-weighted images (KIER et al. 1992; GUINET et al. 1993; STEVENS et al. 1993) (Figs. 18.14, 18.15). On T2-weighted images, dermoids display intermediate to high signal intensity. Sometimes a gravity-dependent fat-fluid level or floating debris can be identified. The dermoid plug protrudes as a rounded nodule or a palm-tree lesion into the dermoid. The chemical shift artifact at the interface between fatty and nonfatty tissue can assist in the diagnosis of a dermoid (TOGASHI et al. 1987). It is, however, a less reliable sign and may be difficult to detect, especially at lower field strengths (KIER et al. 1992; STEVENS et al. 1993). Chemical shift gradient-echo imaging may assist in the depiction of fat (ISHIJIMA et al. 1996). The amount of intralesional

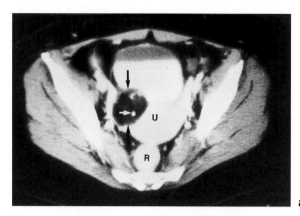

a

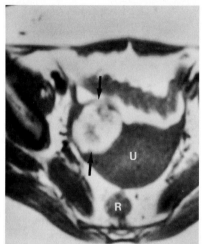

b

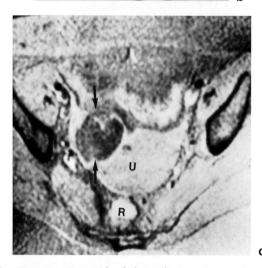

c

Fig. 18.14 a–c. Dermoid of the right ovary. CT (**a**) and transaxial T1-weighted images without (**b**) and with fat saturation technique (**c**). On CT and MRI the density/signal intensity of fat allows the diagnosis of a dermoid (*arrows*). Unlike on CT (**a**), the tiny calcification within the dermoid (*arrowhead*) is missed on the MR images. *U*, Uterus; *R*, rectum

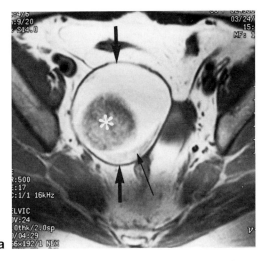
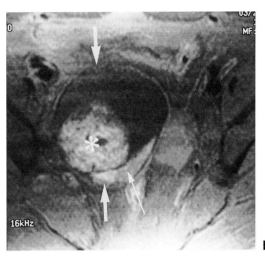

Fig. 18.15 a,b. Dermoid of the right ovary. Transaxial T1-weighted images without (**a**) and with fat saturation (**b**). A well-defined, thin-walled lesion (*arrows*) containing fat shows a mural nodule (*asterisk*), the dermoid plug, and layering (*long arrow*) probably due to debris

fat is variable. HATANAKA et al. (1996) found that in 10% of cases fatty tissue was present only at the edge or within the cyst wall, and in 8% no fat was demonstrated. Calcifications, teeth, or bones are of low signal intensity and may be missed on MRI, in contrast to CT (Fig. 18.14).

Contrast enhancement of the dermoid plug does not necessarily indicate malignancy (YAMASHITA et al. 1995). Extracapsular tumor growth, however, may suggest malignant transformation (BUY et al. 1989).

Differential Diagnosis. Endometriomas display a similar high signal intensity on T1-weighted images, but unlike with dermoids, no loss of signal will occur using fat saturation techniques. Furthermore, the chemical shift artifact is not witnessed in endometrioma (STEVENS et al. 1993). When no or only small amounts of fat are present (8%), dermoids are indistinguishable from cystic or cystic and solid ovarian tumors (HATANAKA et al. 1996; TOGASHI et al. 1987). The rare liposarcoma, or immature teratoma, may contain fat and thus be indistinguishable from mature teratoma. The latter arises in prepubertal girls and young women, and is often associated with a dermoid. At the time of diagnosis advanced tumor stages will be found (SUTTON et al. 1992).

Value of MRI. When a teratoma is suspected on the basis of US, a tailored study with T1-weighted imaging with and without the fat saturation technique will allow definite diagnosis in the vast majority of cases. Fat-containing dermoids are as accurately diagnosed by MRI as by CT, with a sensitivity of 92%–100% and a specificity of 99%–100% (TOGASHI et al. 1991; STEVENS et al. 1993; GUINET et al. 1993; IMAOKA et al. 1993; SCOUTT et al. 1994). Limitations include non-fat-containing dermoids and extremely rare malignant fat-containing neoplasms. Due to the lack of ionizing radiation, MRI should be preferred over CT in young girls.

18.6.2
Cystadenoma

Cystadenomas account for 37%–50% of benign ovarian tumors in the premenopausal phase. Their frequency tends to increase with age and in postmenopausal women they account for the majority of benign ovarian tumors (KOONINGS et al. 1989). Cystadenomas consist of thin-walled unilocular or multilocular cystic lesions filled with serous or mucinous, and sometimes hemorrhagic fluid. Papillary projections within the cyst walls are rare and should principally arouse suspicion of a borderline malignancy (OUTWATER and DUNTON 1995). Calcified psammomatous bodies are a typical feature of serous cystadenomas. Mucinous cystadenomas are less common than serous cystadenomas, often larger and multiloculated, but rarely bilateral (5%). Rupture of a mucinous benign or malignant tumor can result in pseudomyxoma peritonei.

MRI Findings. Cystadenomas are characterized by large (often larger than 10 cm) well-circumscribed

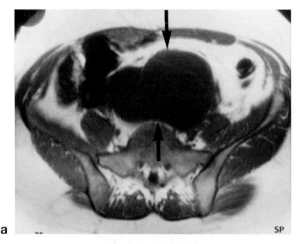

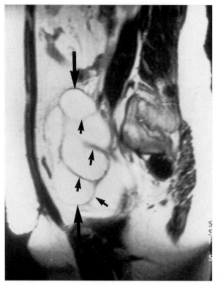

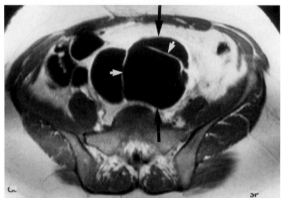

Fig. 18.16 a–c. Serous cystadenoma of the left ovary. Transaxial T1-weighted (a) and contrast-enhanced T1-weighted (b) images and sagittal T2-weighted image (c). An ovarian lesion (*arrows*) 10 cm in diameter displays waterlike signal intensity. The contrast-enhanced T1-weighted image and the T2-weighted image allow superior definition of the multicystic character with demonstration of thin septa (*arrowheads*) and no mural nodules or solid structures (b, c). It is often impossible to differentiate a serous from a mucinous cystadenoma. (Courtesy of A. Heuck, Munich)

cystic tumors with thin gadolinium-enhancing walls and septations (<3 mm).

Serous cystadenomas typically consist of unilocular lesions (sometimes they are multilocular), often with waterlike contents (Fig. 18.16). On T1-weighted images they display similar or higher signal intensity than water. On T2-weighted images their high signal intensity contents can be separated by thin septa of low signal intensity.

Mucinous cystadenomas are multilocular cystic lesions with a broad spectrum of signal intensities. They are filled with waterlike and/or mucinous contents, often also with hemorrhage or layering. Multiple cysts of different signal intensities within one large lesion are a typical finding (Fig. 18.17). Mucinous cystadenomas show intermediate signal on T1-weighted images and high or medium signal on T2-weighted images, depending on the mucinous character. When hemorrhage is present, blood products may be identified. In this case, the signal in-

tensity on T1-weighted images is almost always less than that of fat or blood; a distinctly low signal intensity on T2-weighted images, as in endometrioma, is not found (OUTWATER and DUNTON 1995).

Differential Diagnosis. Serous and mucinous cystadenomas can display similar MRI findings. Furthermore, there is an overlap in imaging characteristics in cystadenoma, borderline tumor, and cystadenocarcinoma (GHOSSAIN et al. 1991; YAMASHITA et al. 1995). Microscopic foci of cancer arising in a cystadenoma will invariably be missed by MRI. On the other hand, the presence of papillary vegetations or focal wall thickening is highly suggestive of malignancy. Nodules in unilocular cystadenoma very likely represent borderline tumors (OUTWATER and DUNTON 1995). Endometrioma may resemble mucinous cystadenoma, especially when complicated by hemorrhage. Blood products are more

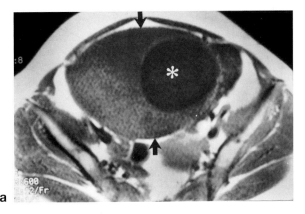 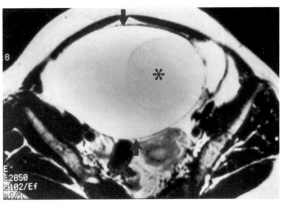

Fig. 18.17 a,b. Mucinous cystadenoma. Transaxial T1-weighted image (**a**) and T2-weighted image (**b**). On the T1-weighted image a large thin-walled cystic lesion (*arrows*) demonstrates a signal intensity slightly higher than that of

water. Furthermore, a thin-walled internal cystic area (*asterisk*) with a different signal intensity on both sequences can be identified

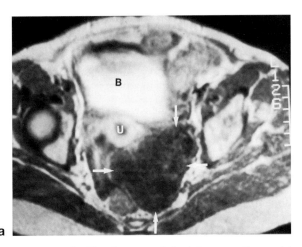 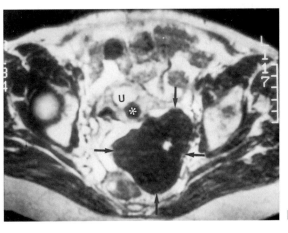

Fig. 18.18 a,b. Fibrothecoma of the left ovary. Transaxial contrast-enhanced T1-weighted image (**a**) and transaxial T2-weighted image (**b**). A large left adnexal mass (*arrows*) displays low signal intensity on both sequences. The signal

intensity on the T2-weighted image (**b**) is similar to that of the mural uterine fibroid (*asterisk*) and thus allows the diagnosis of a stromal tumor. *U*, Uterus; *B*, bladder

evident on both T1- and T2-weighted imaging in cases of endometrioma, and walls in endometrioma tend to be thicker and more irregular than in cystadenoma.

Hydrosalpinx can also display multiloculated, thin-walled, cystic uni- or bilateral lesions. However, in contrast to cystadenomas these cysts communicate and their origin from the tubal angle can be demonstrated on multiplanar imaging.

18.6.3
Fibroma, Fibrothecoma

Fibromas and fibrothecomas are rare solid tumors composed of fibrocytes and varying amounts of

stromal cells. They account for 3%–4% of all ovarian tumors and 10% of solid adnexal masses. They are typically unilateral (90%) lesions that occur in peri- and postmenopausal women. In one-third of cases, fibromas are found in association with ascites. The triad of benign ovarian fibroma, ascites, and pleural effusion constitutes Meigs' syndrome, which can be associated with elevated CA-125 levels (TIMMERMAN et al. 1995). In the basal cell nevus syndrome, numerous basal cell carcinomas are associated with abnormalities of bones, eyes, brain, and tumors, including ovarian fibromas (CARTER and LIN 1993).

MRI Findings. Small fibromas and fibrothecomas are solid lesions with intermediate to low signal on

T1- and low signal on T2-weighted images, similar to nondegenerative uterine fibroids (WEINREB et al. 1990) (Fig. 18.18). Large lesions, however, can display an inhomogeneous signal as they may have mixed solid and cystic components. Contrast-enhanced T1-weighted images show no or little inhomogeneous enhancement.

Differential Diagnosis. The signal intensity is fairly characteristic of fibroids/fibrothecoma. Broad ligament and pedunculated uterine fibroids may mimic ovarian fibroids. If the ipsilateral ovary is separated from the lesion, a uterine origin should be favored. Furthermore, large uterine fibroids are often not of very low signal intensity on T2-weighted images (OUTWATER and DUNTON 1995). Fibromas/fibrothecomas with large cystic or regressive areas or inhomogenoeus contrast enhancement cannot be reliably differentiated from other solid ovarian lesions. Dysgerminoma, metastases, serous adenofibroma, and nondifferentiated ovarian carcinoma should be included in the differential diagnosis.

Value of MRI. Similar to uterine fibroids, many fibromas/fibrothecomas can be reliably diagnosed by MRI due to their signal characteristics. In the presence of a pedunculated uterine or broad ligament, fibroid surgery may be postponed or obviated (OUTWATER and DUNTON 1995; CURTIS et al. 1993).

18.7
Malignant Ovarian Neoplasms

Malignant ovarian neoplasms account for 10%–15% of all ovarian tumors. They derive from one of the three histologic elements: coelomic epithelial, germ, and stromal cells. The surface coelomic epithelium gives rise to ovarian cancer, which accounts for the vast majority of all ovarian neoplasms (85%–90%). The remaining 10%–15% consist of stromal and germ cell ovarian neoplasms (YOUNG et al. 1993). The latter affect primarily infants and young women and are responsible for the majority of ovarian malignancies in this age group. Ovarian metastases account for 5%–8% of all ovarian tumors. Primaries with common sites in the ovaries include those of the breast, gastrointestinal tract, and endometrium and melanoma. Extremely rarely, the ovary may be involved by lymphoma.

18.7.1
Primary Malignant Ovarian Tumors

18.7.1.1
Epithelial Ovarian Cancer

Although ovarian cancer ranks second in incidence among gynecologic cancers, it causes more deaths than endometrial and cervical cancer combined (BORING et al. 1994). Its incidence rises until menopause, at which it is about 50 cases per 100 000 women annually. Women with nulliparity, late parity, or low parity are considered at risk for ovarian cancer. Furthermore, familial ovarian cancer may contribute to 5%–10% of all cases (YOUNG et al. 1993).

Ovarian cancer is believed to originate from inclusion bodies within the ovary, which are influenced by growth factors and may become malignant due to errors of replication of DNA (TAYLOR and SCHWARTZ 1994). Epithelial carcinomas of the ovary account for the vast majority (85%–90%) of ovarian malignancies (YOUNG et al. 1993). In order of decreasing frequency, malignant epithelial tumors comprise serous ovarian cancers, undifferentiated carcinoma, endometrioid tumors, mucinous ovarian cancers, clear cell tumors, and mixed epithelial tumors (YOUNG et al. 1993). Ovarian cancers are classified as invasive cancers with different degrees of differentiation (I–III, unclassified) and borderline tumors (cancers of low malignant potential) (GERSHENSON and SILVA 1990; YOUNG et al. 1993). Between 20% and 25% of ovarian cancers are serous and mucinous borderline tumors, and these have a better prognosis than other ovarian cancers (TAYLOR and SCHWARTZ 1994). Primary peritoneal adenocarcinoma occurs primarily in older women. It is thought to originate from ovarian surface epithelium, cannot be differentiated histologically and clinically from ovarian carcinomas, and can occur with no or minimal ovarian involvement (ALTARAS et al. 1991; WHITE et al. 1985). Endometrioid and clear cell carcinomas can be associated with synchronous carcinoma of the uterus or pelvic endometriosis (DEPRIEST et al. 1992; OUTWATER and DUNTON 1995).

The most useful tumor marker in ovarian cancer is CA-125 (TAYLOR and SCHWARTZ 1994). Studies have shown that CA-125 levels are elevated (>35 U/ml) in 80%–85% of patients with epithelial ovarian cancer. In stage I disease, however, CA-125 is elevated in fewer than 50% of cases (JACOBS and BAST 1989). The greatest problem of CA-125 determination in primary ovarian cancer is its lack of specificity. Elevated levels are not only found in malignancy: they can also be associated with fibroids, pregnancy, menstruation, endometriosis, and liver disease with or without ascites.

MRI Criteria for Malignant Ovarian Lesions. The criteria most useful for prediction of malignancy include lesion size (>4 cm), thickness (>3 mm) of the walls and septa, and internal structure, including papillary projections, nodularity, various degrees of solid components, necrosis, and hemorrhage (STEVENS et al. 1991; SCOUTT et al. 1994; SICA et al. 1992; YAMASHITA et al. 1995; KOMATSU et al. 1996)

(Fig. 18.19). If an ovarian lesion is mixed cystic and solid (Fig. 18.20) or cystic with mural nodules (dermoid excluded), or if it shows thick and/or irregular walls or septations, or if it is solid with areas of necrosis, there is a high probability of malignancy (STEVENS et al. 1991; SICA et al. 1992).

Furthermore, ancillary findings indicating malignancy are pelvic organ and pelvic sidewall invasion, peritoneal, omental (Fig. 18.21), or mesenteric involvement, massive ascites, and lymphadenopathy (STEVENS et al. 1991; KOMATSU et al. 1996). The combination of tumor size and architecture and ancillary signs improves prediction of malignancy and, for contrast-enhanced T1-weighted imaging, yields an accuracy of 89%–95% (KOMATSU et al. 1996; STEVENS et al. 1991).

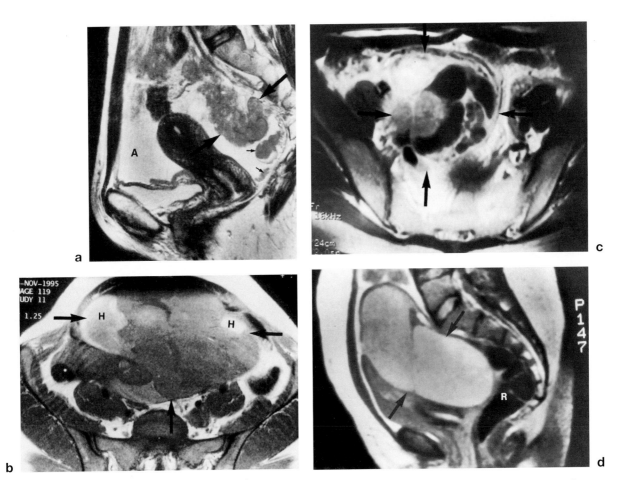

Fig. 18.19 a–d. Spectrum of findings in ovarian cancers. Sagittal T2-weighted image (**a**), transaxial T1-weighted image (**b**), transaxial contrast-enhanced T1-weighted image (**c**), and sagittal T2-weighted image (**d**). The images are from different patients with different types of epithelial ovarian cancer. **a** Ascites (*A*), peritoneal implants (*small arrows*), and predominantly solid ovarian tumor (*arrows*) in a patient with an undifferentiated ovarian cancer. **b** A large cystic and solid ovarian tumor (*arrows*) with hemorrhage (*H*) in a patient with endometrioid ovarian cancer. **c** Mixed solid and cystic architecture (*arrows*) in a patient with papillary serous adenocarcinoma. **d** A large multiseptate cystic lesion (*arrows*) which at histology showed microscopic foci of ovarian cancer within a cystadenoma. *R*, Rectum. (**a**, **b**, Courtesy of A. Heuck, Munich)

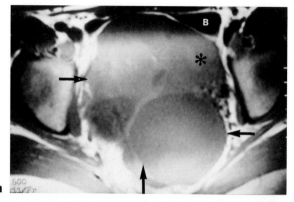

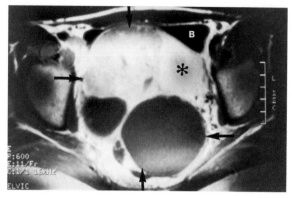

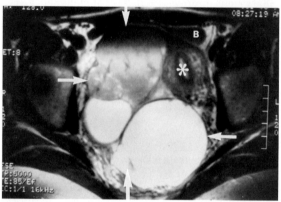

Fig. 18.20 a–c. Ovarian cancer. Transaxial T1-weighted image (a), transaxial contrast-enhanced T1-weighted image (b) and T2-weighted image (c). A solid and cytic lesion of the right ovary (arrows) is displacing the uterus (asterisk) and compressing the urinary bladder (B). The internal architecture of the lesion is better appreciated on the contrast-enhanced and T2-weighted images (b, c)

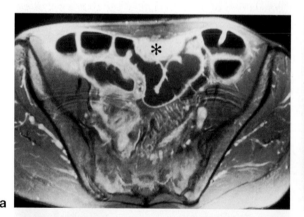

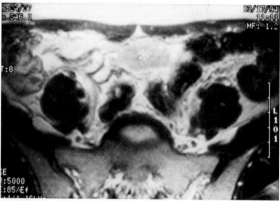

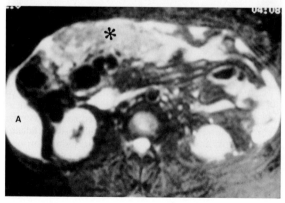

Fig. 18.21 a–c. Omental implants. Transaxial fat-saturated T1-weighted image after gadolinium enhancement (a), T2-weighted image (b), and fat-saturated T2-weighted image (c) in three different patients. Nodular omental implants (asterisk, a and b) and omental cake (asterisk, c) are typically located between the abdominal wall and bowel loops. (a Courtesy of A. Heuck, Munich)

Papillary projections in uni- or multilocular cystic lesions, often appreciated only on contrast-enhanced images, are highly suspicious of malignancy and are often found in borderline tumors (Fig. 18.7).

Ascites alone is nonspecific and is also found in 33% of patients with benign ovarian lesions (Scoutt et al. 1994). Absence of ascites in the cul-de-sac in the presence of general ascites, however, has been described as a sign of malignancy (Walkey et al. 1988).

Differential Diagnosis. In general, one should keep in mind that there is an overlap of imaging findings in benign and malignant ovarian lesions.

Like ovarian cancer, cystadenoma may display papillary projections, though it does so less frequently (9% of cases) (Ghossain et al. 1991). On the other hand, microscopic foci of cancer arising within a benign cystadenoma cannot be detected by MRI. Rare benign tumors, e.g., dysgerminoma, degenerative fibrothecoma, cystadenofibroma, or Brenner tumor, can mimic malignant tumors. The various histologic types of epithelial cancer cannot be differentiated, nor can metastases confidently be differentiated from primary ovarian cancer. A clinical history of bilateral solid tumors with necrosis favors the diagnosis of metastases. Concomitant ovarian cancer and endometrial cancer of the uterus cannot be differentiated from metastases of the latter. Imaging findings of thick walls and septations occur in both endometrioma and ovarian cancer. Endometriomas are found in younger patients (25–

40 years), often with a history of infertility; furthermore, endometriomas are rarely larger than an orange (Togashi 1993b). Ovarian abscesses display a complex structure similar to ovarian cancer. Ectopic ovarian pregnancy may present as a rapidly growing ovarian tumor, mimicking ovarian cancer (Kuhl et al. 1995).

18.7.1.1.2
STAGING

Staging of ovarian cancer is based on the extent and location of disease found at exploratory laparotomy (Young et al. 1993). The FIGO classification is the most commonly used staging system (FIGO 1987). An MRI modified staging system is summarized in Table 18.1 (Forstner et al. 1995b).

Knowledge of the pathways of tumor spread is crucial for image interpretation and staging of ovarian cancer. Epithelial ovarian cancer disseminates primarily by surface shedding and lymphatic spread, and less commonly hematogenously. It spreads locoregionally by growing continuously on the surfaces of the pelvic organs involved, including the serosal surface and musculature of the uterus, the bladder, the sigmoid colon, and the pelvic sidewalls. Peritoneal implants are disseminated throughout the lymphatic vessels of the peritoneum. Due to the hemodynamics of peritoneal fluid, the sites most often involved are the right subphrenic space including the diaphragm, the liver surface, and Morison's pouch. Further implants are located within the omentum (more often the infracolic omentum), paracolic gutters, cul-de-sac, and peritoneal bowel surfaces

Table 18.1. Modified FIGO staging of ovarian cancer for MRI

Stage	MRI findings[a]
Stage I	Tumor limited to the ovaries
IA	Limited to one ovary, no ascites (intact capsule and no tumor on the external surface)
IB	Limited to both ovaries, no ascites (as in stage IA)
IC	Stage IA or IB with ascites (or with tumor on surface). Capsule ruptured, peritoneal washing positive for malignant cells
Stage II	Growth involving one or both ovaries, pelvic extension
IIA	Extension and/or metastases to the uterus and/or fallopian tubes
IIB	Extension to other pelvic tissues
IIC	Tumor either stage IIA or IIB with ascites (as in stage IC)
Stage III	Tumor involving one or both ovaries, peritoneal implants (including liver surface, small bowel, and omentum) outside the pelvis and/or implants of retroperitoneal or inguinal lymph nodes
IIIA	Tumor grossly limited to the true pelvis (includes microscopic seeding of abdominal peritoneum)
IIIB	≤2 cm implants of abdominal peritoneal surfaces
IIIC	>2 cm implants of abdominal peritoneal surface and/or retroperitoneal or inguinal lymph nodes
Stage IV	Growth involving one or both ovaries, distant metastases, parenchymal liver metastases

[a] Additional staging criteria used in histopathologic and surgical staging in parentheses.

(BUY et al. 1988; YOUNG et al. 1993; CHOU et al. 1994) (Figs. 18.22, 18.23).

The main pathway of lymphatic spread includes the external iliac and hypogastric and para-aortic nodes between the bifurcation and the renal hilum. Drainage to external and inguinal nodes via the broad ligament accounts for rare inguinal node metastases. At surgery lymph node dissemination is dependent on the stage: in stages I and II up to 14% of lymph nodes may be positive while in stages III and IV the figure reaches up to 64% (BURGHARDT

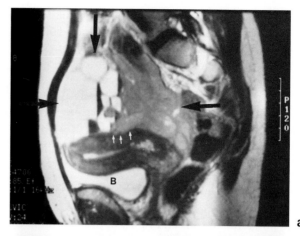

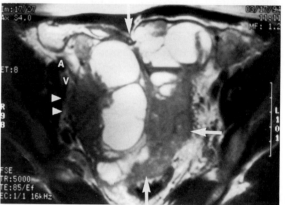

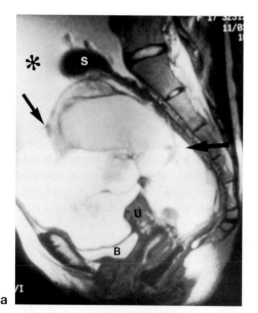

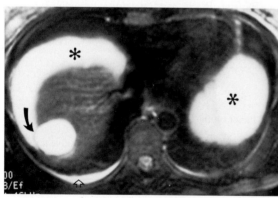

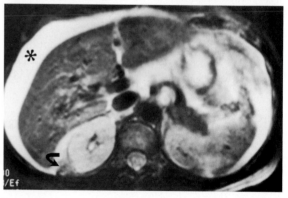

Fig. 18.22 a,b. Serous papillary borderline cancer in a 17-year-old female. Sagittal T2-weighted image (a) and transaxial fat-saturated T2-weighted image at the level of the dome of the liver (b). A large predominantly cystic lesion (*arrows*) with papillary projections occupies the pelvis and displaces the urinary bladder (*B*) and rectum. Ascites (*asterisk*) can be clearly distinguished from the lesion (a) and is present throughout the abdomen (b). A cystic liver surface implant (*curved arrow*) is demonstrated (b). Pleural effusion is indicated by the *open arrow*. *S*, Sigmoid colon. *U*, uterus

Fig. 18.23 a–c. Imaging findings in a patient with Figo stage IIIc ovarian cancer. Sagittal T2-weighted image (a), transaxial T2-weighted image (b), and transaxial fat-saturated T2-weighted image (c). The uterus is displaced by a large mixed solid and cystic ovarian mass with multiple fluid-hemorrhage levels. The irregularity at the uterine interface (*small white arrows*) represents uterine surface implants (a). Right pelvic sidewall invasion (*arrowheads*) can be suggested when the tumor encases the iliac vessels (*A, V*) or reaches behind them (b). Peritoneal implants in Morison's pouch (*curved arrow*) can be easily identified due to surrounding ascites (*asterisk*). *B*, Bladder

et al. 1984). Furthermore, pelvic lymph nodes are more often involved than para-aortic nodes (BURGHARDT et al. 1991).

Hematogenous spread occurs late and includes, in order of decreasing frequency, liver, lung, pleura, kidneys, bone, adrenals, bladder, spleen, and brain (YOUNG et al. 1993). At the time of the initial diagnosis of ovarian cancer, parenchymal liver metastases are extremely rare and patients are more likely to present liver surface metastases (WALKEY et al. 1988).

18.7.1.1.3
PREDICTION OF RESECTABILITY

Cytoreductive surgery including abdominal hysterectomy, bilateral salpingo-oophorectomy, resection of the infracolic omentum, and meticulous biopsies or resections of pelvic and abdominal peritoneal sites and lymph nodes has been established as the mainstay for the treatment of patients with ovarian cancer. Debulking is generally considered optimal or successful when no residual tumor larger than 2 cm in diameter is left after the initial staging laparotomy (YOUNG et al. 1993). Data show that only this patient group will benefit from surgery in terms of response to chemotherapy and survival (YOUNG et al. 1993). Sites considered nonoptimally resectable include lesions larger than 2 cm on the diaphragm, the liver surface [including the gallbladder fossa and porta hepatis (Fig. 18.24)] and liver parenchyma, pleura, mesentery, omental lesions with attachment of the spleen, and para-aortic lymph nodes above the level

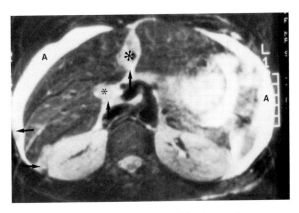

Fig. 18.24. Peritoneal metastasis with signs of nonresectability. Transaxial T2-weighted image of the upper abdomen. Multiple peritoneal implants (*arrows*) are demonstrated in Morison's pouch, at the diaphragm, and at the liver surface. Implants located at the porta hepatis (*asterisk*) and the interlobar fissure (*asterisk*) are considered nonoptimally resectable

of the renal hilum (NELSON et al. 1993; FORSTNER et al. 1995a). MEYER et al. (1995) reported that reference to other factors, e.g., ascites or CA-125, does not improve prediction, and also suggested a scoring system. First MRI data show promising results for prediction of cancer nonresectability, with predictive values of more than 90% (FORSTNER et al. 1995a).

18.7.1.1.4
VALUE OF MRI

Due to its multiplanar capability, MRI is superior to CT in defining the ovarian origin of large pelvic lesions (Fig. 18.25) and in the differentiation between a cystic tumor and ascites. Contrast-enhanced MRI has been found to be superior to transvaginal US in the characterization and differentiation of adnexal lesions (YAMASHITA et al. 1995). Furthermore it has been found useful in the prediction of malignancy, displaying an accuracy of 83%–95% (STEVENS et al. 1991; SCOUTT et al. 1994; THURNHER et al. 1990; YAMASHITA et al. 1995).

Not all patients with suspected ovarian cancer require preoperative imaging. In suspected advanced disease the role of imaging lies in roadmapping for the oncologist surgeon (NIH Consensus Conference 1995). MRI is superior to CT in the depiction of pelvic peritoneal implants; however, using MRI it is difficult to differentiate small (<1 cm) peritoneal implants, especially in the absence of ascites (SEMELKA et al. 1993; FORSTNER et al. 1995a,b; Low et al. 1995). Delayed contrast-enhanced spoiled gradient-recalled MRI has been described to improve depiction of peritoneal lesions over T2-weighted imaging (Low and SIGETI 1994; Low et al. 1995).

Although the performance of MRI in staging is only moderate and comparable to CT, with an accuracy of 78%, MRI may play a role in the prediction of tumor nonresectability in advanced ovarian cancer (FORSTNER et al. 1995a; MEYER et al. 1995).

18.7.1.2
Nonepithelial Ovarian Malignancies

18.7.1.2.1
MALIGNANT GERM CELL TUMORS

Although germ cell ovarian malignancies account for less than 5% of all ovarian malignancies, their clinical importance is based on the typical age distribution. In women younger than 20 years, they represent approximately two-thirds of all ovarian

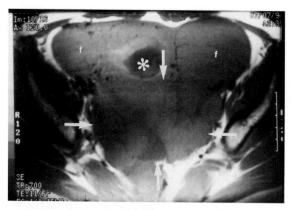
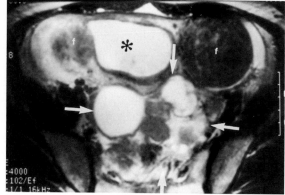

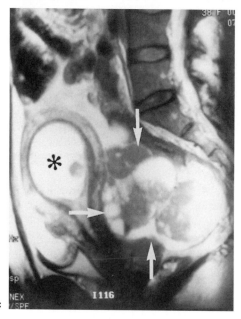

Fig. 18.25 a–c. Value of MRI in further characterizing complex ovarian lesions. Transaxial T1-weighted image (**a**), T2-weighted image (**b**), and sagittal T2-weighted image (**c**). Ascites and a huge pelvic mass were sonographically detected in this pregnant patient (15 weeks of pregnancy). MRI demonstrates a solid and cystic ovarian lesion (*arrows*) which proved to be serous adenocarcinoma at surgery. In addition, the uterine enlargement is due to pregnancy (*asterisk*) and uterine fibroids (*f*)

malignancies. They are solid tumors, sometimes containing calcifications, with rapid and predominantly unilateral growth (BRAMMER et al. 1990). Malignant germ cell tumors comprise, in order of decreasing frequency, dysgerminoma, immature teratoma, endodermal sinus tumor, and embryonal carcinoma.

Dysgerminoma is typically unilateral and spreads via the lymphatics. Elevation of serum beta-hCG may be observed (TANAKA et al. 1994). Although dermoids coexist with all malignant germ cell tumors, they are most frequently encountered with immature teratomas (BRAMMER et al. 1990). Endodermal sinus tumor and embryonal carcinoma are highly aggressive and metastasize hematogenously (YOUNG et al. 1993). The latter is rare, and associated with elevation of beta-hCG and alpha-fetoprotein levels.

MRI Findings. Solid tumors in young females should arouse suspicion of a malignant germ cell tumor.

Dysgerminomas tend to be well-delineated, solid, multilobulated lesions with low signal intensity on T1-weighted images and high signal intensity on T2-weighted images, similar to seminoma of the testis. Areas of necrosis and hemorrhage appear as cystlike locules. Intralesional septa display distinct contrast enhancement (TANAKA et al. 1994).

Immature teratomas are often associated with a dermoid cyst (Fig. 18.26). Scattered calcifications, which are difficult to verify on MRI, have been described as characteristic of immature teratomas (BRAMMER et al. 1990). Inhomogeneous signal intensity on T2-weighted images, with cysts, large areas of necrosis, or hemorrhage, may favor the

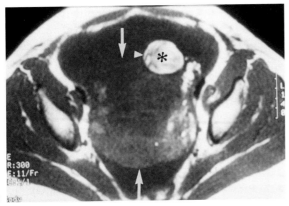

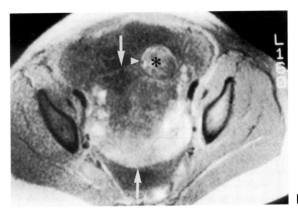

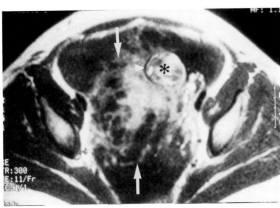

Fig. 18.26 a–c. Malignant teratoma. Transaxial T1-weighted image without (a) and with fat saturation (b) and contrast-enhanced T1-weighted image (c). A large pelvic mass is identified (*arrows*), which is best appreciated on the contrast-enhanced image (c) with demonstration of ill-defined margins and irregular enhancing solid and weblike cystic areas. An intralesional nodule (*asterisk*) seen on all sequences contains fat and shows a chemical shift artifact (*arrowhead*), suggesting a dermoid. Although dermoids can be associated with all malignant germ cell tumors, they are most frequently encountered in conjunction with malignant teratomas

diagnosis of endodermal sinus tumor or embryonal carcinoma (GERSHENSON 1985).

Differential Diagnosis. Dermoid and granulosa cell tumor have to be considered in the differential diagnosis of malignant germ cell tumors.

18.7.1.2.2
GRANULOSA CELL TUMORS

Granulosa cell tumors are neoplasms of generally low-grade malignancy and account for less than 5% of ovarian malignancies. Due to estrogen secretion they can be associated with postmenopausal bleeding. An increased incidence of concomitant endometrial cancer has been noted (YOUNG et al. 1993). The rare juvenile type becomes clinically apparent by virtue of precocious feminization (JABRA et al. 1993). Tumor spread follows the pathways of epithelial ovarian cancer (MACSWEENEY and KING 1994).

MRI Findings. Granulosa cell tumors appear as large well-defined lesions with solid, cystic, and often hemorrhagic components. The findings are not specific (CARRINGTON 1991; NESTE et al. 1996). Pre-

cocity associated with an ovarian tumor suggests the diagnosis of a granulosa cell tumor.

18.7.1.2.3
LYMPHOMA

Although the ovaries are not infrequently found to be involved by malignant lymphoma at biopsy, enlargement of the ovaries is rare. Less than 1% of patients with a lymphoma initially present with uni- or bilateral ovarian masses (MONTERROSO et al. 1993). Primary lymphoma of the ovary without lymph node or bone marrow involvement is extremely rare. The vast majority (95%) of ovarian lymphomas present manifestations of systemic spread of B-cell neoplasms (typically of Burkitt's lymphoma) to the ovaries (MONTERROSO et al. 1993). Furthermore bilateral involvement has been reported as a sign of systemic involvement (MONTERROSO et al. 1993).

MRI Findings. Lymphomas appear as uni- or, more commonly, bilateral solid tumors with intermediate signal on T1-weighted images and high to intermediate signal intensity on T2-weighted images. Hemorrhagic components may be seen on the latter images.

Gadolinium-enhanced images display enhancing lesions, often with necrosis.

Differential Diagnosis. Metastases, germ cell tumors, and ovarian cancer can display similar imaging characteristics. Germ cell tumors typically occur in infancy and young women. In cases with bilateral involvement, a history of malignant lymphoma (especially B-cell lymphoma), or disseminated systemic lymphomatous spread, the diagnosis of lymphoma of the ovaries is warranted.

18.7.2
Metastases

Krukenberg tumors account for 5%–8% of all ovarian tumors. Metastases to the ovaries derive, in order of decreasing frequency, from colon, stomach, breast, lung, and pancreatic primaries. The majority (60%–80%) are bilateral and, unlike in cases of primary ovarian cancer, the ovaries often retain their shape (HALE 1968; HA et al. 1995). Initially, metastases tend to be solid; however, subsequent enlargement, necrosis, and hemorrhage occur (HA et al. 1995). Calcifications may indicate a colonic origin.

MRI Findings. Metastases should be suspected in cases of bilateral (60%–80%) well-delineated oval lesions with central necrosis.

The signal intensity varies on T1-weighted images. T2-weighted images typically show hypointense solid components correlating with collagenous stroma (HA et al. 1995) (Fig. 18.27). Necrosis can be well- or ill-defined and is best differentiated from the enhancing vital tissue on gadolinium-enhanced T1-weighted images (Figs. 18.8, 18.27). Furthermore, well-demarcated, contrast-enhancing intralesional cystic areas within solid lesions have been described (KIM et al. 1996). Completely cystic metastases are rare.

Differential Diagnosis. Bilaterality and solid lesions with necrosis should give rise to a high level of suspicion of metastases. Differential diagnosis includes necrotic fibrothecoma and other solid ovarian tumors, e.g., granulosa cell tumors.

The rare completely cystic metastases cannot be differentiated from other multiseptate lesions, e.g., cystadenoma or cystadenocarcinoma.

18.7.3
Recurrent Ovarian Cancer

Although the initial response to treatment is good, persistence or recurrence of ovarian cancer remains a major clinical problem. This is reflected by the 5-year survival rate for patients with advanced tumor stages of only 17%.

Pelvic recurrences develop after an average of 1.8 years and the rare hematogenous metastases (liver, spleen, lungs, and brain) after an average of 2.5 years (BURGHARDT 1993). The pelvis (commonly the vaginal vault and the cul-de-sac) is the most common site of recurrent tumor, and abdominal peritoneal implants are the next most common form of recurrence (REUTER et al. 1989; YOUNG et al. 1993; FORSTNER et al. 1995a) (Fig. 18.28). The latter are located on the

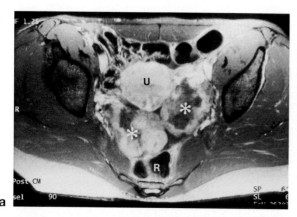
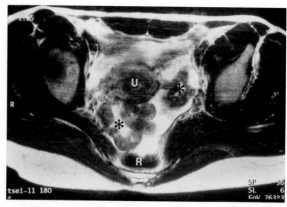

Fig. 18.27 a,b. Bilateral ovarian metastases from breast cancer. Transaxial contrast-enhanced T1-weighted image (**a**) and transaxial T2-weighted image (**b**). Ascites is seen between bilateral lobulated ovarian tumors with enhancing solid structures and an irregular central necrosis (*asterisk*). On the T2-weighted image (**b**) the solid tumor components display low signal intensity. *U*, Uterus; *R* rectum. (Courtesy of A. Heuck, Munich)

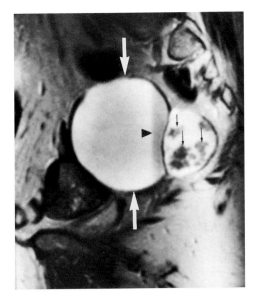

Fig. 18.28. Pelvic ovarian cancer recurrence. Parasagittal T2-weighted image. A multicystic pelvic lesion (*arrows*) with layering due to hemorrhage (*arrowhead*) and papillary projections (*small arrows*) is shown

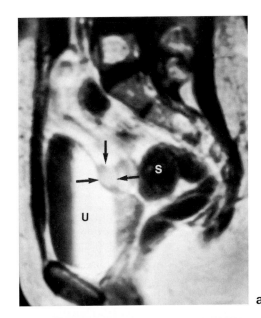

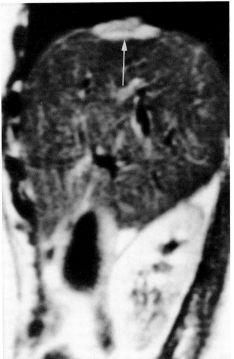

Fig. 18.29 a,b. Peritoneal implants in ovarian cancer recurrence. Sagittal contrast-enhanced T1-weighted (**a**) and sagittal T1-weighted image (**b**) in two different patients. Surface implants (*arrows*) of the urinary bladder (*U*) and a plaquelike metastasis of the dome of the diaphragm (*long arrow*) are clearly depicted. *S*, Sigmoid colon

diaphragm, liver surface, paracolic gutters, small bowel surface, or mesentery (Fig. 18.29). Due to surgical technique, omental recurrence is rare. For the same reason lymph node metastases are demonstrated typically in the para-aortic region, with a frequency of 18%–33% (FORSTNER et al. 1995a; BURGHARDT 1993).

Unlike primary ovarian cancer, recurrent ovarian cancer is not strongly associated with ascites. In one study ascites was found in only 38% of patients with recurrent ovarian cancer, and in the vast majority of these patients only small amounts of fluid were detected. (FORSTNER et al. 1995a). Furthermore, small amounts of ascites were also detected in patients without recurrent disease.

CA-125 determination plays a pivotal role in the follow-up of patients with ovarian cancer. Persistently elevated or rising CA-125 levels are almost invariably indicators of recurrent ovarian cancer (YOUNG et al. 1993). The elevation of this tumor marker, however, may precede the clinical appearance by several months or even by more than a year (KENEMANS et al. 1993). Nevertheless, there are certain problems associated with CA-125 determination, including its lack of specificity in identifying patients who are tumor-free after chemotherapy: normal CA-125 levels can be found in up to 50% of patients with persistent disease during and after chemotherapy (YOUNG et al. 1993).

MRI Findings. Recurrent ovarian cancer most frequently presents as solid enhancing lesions, followed by complex mixed solid (Fig. 18.29) and cystic lesions. Entirely cystic lesions are rare (FORSTNER et al. 1995a).

Lesions display low to intermediate signal intensity on T1-weighted images. T2-weighted images show various signal intensitities depending on the internal architecture. Contrast-enhanced T1-weighted imaging allows superior definition of the internal structure. Furthermore, contrast-enhanced, breath-hold, fast multiplanar spoiled gradient-recalled images, with fat suppression, have shown excellent performance in depicting peritoneal disease (Low et al. 1995). Diffuse peritoneal enhancement presents carcinosis peritonei. The peritoneal thickness may vary from diffuse peritoneal lining of 3–5 mm thickness to plaquelike lesions of more than 10 mm (Low and SIGETI 1994). Omental caking is usually only found in patients receiving primary chemotherapy.

Differential Diagnosis. Not every solid lesion in a postoperative patient represents recurrence (Fig. 18.30). The combination of tumor markers and a baseline study aids in the differentiation. Bowel loops or tracked ascites may mimic recurrent disease (FORSTNER et al. 1995a). Benign forms of peritoneal thickening, e.g., in endometriosis, bacterial peritonitis, or postoperative changes, cannot be differentiated from diffuse peritoneal tumor spread. Chemical peritonitis following intraperitoneal chemotherapy also results in peritoneal thickening (Low and SIGETI 1994).

Value of MRI. In the postoperative evaluation of patients with ovarian cancer, MRI can be used in conjunction with tumor markers to assess disease progression and response to therapy and its termination. Baseline examinations after surgery or before chemotherapy play a pivotal role, as they allow objective follow-up (JOHNSON 1993). In patients with rising tumor marker levels, MRI helps to delineate the extent of recurrence and thus may aid in therapy planning.

Compared with CT, MRI permits improved assessment of pelvic lesions, especially in the vaginal vault and cul-de-sac (FORSTNER et al. 1995b,c; SEMELKA et al. 1993). However, MRI with the SE technique has limited ability to depict tumors smaller than 2 cm, especially on the small bowel surface, in the mesentery, and in cases of carcinosis peritonei (FORSTNER et al. 1995a; PRAYER et al. 1993). Fast imaging with bowel contrast and delayed gadolinium-enhanced images with fat suppression show promising results in detecting small peritoneal lesions and diffuse peritoneal disease (Low and SIGETI 1994; Low et al. 1995; SEMELKA et al. 1993). Combination of MRI with determination of CA-125 levels and also with immunoscintigraphy has been proposed for the evaluation of patients with suspected ovarian cancer recurrence (FORSTNER et al. 1995a; Low et al. 1995).

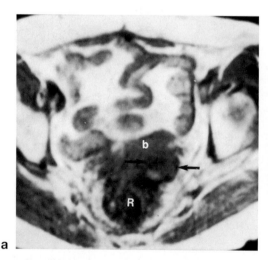
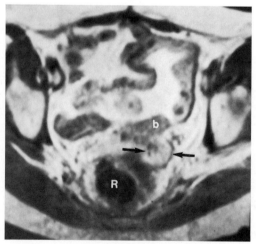

Fig. 18.30 a,b. Ovarian cancer recurrence: false-positive MRI. Transaxial T1-weighted image (**a**) and transaxial contrast-enhanced T1-weighted image (**b**). A lesion (*arrows*) adjacent to the rectum (*R*) and bowel loops (*b*) is demonstrated, and shows contrast enhancement (**b**). As it was not found at surgery, it most likely represented a bowel loop or scar tissue

18.8
Neoplasms of the Fallopian Tube

18.8.1
Benign Fallopian Tube Tumors

Benign fallopian tube tumors are rare, and typically leiomyomas. They can derive from the tubal muscularis or the smooth muscle of the broad ligament.

MRI Findings. Benign fallopian tube tumors appear as solid round to oval adnexal masses of low signal intensity on T1- and T2-weighted images. Foci of high signal intensity on T2-weighted images represent degeneration.

Differential Diagnosis. Ovarian fibroid, fibrothecoma, and pedunculated uterine leiomyoma display the same imaging characteristics as benign fallopian tube tumors, often rendering differential diagnosis impossible.

18.8.2
Primary Malignant Tumors

Primary malignant tumors of the fallopian tube are extremely rare, accounting for only 0.3%–1.1% of all gynecologic cancers. At histology they are most frequently found to be adenocarcinomas. Sarcomas are exceedingly uncommon, with fewer than 50

reported cases in the literature (KAWAKAMI et al. 1993). Carcinoma of the fallopian tube appears as a fusiform swelling. Due to tubal occlusion, tubal carcinoma resembles hydrosalpinx in approximately half of all cases and is often mistaken as such at surgery.

MRI Findings. A small but distinct solid, often lobulated, adnexal mass can be identified (KAWAKAMI et al. 1993). The mass displays homogeneous low signal intensity on T1-weighted images and intermediate to high signal intensity on T2-weighted images. The appearance on the latter is similar to that of uterine myometrium. On contrast-enhanced T1-weighted images homogeneous enhancement is seen, and sometimes small cystic nonenhancing areas in the periphery can be identified. Common associated findings include distension of the uterine cavity and ascites (KAWAKAMI et al. 1993). Hydrosalpinx may be found in 50% of cases and sometimes an intra-luminal mass is displayed (Fig. 18.31). Furthermore, due to hydrosalpinx, fallopian tube cancer can mimic a large ovarian mass with mixed cystic and solid components.

Differential Diagnosis. Primary ovarian tumors cannot be reliably differentiated from malignant tumors of the fallopian tube. In the presence of associated hydrosalpinx, tubal tumors may be misinterpreted as ovarian cancer. However, the cystic area may be recognized as a loop of dilated fallopian tube with the use of multiplanar T2-weighted images. Fibroma,

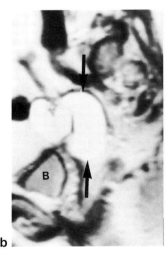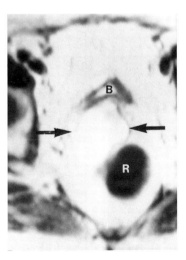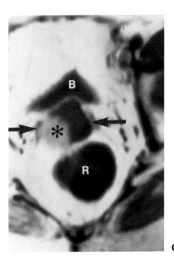

a,b   c

Fig. 18.31 a–c. Fallopian tube carcinoma arising within a hydrosalpinx. Sagittal T2-weighted image (**a**), transaxial T2-weighted image (**b**), and transaxial contrast-enhanced T1-weighted image (**c**). In a patient with a history of hysterectomy the typical finding of a hydrosalpinx (*arrows*) is demonstrated. Within the dilated ampulla a solid lesion (*asterisk*) 2 cm in diameter is best seen on the contrast-enhanced image (**c**). *R*, Rectum; *B*, bladder

the only entirely solid ovarian tumor, displays a very low signal intensity on T2-weighted images.

Value of MRI. The value of MRI in the diagnosis of fallopian tube cancer is limited: correct preoperative diagnosis of primary tubal tumor was made in only 0%–0.3% of the cases according to EDDY et al. (1984) and PFEIFFER et al. (1989).

18.8.3
Metastases

Metastases to the fallopian tubes are usually of ovarian or uterine origin. Hematogenous spread (commonly from breast cancer) is rare.

MRI Findings. As in primary fallopian tube carcinoma, the findings are similar to those of ovarian carcinoma and thus these lesions cannot reliably be differentiated.

18.9
Pelvic Inflammatory Disease

The term pelvic inflammatory disease (PID) encompasses ascending infections (most commonly with *Neisseria gonorrhoeae* or superinfecting anaerobes) from the vagina to the endometrium, fallopian tubes, and pelvic peritoneum. Infections are usually sexually transmitted or occur following surgical procedures or during parturition. Use of an intrauterine devise increases threefold the risk of infection (KAUFMAN et al. 1980; WESTSTROM 1987).

In the course of the infection, exudation and inflammatory reaction lead to acute suppurative salpingitis, which often results in tubal occlusion. Hydrosalpinx and pyosalpinx are characterized by obliteration of the abdominal ostium and dilatation of the fallopian tube. Salpingo-oophoritis may subsequently result, when sealed fimbriae become plastered against the ovary. Finally, tubo-ovarian abscess may be encountered. During chronic infection pus undergoes slow proteolysis and the tubes become transformed into thin-walled, serous hydrosalpinx.

Rupture of a pyosalpinx or tubo-ovarian abscess will cause peritonitis. Occasionally patients will develop Fitz-Hugh-Curtis syndrome due to perihepatitis caused by tracking of fluid into the right paracolic gutter (VITALE ROMO and CLARKE 1992).

Infertility is seen in 25%–60% of women after the second and third episodes of PID (WESTSTROM 1987). Furthermore, 50% of women with ectopic pregnancy report a history of or suffer from PID.

18.9.1
Hydrosalpinx/Pyosalpinx

Obliteration of the fimbriated end of the tube leads to hydrosalpinx. Salpingitis is the leading cause; other etiologies include endometriosis, fallopian tube tumors, and adhesions from prior surgery. Thus serous fluid, blood, or pus may accumulate. As diameters of up to 10 cm are not uncommon, hydrosalpinx may mimic a multiseptate ovarian tumor, e.g., cystadenoma (Fig. 18.32).

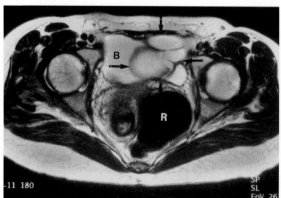
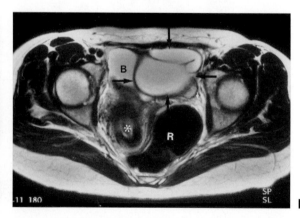

Fig 18.32 a,b. Hydrosalpinx of the left ovary. Transaxial T2-weighted images at the level of the cervix uteri on two consecutive levels (**a, b**). The urinary bladder (*B*) is displaced by a left multicystic adnexal lesion (*arrows*). The latter is composed of multiple thin-walled ovoid or tubular structures with longitudinal septa. *R*, Rectum. Histologically verified fibromuscular polyp of the cervix uteri (*asterisk*). (Courtesy of A. Heuck, Munich)

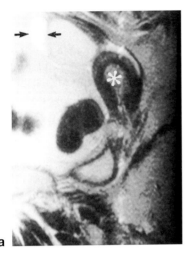
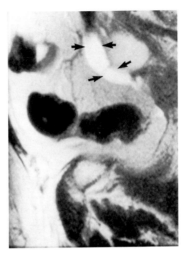

Fig. 18.33 a,b. Hydrosalpinx. Sagittal T2-weighted images at the level of the uterus (a) and 4 cm more lateral (b). A tubular cystic structure (*arrows*) with thin septa is identified lateral to the uterus. There is distension of the uterine cavity (*asterisk*) due to an endometrial cancer (a)

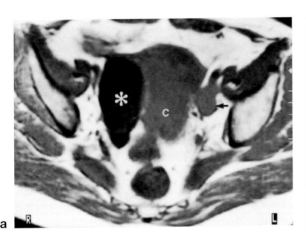
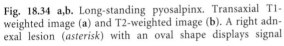
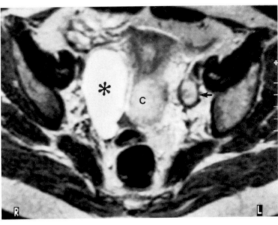

Fig. 18.34 a,b. Long-standing pyosalpinx. Transaxial T1-weighted image (a) and T2-weighted image (b). A right adnexal lesion (*asterisk*) with an oval shape displays signal intensity similar to water. However, pus was found at surgery. C, Cervical cancer. *Arrowhead*, lymph node metastasis

MRI Findings. Tubal enlargement is characterized by a typical extraovarian, tubular tortuous cystic structure with interdigitating septa (Fig. 18.33). The signal intensity on T1-weighted images varies in accordance with the contents, which range from waterlike fluid to proteinaceous or hemorrhagic components. T2-weighted images allow demonstration of low signal intensity septa and the liquid contents. Multiplanar T2-weighted imaging facilitates depiction of the tubal origin and differentiation from dilated bowel loops. On contrast-enhanced T1-weighted images, enhancement of the wall and septa is noted. Any solid component within a dilated tube should suggest the possibility of fallopian tube carcinoma or ectopic pregnancy (KAWAKAMI et al. 1993).

Differential Diagnosis. Hydrosalpinx can mimic multiseptate ovarian cystadenomas: unless the ovary is demonstrated separately, the differentiation can sometimes be difficult. Hydrosalpinx cannot be reliably differentiated from pyosalpinx (Fig. 18.34). Regions of nodularity should arouse suspicion of a primary or metastatic neoplasm or ectopic pregnancy involving the fallopian tube.

18.9.2
Tubo-ovarian Abscess

In the majority of cases, tubo-ovarian abscesses are associated with PID. Use of an intrauterine device gives rise to an increased risk of abscess formation.

Abscesses confined only to the ovaries are rare, and commonly result from inflammatory reactions of adjacent organs, e.g., appendicitis, diverticulitis, or Crohn's disease. Tubo-ovarian abscesses in the post-menopausal period are rare and encountered in patients with diabetes or previous radiation therapy (Rodriguez-de-Velasquez et al. 1995). The vast majority of abscesses are multilocular uni- or bilateral lesions with thick walls and necrotic areas and, inconsistently, air. Solid abscesses are rare.

MRI Findings. MRI demonstrates uni- or bilateral ill-defined complex adnexal masses with central liquid or necrotic areas. The latter may resemble serous fluid, with only mild T2 shortening, or may be hemorrhagic, with T1 shortening. In one study, all abscesses associated with PID were predominantly isointense, or slightly hyperintense, relative to urine (Mitchell et al. 1987). Due to surrounding edema the outer margin of a tubo-ovarian abscess is ill-defined. Increased vascularity within the pelvis associated with inflammatory tissue can lead to a heterogeneous signal intensity of the surrounding fat. Contrast-enhanced T1-weighted images allow superior delineation of the central abscess cavity from the enhancing irregular wall (Fig. 18.35). Associated inflammatory adenopathy may also show contrast enhancement (Stevens et al. 1991).

Differential Diagnosis. The rare solid abscesses cannot be distinguished from solid ovarian tumors. Endometriomas can display the same imaging characteristics as tubo-ovarian abscesses. Ovarian cancer and especially ovarian metastases also present as complex adnexal lesions; however, they are not usually associated with tubal dilatation. If a tubo-ovarian abscess involves adjacent pelvic organs, the site of origin often cannot be reliably defined. Conversely, appendicitis, diverticulitis, and Crohn's disease may result in abscesses involving the adjacent adnexa.

Value of MRI. Endovaginal US is used as the primary imaging modality to show tubal dilatation and/or an adnexal mass. Either MRI or CT can be used when the US study is of limited value or equivocal. MRI findings, however, can only be interpreted in the context of the clinical background.

18.10
Vascular Disorders

18.10.1
Ovarian Torsion

Ovarian torsion is usually associated with tubal torsion and typically occurs within the first three decades of life. Increased intra-abdominal pressure and mobility of the ovaries have been reported to be responsible for torsion. Up to a quarter of torsions occur during pregnancy, typically in the first and second trimesters. Torsion may involve normal ovaries; in the majority of cases the involved adnexa, however, contain an associated ovarian mass, typically functional cysts and dermoids, or

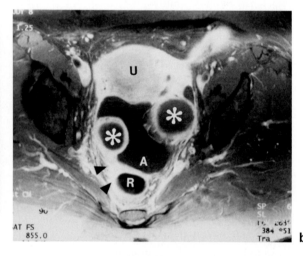

Fig. 18.35 a,b. Bilateral tubo-ovarian abscesses. Consecutive transaxial fat-saturated T1-weighted images at the level of the acetabulum. Bilateral thick-walled cystic adnexal masses (*asterisks*) show ill-defined margins in relation to the surrounding fat. Excessive contrast enhancement along the uterosacral ligament (*arrowheads*) and rectal wall can also be noted (**b**). *R*, Rectum; *A*, ascites; *U*, uterus. (Courtesy of A. Heuck, Munich)

hyperstimulated ovaries in pregnancy (BIDER et al. 1991). In the early stages of ovarian torsion, venous but not arterial flow is cut off from the ovary, resulting in hemorrhagic venous infarction of the ovary and its associated mass. At surgery ovarian enlargement due to edema and hemorrhage is found.

MRI Findings. The MRI appearance depends on the degree of torsion. In patients with extreme abdominal pain, especially if the medical history is remarkable for previous pain attacks, the combination of an ovarian hemorrhagic mass and dilatation of the fallopian tube should arouse suspicion of ovarian torsion.

Hemorrhage shows the imaging characteristics previously described (KIER et al. 1992; OUTWATER et al. 1993). The T1-weighted image may show a high signal intensity ring, as seen in any subacute hematoma. The adnexal mass will display a thick wall which is best seen on T2- or contrast-enhanced T1-weighted images. If arterial occlusion has occurred, contrast-enhanced T1-weighted images will show no enhancement of the mass. Associated findings include deviation of the uterus to the side of torsion, tubal protrusion at the periphery of the mass (Fig. 18.36), dilated vessels within the parametria, and fluid in the cul-de-sac (KIMURA et al. 1994).

Differential Diagnosis. Endometrioma, abscess, and hemorrhagic adnexal lesions may display similar findings. The clinical history and laboratory data will aid in the differential diagnosis.

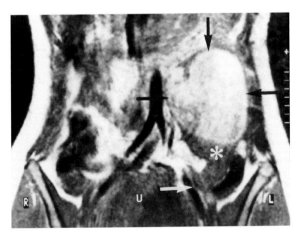

Fig. 18.36. Torsion of a left ovarian dermoid. Coronal T1-weighted image in the mid abdomen. A 12-cm lesion (*arrows*) displays high signal intensity due to fat and hemorrhage. The dilated fallopian tube (*asterisk*) and accompanying vessels are seen at the inferior aspect of the lesion. At surgery complete hemorrhagic infarction of the dermoid and the fallopian tube due to torsion at the level of the iliac vessels (*white arrow*) was found. The uterus (*U*) is enlarged due to pregnancy

Value of MRI. MRI signs are unspecific (KIMURA et al. 1994). Considered in combination with the clinical history, however, the findings may render diagnostic clues. Color Doppler shows absence of flow to the affected ovary (STARK and SIEGEL 1994), but in the event of displacement of the lesion out of the pelvis, US may be of limited value.

18.10.2
Massive Edema of the Ovary

Massive edema of the ovary occurs in the second and third decades of life. It is a rare entity and considered a variant of ovarian torsion resulting from partial or intermittent torsion. Massive interstitial ovarian edema causes unilateral, excessive enlargement (up to 35 cm in diameter) almost exclusively of the right ovary. Clinical symptoms correlate with those of ovarian torsion.

MRI Findings. The imaging findings are not specific; in young patients, however, the clinical symptoms may assist in the diagnosis.

A large pelvic mass with cystic areas and solid portions which display a heterogeneously high signal intensity on T2-weighted images has been described, as well as heterogeneous contrast enhancement (LEE et al. 1993). Ascites is an associated finding.

Differential Diagnosis. Ovarian cancer may resemble massive edema of the ovary.

18.10.3
Ovarian Vein Thrombosis

Ovarian vein thrombosis is a complication in the puerperal period and encountered most frequently after cesarean section. It usually presents as a sequela of postpartal infection, hypercoagulability, or trauma (DUNNIHOO et al. 1991). Although rare, it still represents an important differential diagnostic problem in patients with prolonged fever in the puerperal period. The clinical symptoms are non-specific and include fever, chills, vomiting, and often right-sided pain, as the majority of ovarian vein thromboses occur on the right side.

MRI Findings. In the postpartum period the ovarian veins are usually enlarged and well depicted. The SE images demonstrate enlargement of the ovarian vein (in 90% of cases on the right side) with high signal intensity on both T1- and T2-weighted images (MARTIN et al. 1986; SAVADER et al. 1988). MR venography allows direct visualization of the occlusion of the vein. Furthermore, transaxial gradient-echo images can be used to image the ovarian veins. Thrombi can be identified as low signal intensity filling defects within the ovarian vein or inferior vena cava (ARRIVE et al. 1991).

Differential Diagnosis. Due to its course, dilatation of the ureter may be misinterpreted as ovarian vein thrombosis; however, hydronephrosis and the signal intensity allow the exclusion of thrombosis.

Value of MRI. US, particularly color Doppler US, is a valuable imaging tool, especially in thin patients. When the US study is of limited value or equivocal (as is often the case in obese patients the postoperative or postpartal period), MRI can be used as an alternative to CT. MRI should be used as the modality of choice in pregnancy, given the restricted value of US.

18.11
Ectopic Pregnancy

Ectopic pregnancy describes an implantation of the fetus at any site other than a normal uterine location. More than 95% of ectopic pregnancies occur in the fallopian tubes, with approximately 75%–80% located in the ampulla. PID with chronic salpingitis is the most important risk factor and is found in 35%–50% of patients with ectopic pregnancy. Furthermore, patients who are pregnant with an intrauterine device in place, who have previously undergone tubal reconstructive surgery, or who are pregnant by in vitro fertilization are prone to ectopic pregnancy.

MRI Findings. MRI findings are nonspecific and may simulate ovarian cancer (KUHL et al. 1995). In a patient suspected of ectopic pregnancy the combination of an adnexal mass and intraperitoneal hemorrhage indicates tubal rupture.

Value of MRI. US is used as the primary imaging modality in suspected ectopic pregnancy. MRI may be used when US is of limited value or yields equivocal findings; however, in most cases it is not needed since laparoscopy or laparotomy will in any case be performed for therapeutic purposes.

Acknowledgements. We would like to thank Prof. H. Hricak, MD, PhD, University of California San Francisco, for the figures which she contributed. We also wish to express our appreciation of the contributions made by PD Dr. A. Heuck, MD and Sebastian Lins, University of Munich.

References

Alpern MB, Sandler MA, Madrazo BL (1984) Sonographic features of parovarian cysts and their complications. AJR 143:157–160

Altaras MM, Aviram R, Cohen I, Cordoba M, Weiss E, Beyth Y (1991) Primary peritoneal papillary serous adenocarcinoma: clinical and management aspects. Gynecol Oncol 40:230–236

Arrive L, Menu Y, Dessarts I, et al. (1991) Diagnosis of abdominal venous thrombosis by means of spin-echo and gradient-echo MR imaging: analysis with receiver operating characteristic curves. Radiology 181:661–668

Bider D, Mashiach S, Dulitzky M, Kokia E, Lipitz S, Ben Raphael Z (1991) Clinical, surgical and pathologic findings of adnexal torsion in pregnant and nonpregnant women. Obstet Gynecol 173:363–366

Boring CC, Squires ST, Tong T, Montgomery S (1994) Cancer statistics. CA Cancer J Clin 44:7–26

Brammer HM, Buck JL, Hayes WS, Sheth S, Tavassoli FA (1990) Malignant germ cell tumors of the ovary: radiologic pathologic correlation. Radiographics 10:715–724

Burghardt E (1993) Epithelial ovarian cancer. Recurrence. In: Burghard E (ed) Surgical gynecological oncology. Thieme, Stuttgart, p 494

Burghardt E, Pickel H, Stettner H (1984) Management of advanced ovarian cancer. Eur J Gynaecol Oncol 3:155–163

Burghardt E, Girardi F, Lahousen M, Tamussino K, Stettner H (1991) Patterns of pelvic and paraaortic lymph node involvement in ovarian cancer. Gynecol Oncol 40:103–106

Buy JN, Moss AA, Ghossain MA, et al. (1988) Peritoneal implants from ovarian tumors: CT findings. Radiology 169:691–694

Buy JN, Ghossain MA, Moss AA, et al. (1989) Cystic teratoma of the ovary: CT detection. Radiology 171:697–701

Buy JN, Ghossain MA, Sciot C, et al. (1991) Epithelial tumors of the ovary: CT findings and correlation with US. Radiology 178:811–818

Carrington BM (1991) The adnexae. In: Hricak H, Carrington BM (eds) MRI of the pelvis: a text atlas. Martin Dunitz, London, p 185

Carter DM, Lin AN (1993) Basal cell carcinoma. In: Fitzpatrick TB, Eisen AZ, Wolff K, Freedberg IM, Austen KF (eds) Dermatology in general medicine, vol I. McGraw Hill, New York, pp 848–854

Chou LK, Liu GC, Su JH, et al. (1994) MRI demonstration of peritoneal implants. Abdom Imaging 19:95–101

Coleman BG (1992) Transvaginal sonography of adnexal masses. Radiol Clin North Am 30:677–690

Curtis M, Hopkins MP, Zarlingo P, Martino C, Graciansky-Lengyl M, Jenison EL (1993) Magnetic resonance imaging to avoid laparotomy in pregnancy. Obstet Gynecol 82:833–836

DePriest PD, Banks ER, Powell DE, et al. (1992) Endometrial carcinoma of the ovary and endometriosis: the association in postmenopausal women. Gynecol Oncol 47:71–75

Dunnihoo D, Gallaspy J. Wise R, Otterssen W (1991) Postpartum ovarian vein thrombophlebitis: review. Obstet Gynecol Surv 46:415–427

Eddy GL, Copeland LJ, Gerhenson DM, et al. (1984) Fallopian tube carcinoma. Obstet Gynecol 64:546–552

Farquhar CM, Birdsall M, Manning P, Mitchell JM (1994) Transabdominal versus transvaginal ultrasound in the diagnosis of polycystic ovaries in a population of randomly selected women. Ultrasound Obstet Gynaecol 4:54–59

FIGO (1987) Changes in definition of clinical staging for carcinoma of the cervix and ovary. Am J Obstet Gynecol 156:236

Filly RA (1993) Ovarian masses. What to look for. What to do. In: Callen P (ed) Ultrasonography in obstetrics and gynecology, 3rd edn. W.B. Saunders, Philadelphia, pp 625–640

Fleischer AC, Kepple DM, Vasquez J (1992) Conventional and color Doppler transvaginal sonography in gynecologic infertility. Radiol Clin North Am 30:693–702

Forstner R, Hricak H, Powell CB, Aziizi L, Frankel SD, Stern JL (1995a) Ovarian cancer recurrence: value of MR imaging. Radiology 196:715–720

Forstner R, Hricak H, Occhipinti KA, Powell CB, Frankel SD, Stern JL (1995b) Ovarian cancer: staging with CT and MR imaging. Radiology 197:619–626

Forstner R, Chen M, Hricak H (1995c) Imaging of ovarian cancer. J Magn Reson Imaging 5:606–613

Foshager MC, Walsh JW (1994) CT anatomy of the female pelvis: a second look. Radiographics 14:51–66

Fried AM, Rhodes RA, Morehouse R (1993) Endometrioma: analysis and sonographic documentation of 51 documented cases. South Med J 86:297–301

Gambino J, Cohen AJ, Friedenberg RM (1993) The direction of bladder displacement by adnexal masses. Clin Imaging 17:8–11

Gershenson DM (1985) Malignant germ cell tumors of the ovary. Clin Obstet Gynecol 28:824–838

Gershenson DM, Silva EG (1990) Serous ovarian tumors of low malignant potential with peritoneal implants. Cancer 65:578–585

Ghossain MA, Buy JN, Ligneres C, et al. (1991) Epithelial tumors of the ovary: comparison of MR and CT findings. Radiology 181:863–870

Ginburg J, Havard CWM (1976) Polycystic ovary syndrome. BMJ 2:737–740

Goldstein SR, Subramanyam B, Synder JR, et al. (1989) The postmenopausal cystic adnexal mass: the potential role of ultrasound in conservative management. Obstet Gynecol 73:8–10

Guinet C, Ghossain MA, Buy JN, et al. (1993) Fat suppression techniques in MR imaging of mature teratomas: comparison with CT. Eur J Radiol 17:117–121

Guinet C, Ghossain MA, Buy JN, et al. (1995) Mature cystic teratoma of the ovary: CT and MR findings. Eur J Radiol 20:137–143

Ha HK, Baek SY, Kim SH, Kim HH, Chung EC, Yeon KM (1995) Krukenberg tumor of the ovary-MR imaging features. AJR 164:1435–1439

Hale RW (1968) Krukenberg tumor of the ovaries: a review of 81 records. Obstet Gynecol 23:221–225

Hayes CR, Dietz MJ, King BF, et al. (1992) Pelvic imaging with phased-array coils: quantitative assessment of signal- to noise-ratio improvement. J Magn Reson Imaging 2:321–326

Hatanaka Y, Yamasita Y, Torashima M, Takahahi M (1996) MR appearance of fat distribution in ovarian teratoma: pathologic correlation. Nippon Acta Radiol 56:477–481

Honore LH, O'Hara KE (1980) Serous papillary neoplasms arising in paramesonephric parovarian cysts: a report of eight cases. Acta Obstet Gynecol Scand 59:525–528

Hricak H (1993) Current trends in MR imaging of the female pelvis. Radiographics 13:913–919

Imaoka I, Sugimura K, Okizuka H, et al. (1993) Ovarian cystic teratomas: value of chemical shift fat saturation magnetic resonance imaging. Br J Radiol 66:994–997

Ishijima H, Ihizaka H, Inoue T (1996) Distinguishing between cystic teratomas and endometriomas of the ovary using chemical shift gradient echo magnetic resonance imaging. Australas Radiol 40:22–25

Jabra AA, Fisman EK, Taylor GA (1993) Primary ovarian tumors in the pediatric patient: CT evaluation. Clin Imaging 17:199–203

Jacobs HS (1995) Polycystic ovary syndrome: aetiology and management. Curr Opin Obstet Gynecol 7:203–208

Jacobs IJ, Bast RC (1989) The Ca-125 tumor associated antigen: a review of the literature. Hum Reprod 4:1–12

Johnson RJ (1993) Radiology in the management of ovarian cancer. Clin Radiol 48:75–82

Kaufman DW, Shapiro S, Rosenberg L, et al. (1980) Intrauterine contraceptive device use and pelvic inflammatory disease. Am J Obstet Gynecol 136:159–162

Kawakami S, Togashi K, Kimura I, et al. (1993) Primary malignant tumor of the fallopian tube: appearance at CT and MR imaging. Radiology 186:503–508

Kenemans P, Yedema CA, Bon GG, von Mensdorff-Poully S (1993) CA 125 in gynecological pathology-a review. Eur J Obstet Gynecol Reprod Biol 49:115–124

Kier R (1992) Nonovarian gynecologic cysts: MR imaging findings. AJR 158:1265–1269

Kier R, Smith RC, McCarthy SM (1992) Value of lipid- and water-suppression MR images in distinguishing between blood and liquid within ovarian masses. AJR 158:325–328

Kim JS, Woo SK, Suh SJ, Morettin LB (1995) Sonographic diagnosis of paraovarian cysts: value of detecting a separate ipsilateral ovary. AJR 164:1441–1444

Kim SH, Kim WH, Park KJ, Lee JK, Kim JS (1996) CT and MR findings of Krukenberg tumors-comparison with primary ovarian tumors. J Comput Assist Tomogr 20:393–398

Kimura I, Togashi K, Kawakami A, Takakura K, Mori T, Konishi T (1994) Ovarian torsion: CT and MR imaging appearances. Radiology 190:337–341

Komatsu KI, Konishi I, Mandai M, Togashi K, Kawakami Y, Konishi J, Mori T (1996) Adnexal masses: transvaginal US and Gadolinium-enhanced MR imaging assessment of intratumoral structure. Radiology 198:109–115

Koonings PP, Campbell K, Mishell DR, Grimes DA (1989) Relative frequency of primary ovarian neoplasm: a 10-year review. Obstet Gynecol 74:921–926

Kuhl CK, Heuck A, Kreft BP, Luckhaus S, Reiser M, Schild HH (1995) Combined intrauterine and ovarian pregnancy mimicking malignant ovarian tumor: imaging findings. AJR 165:369–370

Lee AR, Kim KHK, Lee BH, Chin SY (1993) Massive edema of the ovary: imaging findings. AJR 161:343–344

Low RN (1996) MR imaging of peritoneal tumor. MR Pulse 3:18–19

Low RN, Sigeti JS (1994) MR imaging of peritoneal disease: comparison of contrast-enhanced fast multiplanar spoiled gradient-recalled and spin echo sequence. AJR 163:1131–1140

Low RN, Carter WD, Saleh F, Sigeti JS (1995) Ovarian cancer. Comparison of findings with perfluorocarbon-enhanced MR imaging, In-111-CYT-103 immunoscintigraphy, and CT. Radiology 195:391–400

MacSweeney JE, King DM (1994) Computed tomography, diagnosis, staging and follow-up of pure granulosa cell tumour of the ovary. Clin Radiol 49:241–245

Martin B, Mulopulos GB, Bryan PJ (1986) MRI of puerperal vein thrombosis. AJR 147:291–292

Meyer JI, Kennedy AW, Friedman R, Ayoub A, Zepp RC (1995) Ovarian carcinoma: value of CT in predicting success of debulking surgery. AJR 165:875–878

Mitchell DG, Gefter WB, Spritzer LE, et al. (1986) Polycystic ovaries: MR imaging. Radiology 160:425–429

Mitchell DG, Mintz MC, Spritzer CE, et al. (1987) Adnexal masses: MR imaging observations at 1.5T, with US and CT correlation. Radiology 162:319–324

Monterroso V, Jaffe ES, Merino MJ, Medeiros LJ (1993) Malignant lymphoma involving the ovary. A clinicopathologic analysis of 39 cases. Am J Surg Pathol 17:154–170

Nelson BE, Rosenfield AT, Schwartz PE (1993) Preoperative abdominopelvic computed tomographic prediction of optimal cytoreduction in epithelial ovarian carcinoma. J Clin Oncol 11:166–172

Neste MG, Francis IR, Bude RO (1996) Hepatic metastases from granulosa cell tumor of the ovary: CT and sonographic findings. AJR 166:1122–1124

NIH Consensus Conference (1995) Ovarian cancer. Screening, treatment, and follow-up. JAMA 273:491–497

Outwater EK, Dunton CJ (1995) Imaging of the ovaries and adnexa: clinical issues and applications of MR imaging. Radiology 194:1–18

Outwater EK, Mitchell DG (1994) Magnetic resonance imaging techniques in the pelvis. Magn Reson Imaging Clin North Am 2:161–188

Outwater EK, Mitchell DG (1996) Normal ovaries and functional cysts: MR appearance. Radiology 198:397–402

Outwater E, Schiebler ML, Owen RS, Schnall MD (1993) Characterization of hemorrhagic adnexal lesions with MR imaging: blinded reader study. Radiology 186:489–494

Pfeiffer P, Mogensen H, Amtrup F, Honore E (1989) Primary carcinoma of the fallopian tube: a retrospective study of patients reported to Danish Cancer Registry in a five-year period. Acta Oncol 28:7–11

Prayer L, Kainz C, Kramer J, et al. (1993) CT and MR accuracy in the detection of tumor recurrence in patients treated for ovarian cancer. J Comput Assist Tomogr 17:626–632

Rulin MC, Preston Al (1987) Adnexal masses in postmenopausal women. Obstet Gynecol 70:578–581

Reuter K, Griffin T, Hunter RE (1989) Comparison of abdominopelvic computed tomography results and findings at second- or third-look laparotomy in ovarian carcinoma patients. Cancer 63:1223–1228

Rodriguez-de Velasquez A, Yoder CI, Velasquez PA, Papanicolaou N (1995) Imaging the effects of diabetes on the genitourinary system. Radiographics 15:1051–1068

Savader SJ, Otero RR, Savader BL (1988) Puerperal ovarian vein thrombosis: evaluation with CT, US, and MR imaging. Radiology 167:637–639

Scheidler J, Henck A, Meier W, Reiser M (1997) MR imaging of pelvic masses: efficacy of the rectal superparamagnetic contrast agent Ferumoxsil. J Magn Reson Imaging (in press)

Scoutt LM, McCarthy SM, Lange R, Bourque A, Schwartz PE (1994) MR evaluation of clinically suspected adnexal masses. J Comput Assist Tomogr 18:609–618

Semelka RC, Lawrence PH, Shoenut JP, et al. (1993) Primary ovarian cancer: prospective comparison of contrast-enhanced CT and pre and post contrast fat suppressed MR imaging, with histologic correlation. J Magn Reson Imaging 3:99–106

Sheth S, Fishman EK, Buck JL, et al. (1988) The sonographic appearance of ovarian teratomas: correlation with CT. AJR 151:331–334

Sica GT, Stevens SK, Hricak H, et al. (1992) Comparison of unenhanced and contrast-enhanced MR images in the evaluation of ovarian lesions. Presented at the 78th Scientfic Assembly and Annual Meeting of the Radiological Society of North America. Chicago

Stark JE, Siegel MJ (1994) Ovarian torsion in prepubertal and pubertal girls, sonographic findings. AJR 163:1479–1482

Stevens SK (1992) The adnexa. In: Higgins CB, Hricak H, Helms CA (eds) Magnetic resonance imaging of the body. Raven Press, New York, pp 865–889

Stevens SK, Hricak H, Stern JL (1991) Ovarian lesions: detection and characterization with Gadolinium-enhanced MR imaging at 1.5T. Radiology 181:481–488

Stevens SK, Hricak H, Campos Z (1993) Teratoma versus cystic hemorrhagic adnexal lesions: differentiation with proton selective fat-saturation MR imaging. Radiology 188:481–488

Sugimura K, Okizuka H, Imaoka I, et al. (1993) Pelvic endometriosis: detection and diagnosis with chemcal shift MR imaging. Radiology 188:435–438

Sugimura K, Okizuka H, Kaji Y, et al. (1996) MRI in predicting the response of ovarian endometriomas to hormone therapy. J Comput Assist Tomagr 20:145–150

Sutton CL, NcKinney CD, Jones JE, Gay SB (1992) Ovarian masses revisited: radiologic and pathologic correlation. Radiographics 12:853–877

Tanaka YU, Kurosaki Y, Nishida M, Michishita N, Kuramato K, Itai Y, Kubo T (1994) Ovarian dysgerminoma: MR and CT appearance. J Comput Assist Tomogr 18:443–448

Taylor JKW, Schwartz PE (1994) Screening for early ovarian cancer. Radiology 192:1–10

Thurnher SA (1992) MR imaging of pelvic masses in women: contrast-enhanced versus unenhanced images. AJR 159:1243–1250

Thurnher S, Hodler J, Baer S, Marincek B, von Schulthess GK (1990) Gadolinium-Dota enhanced MR imaging of adnexal tumors. J Comput Assist Tomogr 14:939–949

Timmerman D, Moerman P, Vergote I (1995) Meig's syndrome with elevated serum CA 125 levels: two case reports and review of the literature. Gynecol Oncol 59:405–408

Togashi K (1993a) Normal pelvic structures. In: Togashi K (ed) MRI of the female pelvis. Igaku-Shoin, Tokyo, pp 29–68

Togashi K (1993b) Endometriosis. In: Togashi K (ed) MRI of the female pelvis. Igaku-Shoin, Tokyo, pp 203–226

Togashi K, Nishimura K, Itoh K, et al. (1987) Ovarian cystic teratomas: MR imaging. Radiology 162:669–673

Togashi K, Nishimura K, Kimura I, et al. (1991) Endometrial cysts of the ovary: MR imaging. Radiology 180:73–78

Vitale Romo L, Clarke P (1992) Fitz-Hugh-Curtis syndrome: pelvic inflammatory disease with an unusual CT presentation. J Comput Assist Tomogr 16:832–833

Walkey MM, Friedman AC, Sohotra P, Radecki PD (1988) CT manifestations of peritoneal carcinosis. AJR 150:1035–1041

Walsh JW, Taylor KJW, Rosenfield AR (1979) Gray scale ultra-sonography in the diagnosis of endometriosis and ad-enomyosis. AJR 132:87–90

Warner M, Fleischer AC, Edell S, et al. (1985) Uterine adnexal torsion: sonographic findings. Radiology 154:773–775

Weinreb JC, Barkoff ND, Megibow A, Demopoulos R (1990) The value of MR imaging in distinguishing leiomyomas from other solid pelvic masses when sonography is inde-terminate. AJR 154:295–299

Weststrom L (1987) Pelvic inflammatory disease: bacteriology and sequelae. Contraception 36:111–128

White PF, Merino MJ, Barwick KW (1985) Serous surface papillary carcinoma of the ovary: a clinical, pathologic, ultrastructural and immunohistochemical study of 11 cases. Pathol Annu 20:403–418

Yamashita Y, Torashima M, Hatanaka Y, et al. (1995) Adnexal masses: accuracy of characterization with transvaginal US and precontrast and postcontrast MR imaging. Radiology 194:557–565

Young RC, Perez CA, Hoskins WJ (1993) Cancer of the ovary. In: De Vita VT, Hellman S, Rosenberg SA (eds) Cancer. Principles and practice of oncology, vol I. Lippincott, Philadelphia, pp 1226–1263

Zawin M, McCarty S, Scoutt L, Comite F (1989) Endome-triosis: appearance and detection at MR imaging. Radiol-ogy 171:693–696

19 Uterus and Vagina

A. Heuck and J. Scheidler

19.1
Introduction

Magnetic resonance (MR) imaging has proved to be a most valuable diagnostic tool for study of the female pelvis. As documented by numerous studies during the last decade, MR imaging offers a completely noninvasive assessment of normal anatomy, congenital anomalies, and benign and malignant disease of the uterus. For most conditions it has proved superior to clinical examination, ultrasonography (US), and computed tomography (CT).

Continuing advances in MR imaging of the pelvis – including the development of new pulse sequences and coil techniques, the use of gadolinium chelates as paramagnetic contrast media, and the increasing experience of radiologists – have further improved the potential of MR imaging as a problem-solving modality and have helped to establish its immediate and cost-effective impact on treatment alternatives (Schwartz et al. 1994; Hricak et al. 1996).

In the evaluation of uterine and vaginal malignancies, MR imaging is increasingly advocated as the primary imaging modality due to its inherent tissue characterization properties and multiplanar imaging capabilities, which are recognized as invaluable tools in pretherapeutic staging. In benign disease of the uterus, however, US remains the most appropriate initial imaging procedure, and MR imaging is reserved for those patients in whom US is suboptimal or equivocal.

19.2
MR Imaging Techniques

19.2.1
MR Imaging Coils

Commonly MR imaging of the pelvis is performed by use of a standard body coil. However, the use of phased-array coils significantly improves the signal-to-noise (S/N) ratio by a factor of 2–3.5 (Gauger et al. 1996), allowing for excellent image quality with a reduced field of view (FOV) down to 16 cm and slice thickness as low as 4 mm. The image resolution is very high and approaches $0.60\,mm^2$ pixel size. Early technical problems of phased-array coils such as increased motion and ghosting artifacts due to very high signal intensity in the near field have been almost completely resolved. However, very obese patients or those with protuberance of the abdomen due to tumor or ascites may not be suited for phased-array coil imaging.

Endorectal coil imaging may be applied to study cervical cancer. It allows excellent S/N levels with a reduction of the FOV to below 16 cm. Endorectal coil images provide excellent details of the anatomy of the cervix, including tumor presence and extent, as well as the parametrial space (Baudouin et al. 1992). However, no definitive study has yet proven advan-

A. Heuck, MD, Department of Diagnostic Radiology, Klinikum Großhadern, Ludwig-Maximilians University, Marchioninistrasse 15, D-81377 München, Germany
J. Scheidler, MD, Department of Diagnostic Radiology, Klinikum Großhadern, Ludwig-Maximilians University, Marchioninistrasse 15, D-81377 München, Germany

tages of endorectal coils over phased-array or body coils.

19.2.2
Pulse Sequences and Imaging Planes

T1- and T2-weighted images are both necessary for the evaluation of the uterus. T1-weighted images provide the required contrast between the uterus, the surrounding fatty tissue, and the ovaries. They also allow for the best contrast for imaging lymph nodes. Heavily T2-weighted images are essential for depicting the normal zonal anatomy as well as pathologic changes of the uterus and vagina. However, conventional T2-weighted spin-echo (SE) imaging is time-consuming and often degraded by motion artifacts.

T2-weighted turbo spin-echo (TSE) or fast spin-echo (FSE) sequences provide anatomic and pathologic information superior to that provided by conventional SE sequences. TSE sequences allow higher S/N ratios and a significant decrease in imaging time (by a factor of 3–4), leading to a considerable reduction of motion artifacts (NGHIEM et al. 1992; HEUCK et al. 1994a). Today, in many centers TSE sequences have fully replaced conventional SE sequences.

Fast and ultrafast T1-weighted gradient-recalled echo (GRE) images should be used when contrast-enhanced dynamic imaging is required, e.g., in the diagnosis and staging of endometrial carcinoma. Usually a FLASH type fast multiple-section GRE sequence provides a temporal resolution of 15–18 s, which can be considered sufficient for dynamic imaging in most instances. With ultrafast turbo-FLASH type sequences the temporal resolution may be further increased.

Short tau inversion recovery (STIR) sequences provide two general features: (a) robust fat suppression and (b) positive T1 and T2 contrast. By suppressing the normally intense signal from fat, STIR sequences greatly increase the conspicuity of structures or lesions that are surrounded by fat such as the parametria or lymph nodes. Due to sequence properties, T1 contrast and T2 contrast are additive with STIR imaging, thus enhancing the contrast between lesions and low-signal fat tissue. Despite these properties. STIR sequences have not yet been shown to be superior to T2-weighted TSE sequences in imaging of the uterus (HEUCK et al. 1995; SCHEIDLER et al. 1998). In addition, STIR cannot necessarily distinguish short T1 fat from short

T1 subacute hemorrhage, as they are both equally suppressed.

Spectral fat saturation techniques have recently been introduced into MR imaging of the body. Early application of these techniques showed inconsistent fat suppression in a considerable percentage of cases, limiting its utility. However, advances in shim procedures have helped to make fat saturation available as a robust technique even in phased-array coil studies. Fat saturation sequences are recommended for the differentiation of fat and hemorrhage, e.g., differentiation of fat-containing teratoma from endometrioma. The impact of T1-weighted fat saturation sequences on the assessment of parametrial involvement in cervical carcinoma is currently under investigation. Preliminary data suggest that contrast-enhanced fat saturation sequences are valuable in the study of parametrial involvement while non-enhanced sequences are not useful. However, the impact of contrast-enhanced T1-weighted fat saturation sequences does not surpass the diagnostic value of T2-weighted TSE sequences (HEUCK et al. 1994c; SCHEIDLER et al. 1998).

A standard protocol for imaging the uterus should always include heavily T2-weighted sequences in the sagittal and axial planes and a T1-weighted sequence in the axial plane (Table 19.1). An additional T2-weighted sequence in the coronal plane may be helpful in some instances. However, it may also be

Table 19.1. Suggested MRI protocols for the uterus and vagina

Indication	Plane	Sequence	Slice thickness
Congenital anomalies	1. Sagittal	T2w TSE (SE)	
	2. Axial	T2w TSE (SE)	
	3. Coronal	T2w TSE (SE) optional	
Adenomyosis, leiomyoma	1. Sagittal	T2w TSE (SE)	
	2. Axial	T2w TSE (SE)	
	3. Axial	T1w TSE (SE)	
Cervical cancer and vaginal cancer	1. Sagittal	T2w TSE (SE)	
	2. Axial	T2w TSE (SE)	
	3. Axial	T1w SE/TSE	
Endometrial cancer	1. Axial	T2w TSE (SE)	
	2. Axial	T1w SE/TSE	
	3. Sagittal	T2w TSE (SE)	
	4. Sagittal	T1w fast dynamic GRE pre, during and post gadolinium	

Reduction of bowel motion by intramuscular or fractionated intravenous administration of glucagon or butylscopolamine. T2w, T2-weighted; T1w, T1-weighted.

advantageous to use off-axis planes perpendicular to or within the long axis of the endometrial cavity or the endocervical canal (BAUMGARTNER and BERNARDINO 1989) to display congenital anomalies or to exactly define the extent of tumor.

Dynamic contrast-enhanced GRE imaging in the sagittal plane has been proven to increase the accuracy of MR imaging in defining the depth of myometrial infiltration in endometrial cancer and is, therefore, strongly recommended for this indication.

19.2.3
Motion Artifact Suppression

Suppression of motion artifacts should be performed whenever possible. If special software to compensate for respiratory motion is available, it should be used. If it is unavailable, a strap band over the pelvis is helpful. Pulsation artifacts should be suppressed by flow compensation techniques. For the reduction of artifacts caused by bowel peristalsis, administration of butylscopolamine or glucagon is recommended unless medically contraindicated.

19.2.4
Contrast Media

19.2.4.1
Intravenous Contrast Media

Intravenous gadolinium chelate contrast media can be of great use in pelvic MR imaging. However, the established indications for the use of gadolinium chelates (such as Gd-DTPA) in MR imaging of the uterus are limited in number: staging of endometrial carcinoma, evaluation of certain cases of advanced cervical carcinoma, and detection of lymph nodes when conventional unenhanced images are inconclusive. In general, gadolinium chelates are nontoxic and well tolerated even in patients with renal insufficiency.

19.2.4.2
Gastrointestinal Contrast Media

Numerous bowel contrast agents are available or under investigation to improve delineation of bowel from abdominal or pelvic organs (HEUCK et al. 1994b; SCHEIDLER et al. 1997b; BROWN 1996; PELS RIJKEN et al. 1994). They can be divided into positive

(e.g., Magnevist oral, Ferriseltz) and negative contrast agents (e.g., oral magnetic particles, ferumoxsil, perfluoroctylbromide). While gastrointestinal contrast media may be of great value in the evaluation of patients with endometriosis and ovarian masses, they are usually not indicated for MR imaging of the uterus.

19.3
Normal Anatomy of the Uterus and Vagina

The uterus, cervix, and upper third of the vagina are formed by fusion of the medial portions of the müllerian ducts (originating from the mesoderm), while the lower two-thirds of the vagina are derived from the sinovaginal bulb (originating from the urogenital sinus).

19.3.1
Uterus

19.3.1.1
Anatomy

The uterus is a pear-shaped organ located posterior to the urinary bladder and anterior to the rectum. It is divided into the fundus, corpus, and cervix and is 7–9 cm in length (corpus 4–6 cm, cervix 2.5–3.2 cm). It varies in size, being largest in women of reproductive age and smallest during childhood and menopause. The fundus, which is part of the body (corpus), lies above the level where the fallopian tubes enter the superolateral corners (cornua). The corpus narrows at the isthmus, which is the region between the corpus and the cervix. The internal os opens into the cervical canal, which ends at the external os, opening into the vagina (Fig. 19.1). The inner mucosal surface of the fundus and isthmus is the same as the endometrium of the corpus.

The anterior and posterior outer surfaces of the uterus are covered by a layer of visceral peritoneum, which continues laterally to form the anterior and posterior leaves of the broad ligament (Fig. 19.1). Anteriorly, the peritoneum is reflected off the uterus and onto the bladder, forming the vesicouterine pouch. Posteriorly, the peritoneum reflects down deeply to the rectum, covering the posterior wall of the uterus and the posterior fornix of the vagina and forming the rectouterine pouch (cul-de-sac, pouch of Douglas). As the anterior peritoneal reflection is

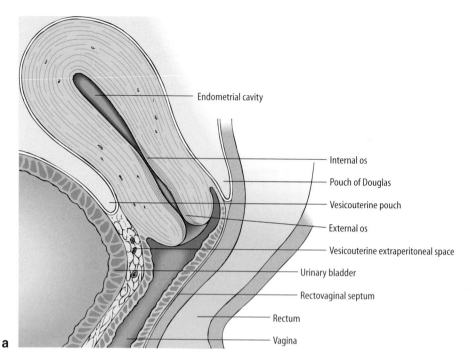

Endometrial cavity

Internal os

Pouch of Douglas

Vesicouterine pouch

External os

Vesicouterine extraperitoneal space

Urinary bladder

Rectovaginal septum

Rectum

Vagina

a

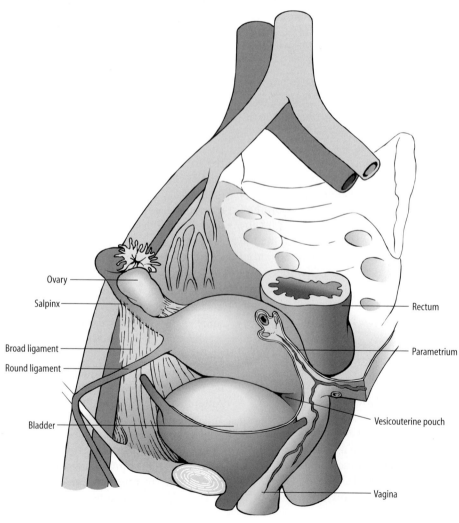

Ovary

Salpinx

Broad ligament

Round ligament

Bladder

Rectum

Parametrium

Vesicouterine pouch

Vagina

b

more cephalad, the anterior wall of the uterus is not completely covered by visceral peritoneum. The insertion of the round ligament is located at the level of the isthmus of the fallopian tubes.

In the central portion of the uterine corpus, the *endometrium* consists of two layers: the superficial functional layer (zona functionalis, including the zona compacta and the zona spongiosa), which undergoes cyclic growth and shedding, and the deep basal layer (zona basalis), which does not undergo cyclic changes.

The uterine *myometrium* is composed of three muscle layers. The innermost subendometrial layer consists of longitudinal and circular fibers. The intermediate layer is the stratum vasculare and contains numerous arcuate veins. The outer subserosal layer is very thin and consists of longitudinal muscle fibers extending from the cervix to the cornua.

19.3.1.2
MR Imaging

On T1-weighted sequences, the uterus is imaged relatively homogeneously, with intermediate to low signal intensity (Figs. 19.2b, 19.3a). On T2-weighted images, four distinct zonal layers can be differentiated in women of reproductive age. These are – from inside out – the endometrium, the junctional zone, a thick intermediate zone, and a thin subserosal zone of the myometrium (Figs. 19.2a,c,d, 19.3b).

The *endometrium* appears uniformly hyperintense on T2-weighted scans and is best shown in the sagittal orientation. Fluid in the endometrial cavity may be displayed with even higher signal intensity unless hemorrhagic; however, in most cases the signal contributions of blood and fluid cannot be clearly separated from the glandular layer. Endometrial thickness varies during the menstrual cycle (Fig. 19.4). The endometrium is usually thinnest just after menses and gradually thickens during the proliferative phase from a width of 3–5 mm to thickness of 6–10 mm at the start of the secretory phase. It is thickest in the mid-secretory phase, with a width up to 14 mm (McCARTHY et al. 1986; DEMAS et al. 1986; HEUCK and LUKAS 1997). In women taking oral contraceptives the endometrium does not cycle and re-

mains thin (1–3 mm). In postmenopausal women, due to the lack of cyclic hormonal stimulation, it atrophies with an average thickness of 2–3 mm. However, in women taking exogenous hormones, the appearance is similar to that in women of reproductive age (DEMAS et al. 1986; McCARTHY et al. 1986).

The *junctional zone* represents the inner, subendometrial or basal layer of the myometrium and is shown as a discrete low signal intensity region (Figs. 19.2a, 19.3b). It has a lower water content and a higher degree of smooth muscle cellularity than the intermediate zone, which accounts for the different MR signal intensity of the two layers. The junctional zone normally measures less than 12 mm in width, with an average of about 5 mm (REINHOLD et al. 1993). The interface with the endometrium is sharp, but that with the intermediate zone of the myometrium is less clearly defined. In postmenopausal women, the junctional zone is usually absent or may be incomplete (Fig. 19.5).

The *intermediate zone* or stratum vasculare of the myometrium displays a relatively diffuse intermediate to high signal intensity on T2-weighted images during the early proliferative phase (Fig. 19.4). Towards and in the secretory phase of the cycle, the myometrial signal and thickness increase due to increasing interstitial fluid content and vascular flow. Flow in the arcuate uterine vessels is normally not sufficient to produce signal voids. Maximum signal intensity in the intermediate zone is found in the mid-secretory phase, when the junctional zone still displays low signal intensity. Similar changes are observed in women using oral contraceptives. In postmenopausal women, the myometrium no longer shows cyclic changes and progressively decreases in signal intensity and in diameter. Therefore, the zonal anatomy of the uterus becomes indistinct and the uterus atrophies (Fig. 19.5).

The *outer subserosal layer* may be seen on high-resolution T2-weighted images as a thin dark line (Figs. 19.2a, 19.3b) which does not undergo noticeable changes within the menstrual cycle.

With the intravenous application of gadolinium chelates the myometrium displays early and strong enhancement, while the enhancement of the endometrium is more progressive and moderate. The

Fig. 19.1 a,b. Schematic drawings illustrating the uterus and vagina and their relation to the peritoneal reflections, parametria, and ligaments (adapted from HRICAK and CARRINGTON 1991). **a** The sagittal view demonstrates the anterior (vesicouterine pouch) and posterior (pouch of Douglas) reflections between the uterus, bladder, and rectum. **b** The oblique view demonstrates the position of the uterus in relation to the rectum, bladder, ligaments, parametrium, and peritoneal reflections

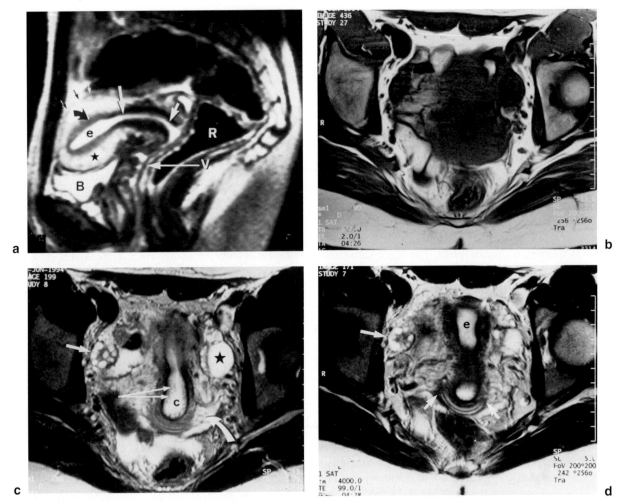

Fig. 19.2 a–d. Normal MR imaging appearance of the anteverted uterus and adjacent structures of the true pelvis. **a** Sagittal T2-weighted FSE image of the anteverted uterus showing the normal zonal architecture. The innermost layer of high signal intensity is the endometrium (*e*). The subendometrial layer of the myometrium or junctional zone is displayed with low signal intensity (*curved arrow*) and the stratum vasculare or intermediate zone (***) of the myometrium displays a diffuse relatively high signal intensity. The subserosal layer can be seen as a thin line of low signal intensity (*small arrows*). The cervix is displayed with its high signal intensity endocervical canal extending from the internal os (*white arrow*) to the external os (*short white arrow*), its low signal intensity inner stroma and its intermediate signal intensity outer stroma. *R*, Rectum; *V*, vagina; *B*, bladder. **b** Axial T1-weighted SE image of an anteverted uterus at the level of the cervix. The uterus displays intermediate to low signal intensity and zonal anatomy cannot be assessed. Also the parametrial plexuses

cannot be delineated from uterine tissue. **c** The axial T2-weighted FSE image at the same level as **b** fully displays the zonal anatomy of the cervix. The endocervical canal (*c*) shows high signal intensity representing mucosa and mucus and is lined by mucosal folds [plicae palmatae (long arrows)]. To the periphery the endocervical canal is surrounded by low signal intensity inner stroma and intermediate signal intensity outer stroma. The parametria display high signal intensity due to the high density of arterial and venous plexuses (*curved arrow*). Note the normal right ovary (*arrow*) and a unilocular cyst (***) of the left ovary. **d** Axial T2-weighted FSE image, 1 cm superior to the level of **b** and **c**. The endometrial cavity (*e*) is surrounded by the low signal intensity band of the junctional zone. At this level the parametria are displayed with intermediate to high signal intensity. Note the normal right ovary (*arrow*) and vaginal fornices attaching to the cervix (*short arrows*)

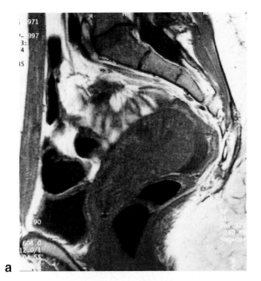

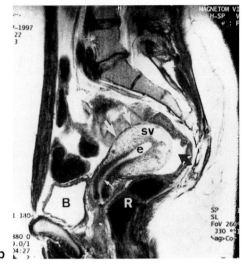

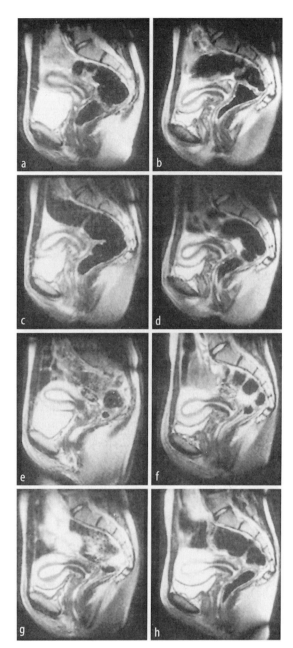

Fig. 19.3 a,b. Normal MR imaging appearance of the retroverted uterus. **a** Sagittal T1-weighted SE image of the pearshaped uterus clearly shows retroversion but the zonal architecture cannot be depicted. **b** The T2-weighted FSE image in the same plane as **a** clearly displays the zonal anatomy: the central endometrial cavity (*e*) with high signal intensity is sharply delineated from a small layer of low signal intensity representing the junctional zone. The intermediate zone [stratum vasculare (*sv*)] of the myometrium is shown with intermediate to high signal intensity and is surrounded by the thin low signal intensity layer of subserosal myometrium (*short arrows*). The appearance of the cervix is dominated by the low signal intensity of the cervical stroma surrounding the high signal intensity line of the endocervical canal (*small arrow*). There is a small amount of fluid in the pouch of Douglas (*short curved arrow*). R, Rectum; B, bladder

Fig. 19.4 a–h. Appearance of the uterus during the menstrual cycle (22-year-old woman); sagittal T2-weighted TSE images. **a** Day 5 of the menstrual cycle (end of menstruation): the endometrium shows moderately high signal intensity (SI) and is small in diameter. **b** In the early proliferative phase (day 8 of the cycle) the endometrium displays higher SI. **c,d** In the later proliferative phase (days 11 and 14 of the cycle) the endometrium becomes thicker and the myometrium higher in SI. **e–g** In the secretory phase (days 17, 19, 21) the endometrium reaches maximum thickness and the SI of myometrium increases further. **h** At day 25 of the cycle the endometrial thickness decreases slightly. (From HEUCK and LUKAS 1997)

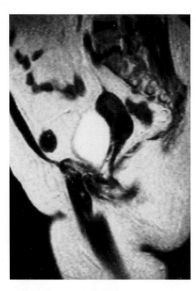

Fig. 19.5. Appearance of the uterus in a postmenopausal woman. The sagittal T2-weighted FSE image shows an atrophied uterus with low signal intensity endometrium and myometrium and indistinct zonal anatomy

junctional zone shows only mild contrast uptake, most likely due to its more compact structure and decreased extracellular space (HRICAK and KIM 1993).

19.3.2
Cervix

19.3.2.1
Anatomy

The cervix is the cylindrical part of the uterus inferior to the isthmus and is connected to the isthmus uteri at the internal os. The junction is demarcated histologically by a change of the epithelium from glandular (corpus) to columnar (cervix). The internal os is connected to the external cervical os by the endocervical canal, which is lined by multiple mucosal folds (plicae palmatae) and measures 8 mm at its widest point. The external os represents the opening between the cervix and the vagina and is marked histologically by the junction of squamous and columnar epithelium.

The cervix is divided by the vaginal fornices into the supravaginal and intravaginal portions. The latter is covered by squamous cell epithelium and is also known as the exocervix or portio. Unlike the uterine myometrium, the cervical stroma is composed predominantly (80%) of fibrous connective tissue and to a lesser degree of smooth muscle (15%)

and elastic tissue. Only in the upper portion of the cervix, next to the internal os, does smooth muscle dominate (60%), forming a sphincter (FERENCZY and WINKLER 1987).

19.3.2.2
MR Imaging

While on T1-weighted images the cervix shows relatively uniform intermediate signal intensity similar to the corpus, its anatomy is best displayed by a combination of sagittal and axial heavily T2-weighted sequences (Figs. 19.2, 19.3). The sagittal orientation allows visualization of the cervix in its whole extent from the internal to the external os including the anterior and posterior lips of the cervix (Figs. 19.2a, 19.3b). The cervix is displayed with a small inner area of high signal intensity representing the endocervical mucosa and mucus, a broad layer of low-signal inner cervical stroma, and a varying layer of slightly higher signal intensity representing the outer cervical stroma (Fig. 19.2a,c,d). The inner dense fibrous stroma is continuous with the junctional zone of the corpus. In the axial plane, depending on the degree of uterine flexion, the cervix may be displayed either as a compact round structure with a target appearance or as a more longitudinal solid structure with the typical zonal anatomy (Fig. 19.2c).

Gadolinium administration leads to enhancement of the inner mucosal epithelium and the paracervical tissue, whereas the cervical stroma shows only minor enhancement.

19.3.3
Parametrium and Pelvic Ligaments

19.3.3.1
Anatomy

The broad ligaments are composed of the anterior and posterior layers of peritoneum as they pass over the fallopian tubes (Fig. 19.1b). These peritoneal layers reflect over the uterus and course laterally to the pelvic side walls. The broad ligament terminates caudally and laterally as the cardinal ligament and superiorly as the suspensory ligament of the ovary. The uterosacral ligaments are covered by peritoneum, passing posteriorly from the cervix to the sacrum and encircling the rectum.

The loose connective tissue adjacent to the lateral margins of the uterine myometrium and within the broad ligament (i.e., between the anterior and posterior peritoneal layers) is referred to as the *parametrium* (Fig. 19.1b). Its lateral margin anteriorly is formed by the uterovesical ligaments. The parametria contain the fallopian tubes, the round ligaments, the uterine and ovarian blood vessels, lymphatics, and portions of the ureters. The round ligaments originate at the uterus close to the cornua and pass through the inguinal canal inferiorly to insert into the labia majora. The uterine arteries pass through the parametria and enter the uterus at the level of the internal os. They branch to form arcuate vessels, which supply the myometrium. In addition, there is uterine blood supply from branches of the ovarian and vaginal arteries. The venous drainage is via the uterovaginal venous plexus, which communicate with the internal iliac veins.

Beside this high vascularity the parametrial connective tissue contains numerous lymphatic vessels. The majority of the lymphatic channels of the uterine body pass through the parametrium to the pelvic side wall and then into the iliac chain of lymph nodes. The fundus is drained via lymphatics accompanying the round ligaments to the superficial inguinal nodes and laterally via the mesovarium to the para-aortic nodes.

19.3.3.2
MR Imaging

The cervix is not directly surrounded by fat tissue but is surrounded by the loose connective tissue of the parametrium with abundant vessels. Thus, as cervix and parametrium both demonstrate medium signal intensity with T1-weighted parameters (Fig. 19.2b), it is difficult to distinguish the two on T1-weighted images. On T2-weighted images, the parametrium shows varying degrees of high signal intensity depending on the density and width of the parametrial arterial and venous plexuses (Fig. 19.2c), which appear as high signal intensity serpiginous structures. Flow in these vessels is usually not sufficient to produce a signal void.

While those ligaments which are composed of peritoneal layers (e.g., broad ligament) normally cannot be clearly delineated on MR images, the fibromuscular round ligament is well defined on T2-weighted images with low signal intensity. It projects anteriorly from the uterine cornua at the superior edge of the broad ligament and courses anteriorly toward the internal inguinal ring.

After intravenous injection of gadolinium chelates, the normal parametrial arterial and venous plexuses display strong enhancement on T1-weighted images, leading to increased contrast between cervical stroma and parametrium but simultaneously to decreased contrast between the plexus and the adjacent fat-containing connective tissue, unless fat-saturated T1-weighted sequences are used.

19.3.4
Vagina

19.3.4.1
Anatomy

The vagina is a fibromuscular sheath extending from the uterus to the vestibule and located between the bladder and urethra anteriorly and the rectum posteriorly. The anterior and posterior walls of the vagina are normally in contact and consist of three layers, the mucosa (squamous epithelium), the muscularis, and the adventitia. The length of the anterior wall is approximately 7.5 cm, and that of the posterior wall approximately 9 cm. The upper third of the vagina encompasses the attachments to the uterine cervix and the anterior and posterior recesses, called the vaginal fornices. The middle third is located at the level of bladder base, and the lower third posterior to the urethra.

The paracolpium is the connective tissue adjacent to the vagina encompassing the vascular supply (via branches of the uterine, middle rectal, inferior vesical, and internal pudendal arteries), venous drainage (via the uterine and vaginal plexus), and lymphatics. Lymphatic drainage of the lower vaginal third is to the external iliac and deep inguinal nodes and that of the upper two-thirds is to the internal iliac and common iliac nodes.

19.3.4.2
MR Imaging

On T1-weighted scans the vagina is demonstrated with intermediate signal intensity, similar to the cervix and corpus uteri, the urethra, and the rectal wall. The vaginal anatomy is best displayed on sagittal and axial T2-weighted images. The muscular wall of the vagina is shown as a low signal intensity structure between the rectovaginal septum posteriorly and the urethra and the bladder anteriorly. The vagina is usually collapsed with the high signal intensity inner mucosal surfaces apposed. Within the vaginal lumen there may be a thin layer of very high signal intensity fluid between the mucosal surfaces. In the axial plane, the upper third of the vagina is characterized by depiction of the fornices (Fig. 19.6a), the middle third displays the anterior and posterior walls tightly apposed (Fig. 19.6b), and the lower third appears H-shaped and in close relation to the urethra (Fig. 19.6c).

Variations in the appearance of the vagina with the menstrual cycle have been observed (HRICAK et al. 1988b). While there is excellent contrast between the low signal intensity muscular wall and the high signal intensity central mucosa during the early proliferative phase, there is less contrast between the two layers and luminal mucus in the secretory phase.

The perivaginal venous plexus lies beyond the muscular wall of the vagina within the paracolpium. This plexus is seen as a ring-like high signal intensity area extending from the urethra to the anterior rectal wall and surrounding the entire vagina.

After intravenous administration of gadolinium, both the muscular wall and the mucosa of the vagina are enhanced. A low signal intensity central line which is observed in some patients may represent the inner epithelium of the vagina. The perivaginal plexus usually enhances strongly, similar to other low-flow venous structures.

19.4
Pathology of the Uterus and Vagina

19.4.1
Congenital Malformations

Congenital malformations of the reproductive tract occur in up to 15% of women and result from developmental disorders of the müllerian ducts (SORENSEN 1988). They present with a spectrum of findings ranging from agenesis to duplications and

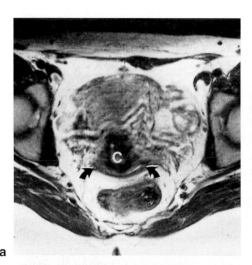

a

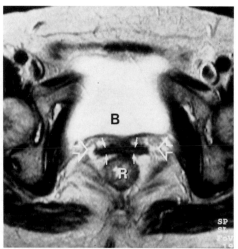

b

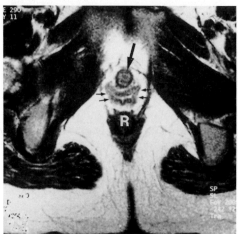

c

Fig. 19.6 a–c. Normal appearance of the vagina on axial T2-weighted FSE images. **a** Upper third of the vagina: the vaginal fornices (*curved arrows*) are in close relation to the uterine cervix (*c*). **b** Middle third of the vagina: the anterior and posterior vaginal wall is displayed with low signal intensity (*small arrows*); the higher signal intensity of the central portion reflects mucosal surfaces. The paracolpium (*open arrows*) displays high signal intensity. *B*, Bladder; *R*, rectum. **c** Lower third of the vagina. The low signal intensity vaginal wall is H-shaped (*small arrows*) and can be clearly delineated from the urethra (*arrow*) and rectum (*R*)

minor contour abnormalities. Müllerian duct anomalies (MDAs) may be clinically silent; however, they may be associated with menstrual disorders, preterm delivery, infertility, or multiple spontaneous abortions. In MDAs renal abnormalities are a frequent additional finding.

For a long time hysterosalpingography (HSG), in combination with hysteroscopy or surgery, has been the main diagnostic procedure to evaluate congenital abnormalities. Ultrasonography (US), especially with an endovaginal approach, has more recently been established as a complementary imaging modality to HSG (MALINI et al. 1984). US of the uterus performed during saline instillation in the uterine cavity (hysterosonography) has even been suggested as an alternative to HSG in the evaluation of MDAs (RANDOLPH et al. 1986).

MR Imaging. MR imaging has emerged as a precise noninvasive modality in the diagnosis and classification of congenital malformations of the uterus that is used as an adjunct or as an alternative to hysterosalpingography, US, and laparoscopy (FORSTNER and HRICAK 1994; CARRINGTON et al. 1990). For tissue characterization T1- as well as T2-weighted imaging should be performed. T2-weighted imaging in two planes, preferably transaxial and sagittal, is recommended for proper classification of the abnormality.

According to the classification suggested by BUTTRAM and GIBBONS (1979), MDAs are divided into six different groups (Table 19.2), which can be clearly differentiated with MR imaging.

Class I: Agenesis (segmental or complete) and hypoplasia. Failure of normal development of müllerian ducts leads to agenesis or hypoplasia. In complete agenesis all structures of the müllerian ducts have not been developed. In segmental agenesis, each part of the müllerian ducts may be affected separately or in combination. The most common anomaly in this group is the Mayer-Rokitansky-Küster-Hauser syndrome, with an incidence of 1:5000. It comprises vaginal agenesis with a spectrum of uterine anomalies ranging from normal to a rudimentary uterus (Fig. 19.7). It is associated with

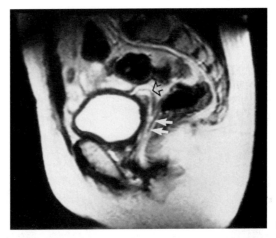

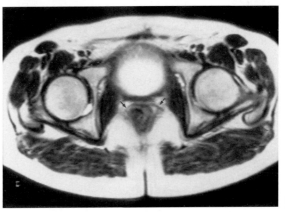

Table 19.2. Classification of müllerian duct anomalies (suggested by BUTTRAM and GIBBONS 1979)

Class I: agenesis or hypoplasia
A. Vaginal
B. Cervical
C. Fundal
D. Tubal
E. Combined

Class II: Unicornuate
A1. Rudimentary horn contains endometrium. Horn may (a) or may not (b) communicate with main uterine cavity
A2. Rudimentary horn without endometrium
B. No rudimentary horn

Class III: Uterus didelphys

Class IV: Bicornuate
A. Complete – division down to internal os
B. Partial
C. Arcuate

Class V: Septate
A. Complete down to internal/external os
B. Incomplete

Class VI: Diethylstilbestrol (DES)-related abnormalities

Fig. 19.7 a,b. Mayer-Rokitansky-Küster-Hauser syndrome in an 18-year-old woman. **a** Sagittal T2-weighted FSE image demonstrating hypoplasia of the uterine body (*open arrow*) and an incomplete vaginal agenesis. Note incomplete upper third of vagina (*arrows*). **b** Axial T2-weighted FSE image below the level of the upper third of the vagina demonstrating rectovaginal fascia (*small arrows*), but no vaginal wall

unilateral renal (50%) and skeletal (12%) anomalies (KOTLUS ROSENBERG et al. 1986).

On MR imaging hypoplasia is characterized by a small uterus with a small endometrial cavity, an abnormally low signal intensity of the myometrium, and poor differentiation of the zonal anatomy. The vagina is also small in diameter and shortened in

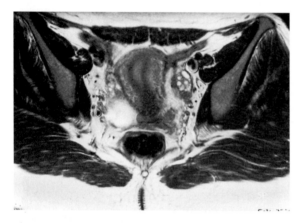

Fig. 19.8. Unicornuate uterus. The axial T2-weighted FSE image shows a "banana-shaped" uterus with a normal right and without a rudimentary left horn, indicating a nondevelopmental subtype. The endometrial and myometrial widths are normal; the endometrium displays a relatively low signal intensity

length without demonstration of high signal intensity mucosa on T2-weighted images.

Class II: Unicornuate uterus. Unicornuate uterus results from nondevelopment or incomplete development of one müllerian duct and accounts for about 13% of congenital anomalies (BUTTRAM and GIBBONS 1979). Two subtypes of unicornuate uterus are recognized, one with (incomplete development) and one without a rudimentary second horn (nondevelopment). The majority of class II anomalies include a unicornuate uterus with a rudimentary horn, which may or may not contain endometrium and communicate with the main uterine cavity. In up to 44% of cases unicornuate uterus can be associated with ipsilateral renal agenesis or renal anomalies.

On T2-weighted MR images of unicornuate uterus with a rudimentary horn the latter may be frequently seen as an asymmetric structure with the typical signal intensity of myometrium, which either does or does not contain high signal intensity endometrium (Fig. 19.8). In nondevelopmental unicornuate uterus the banana-shaped uterine cavity is characteristic and endometrial and myometrial width is normal.

Class III: Uterus didelphys. This rare anomaly results from normal development but nonfusion of the müllerian ducts. Two separate, normal-sized uteri each with a complete corpus and cervix are found. In

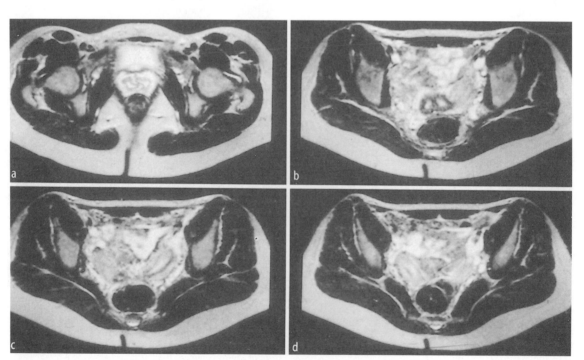

Fig. 19.9 a–d. Uterus didelphys. Axial T2-weighted SE images showing two separate vaginal lumina (**a**) and cervices (**b**) as well as two completely separate uterine horns (**c** and **d**). (From HEUCK and LUKAS 1997)

75% of cases an upper vaginal septum in a sagittal orientation is found. Additional transverse septa may occur and can cause obstruction.

T2-weighted MR images demonstrate two clearly separate corpora uteri, cervices, and sagittally oriented vaginal septum (Fig. 19.9). The endometrial and myometrial width and signal intensities of both uterine bodies are not altered.

Class IV: Bicornuate uterus. Bicornuate uterus is the result of partial failure of müllerian duct fusion. The resulting septum is composed of myometrium and open surgery is required for correction. In complete bicornuate uterus the septum extends at least to the internal os (bicornuate unicollis uterus). It may, however, extend to the external os, dividing the endocervical canal into two lumina (bicornuate

bicollis uterus). Cases with a muscular septum found in the fundus or upper corpus are considered as incomplete bicornuate uterus. Arcuate uterus represents the mildest form of the bicornuate anomaly with slight prominence of the fundal myometrium or a small rudimentary muscular septum.

Differentiation between bicornuate and septate uterus is of paramount importance because these anomalies require different treatment. Bicornuate uterus is treated by transabdominal surgical resection of the muscular septum, whereas septate uterus can be treated less invasively by endoscopic techniques.

On MR imaging the bicornuate anomaly is characterized by a concave surface of the fundus or a fundal notch (Fig. 19.10). In arcuate uterus, the fundal surface is flattened or only slightly concave (Fig. 19.11). The intercornual distance may be increased in bicornuate uterus and the endometrial width and myometrial width display a normal ratio. The muscular septum is displayed with a signal intensity similar to myometrium in T1- and T2-weighted sequences (Fig. 19.10). Its distal portion may be composed of muscular and fibrous elements. The sensitivity and specificity of MR imaging for the diagnosis of bicornuate uterus and its differentiation from septate uterus have been reported to be as high as 100% (PELLERITO et al. 1992). Therefore, MR imaging can be considered as the method of choice to distinguish between class IV and V anomalies.

Class V: Septate uterus. Septate uterus is the most common müllerian duct anomaly and results from failure of resorption of the fibrous midline septum after complete fusion of the ducts. The septum divides the uterine body completely if it reaches to the

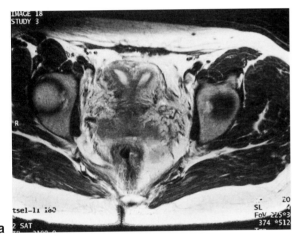

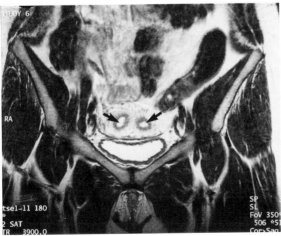

Fig. 19.10 a,b. Bicornuate uterus (uterus bicornuate bicollis). **a** Axial T2-weighted FSE image demonstrating two uterine cornua and two endometrial cavities separated by myometrium (subendometrial and intermediate zone). **b** The coronal T2-weighted FSE image displays a myometrial wall between two endometrial cavities (*arrows*)

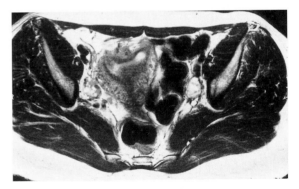

Fig. 19.11. Arcuate uterus. Axial T2-weighted FSE image showing a rudimentary muscular septum in the region of the uterine fundus, leading to a "heart-shaped" appearance of the endometrial cavity. The outer fundal contour is only slightly concave

internal os, and partially when it ends above the internal os. Septate uterus is associated with a ca. 90% incidence of spontaneous abortions or preterm labor, possibly due to inadequate vascular supply within the septum to support implantation or due to septal endometrial incompetence. Unlike in cases of bicornuate uterus, treatment of septate uterus is by hysteroscopic metroplasty.

T2-weighted MR images obtained in the oblique coronal orientation (along the axis of the uterine cavity) allow for proper depiction of a low signal intensity fibrous septum within the cavity in the presence of a widely normal fundal contour and intercornual distance (Fig. 19.12). While HSG and US are limited in their ability to characterize the fibrous nature of the septum, MR imaging provides a very accurate assessment.

Class VI: DES-related anomalies. Diethylstibestrol (DES) is a synthetic estrogen that was widely used until the 1970s in the treatment of abortions, preterm labor, preeclampsia, and diabetes. Structural anomalies of the genital tract have been observed in up to two-thirds of females exposed to DES in utero (VAN GILS et al. 1989). Anomalies include uterine hypoplasia, T-shaped uterine cavities, and irregular constrictions and ridges of the uterus and vagina. In addition, abnormal fallopian tubes and hydrosalpinges have been described.

MR imaging findings include abnormalities of uterine size and shape. The length of the uterine cavity is often less than 3.3 cm and the cervix is also shortened. Sometimes a T-shaped endometrial cavity can be demonstrated. Uterine constrictions may be identified by focal widening of the junctional zone; however, irregular margins of the uterine cavity cannot be demonstrated by MR imaging.

19.4.2
Diseases of the Uterine Body

19.4.2.1
Adenomyosis

In adenomyosis, a progressive and disabling disease of reproductive-age women, heterotopic endometrial glands and stroma are present within the myometrium, at least 2.5 mm from the endometrial basis and extending at least one-third of the thickness of the uterine wall (HENDRICKSON and KEMPSON 1980). These endometrial islands are associated with hyperplasia of the adjacent smooth muscle of the myometrium. Adenomyosis may spontaneously evolve from downward growth of basalis endometrium, but numerous other causes, including hyperestrogenemia and postpregnancy implantation, are discussed. In contrast to endometriosis, the heterotopic endometrial glands in adenomyosis do not respond to hormonal stimulation and they do not undergo the full cyclic changes of normally functioning endometrium.

The incidence of adenomyosis is reported to be 15%–27% (KILKKU et al. 1984; HENDRICKSON and KEMPSON 1980), with predominance of multiparous women; the most common age at presentation is the fourth and fifth decades. Clinically, the diagnosis is difficult to establish because symptoms are variable and often similar to those of patients with leiomyoma. Patients frequently present with menorrhagia or dysmenorrhea, pelvic pain, and enlarged uterus. However, about 50% of patients with adenomyosis are asymptomatic.

Ultrasonography and CT have generally not permitted the specific diagnosis of adenomyosis, both showing nonspecific enlargement of the uterus.

MR Imaging. There are two forms of adenomyosis that can be differentiated pathologically and on MR imaging, a diffuse and a focal type. *Diffuse adenomyosis* is most commonly depicted on T2-weighted images as thickening of the hypointense junctional zone, which should not exceed 6 mm in normal patients (ASCHER et al. 1994). A junctional zone thickness of 12 mm or greater accurately allows the diagnosis of adenomyosis (REINHOLD et al.

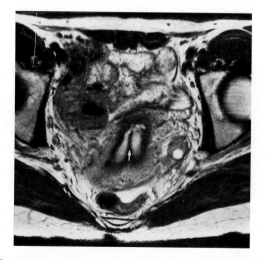

Fig. 19.12. Septate uterus in posterior flexion. On the axial T2-weighted FSE image there is a low signal intensity fibrous septum (*arrow*) extending from the fundus to the uterine isthmus

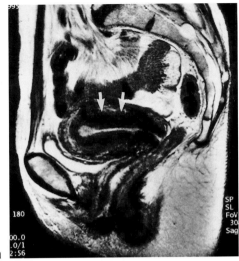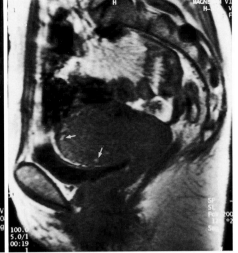

Fig. 19.13 a,b. Diffuse adenomyosis. **a** The sagittal T2-weighted FSE image displays thickening of the low signal intensity junctional zone up to 18 cm (*arrows*). This finding is consistent with diffuse muscular overgrowth in adenomyosis.

b The sagittal T1-weighted SE image does not allow differentiation of uterine zonal architecture; however, the small foci of high signal intensity (*arrows*) are thought to represent focal hemorrhage

1996). The thickening of the junctional zone extends segmentally or diffusely and to varying degrees through the myometrium to the periphery (Figs. 19.13, 19.14). Adenomyosis is usually poorly defined from the myometrium and may contain foci of high signal intensity consistent with islands of endometrial glands (Fig. 19.14). When these foci display high signal intensity on both T1- and T2-weighted images, they are thought to represent hemorrhage (Fig. 19.13b). Adenomyosis does not enhance appreciably after intravenous administration of gadolinium chelates (ASCHER et al. 1994). Coincident endometriomas are often present (TOGASHI et al. 1988; TOGASHI 1993). Diffuse adenomyosis can be accurately distinguished from leiomyoma by its specific MR imaging characteristics.

Focal adenomyosis can be observed as a low signal intensity mass within the myometrium which at first glance appears similar to a leiomyoma and therefore is sometimes referred to as "adenomyoma." Characteristic findings of focal adenomyosis are an elliptical contour, a poorly circumscribed or irregular margin due to interdigitation with normal myometrium, and eventually foci of high signal intensity; if adenomyosis is extensive, a distortion of the endometrial cavity may occur (Fig. 19.14). In contrast, typical findings in leiomyoma consist of a rounded contour with sharply defined margins due to a pseudocapsule, which is created by compression of the surrounding myometrium. Numerous dilated veins that often accompany leiomyomas are not observed in adenomyosis.

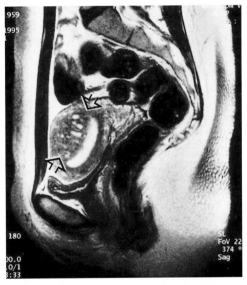

Fig. 19.14. Focal adenomyosis. On the sagittal T2-weighted FSE image focal adenomyosis appears with relatively low signal intensity, elliptical in configuration and with indistinct margins (*open arrows*). It contains multiple foci of high signal intensity

Magnetic resonance imaging is the most accurate noninvasive method in detecting and differentiating adenomyosis (TOGASHI et al. 1988, 1989a; MARK and HRICAK 1987; ASCHER et al. 1994; REINHOLD et al. 1996), with reported accuracy as high as 90%. It is generally found to be superior to transvaginal US (ASCHER et al. 1994), although in cases with diffuse adenomyosis US approaches the accuracy of MR imaging. Differentiation of adenomyosis from other causes of pelvic pain and bleeding, such as leiomyomas or endometriosis, is of particular importance for proper and cost-effective patient management, because the former can be treated only with hysterectomy, whereas leiomyoma can be treated with medication and possibly myomectomy. MR imaging is, therefore, the preferred imaging

modality after sonographic screening for obvious leiomyomas in this clinical setting.

19.4.2.2
Leiomyomas

Uterine leiomyomas (fibroids) are found in up to 25%–40% of women of childbearing age

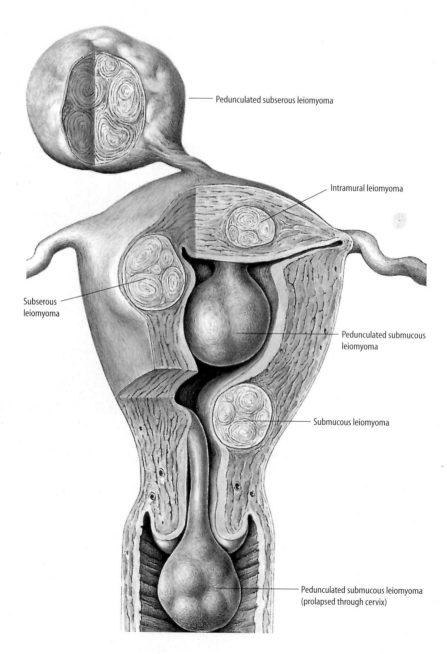

Fig. 19.15. The various types of uterine leiomyoma

(HENDRICKSON and KEMPSON 1980; COTRAN et al. 1989), being the most common benign tumors of the uterus in women over 35 years old. They are composed of smooth muscle and a variable amount of fibrous tissue and are surrounded by a pseudocapsule of areolar tissue. Blood supply is provided by one or two large vessels.

Leiomyomas may undergo secondary changes which should be familiar to the radiologist as they may be causes of misinterpretation. Hyaline degeneration may occur as small focal or as extensive changes within the tumor. Coalescence of focal hyaline degeneration and liquefaction may result in cystic degeneration. During periods of rapid growth, e.g., induced by hormonal stimulation during pregnancy, leiomyomas may show infarction and necrosis (so-called red degeneration). Calcifications can be found in tumors of poor vascular supply, especially in elderly women. Sarcomatous changes in myomas are rare.

Leiomyomas may be solitary or multiple and over 90% are found in the uterine corpus. Five percent arise in the cervix and a smaller number are found in the broad ligament.

Depending on their position relative to the uterine wall, leiomyomas are classified into three types: the *intramural* myoma, which is confined to the myometrium; the *submucosal* tumor, which projects into the uterine cavity, distorting the endometrium and the contour of the cavity; and the *subserosal* leiomyoma, which projects off the peritoneal surface of the uterus (Fig. 19.15). Either the subserosal or the submucosal myoma may be sessile or pedunculated and the latter can become prolapsed through the cervix.

Submucosal leiomyomas, which account for 5%–10% of fibroids, most often come to clinical attention because of infertility, recurrent abortion, and other clinical symptoms such as abnormal uterine bleeding, pelvic pain, and bladder or rectal pressure. Intramural leiomyomas may be associated with the same symptoms, while pedunculated subserosal fibroids may undergo torsion, causing acute abdominopelvic pain.

Clinical diagnosis of leiomyoma is presumptive and is made by abdominal and bimanual palpation. However, preoperative clinical diagnosis of leiomyoma could be confirmed by pathologic examination in only 84% of cases, and 30% of the pathologically identified tumors were not diagnosed preoperatively (LEE et al. 1984). Extensive degenerative changes in leiomyomas may lead to softening of the mass and lead to clinical and sonographic misdiagnosis of pregnancy or ovarian cyst.

Treatment depends on symptoms and the size and location of fibroids. Asymptomatic patients with small leiomyomas may be managed expectantly. Administration of gonadotropin-releasing hormone analogs reduces estrogen function and results in shrinkage of many tumors. Small submucosal tumors may be treated by hysteroscopic excision, whereas intramural lesions are treated by myomectomy.

MR Imaging. On T2-weighted MR images leiomyomas are displayed as well-circumscribed, rounded masses of variable size and predominantly low signal intensity with sharp margins delineating them from adjacent tissue.

Nondegenerative leiomyomas demonstrate almost homogeneous low signal intensity on T2-weighted images (Fig. 19.16) with contrast to the surrounding myometrium of −44% ± 16% and to the endometrium of −54% ± 14% (HRICAK et al. 1986a). On T1-weighted images they are displayed with intermediate signal intensity, often being indistinguishable from adjacent uterine tissues (contrast to myometrium −16% ± 11% and to endometrium −6% ± 12% signal intensity).

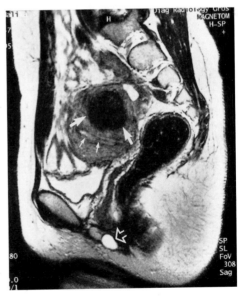

Fig. 19.16. Intramural leiomyoma. On the sagittal T2-weighted FSE image the nondegenerated myoma (*arrows*) can be clearly distinguished from the normal myometrium by its homogeneous low signal intensity. The endometrial cavity (*small arrows*) is flattened by the mass effect of the myoma. Note also the high signal intensity Bartholin cyst in the labia majora (*open arrow*)

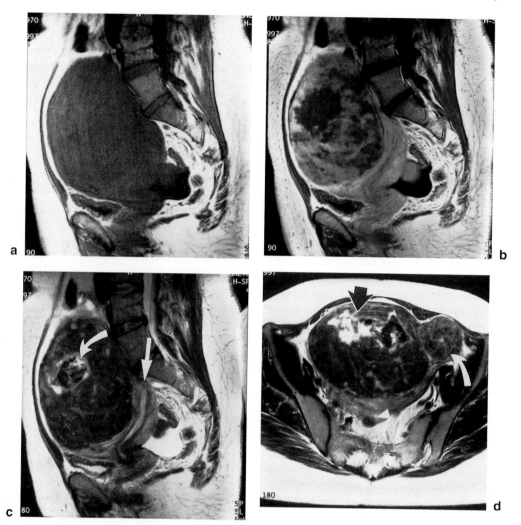

Fig. 19.17 a–d. Degenerative intramural leiomyoma. **a** On the sagittal T1-weighted SE image the uterus is markedly enlarged but the leiomyoma cannot be readily delineated due to low contrast. **b** After administration of a contrast agent (gadolinium chelate) a large well-defined mass, originating from the anterior uterine wall, can be delineated. Viable parts of the leiomyoma display heterogeneous enhancement, whereas necrotic areas do not enhance. **c** On the corresponding T2-weighted FSE image the leiomyoma displays predominantly low signal intensity. In the area of degeneration and necrosis, areas of high signal intensity can be appreciated (*curved arrow*). The tumor can be clearly delineated from the vertically oriented uterus (*arrow*). **d** The axial T2-weighted FSE image shows the large leiomyoma with central degeneration and necrosis (*arrow*), an adjacent intermediate (*curved arrow*), and a small nondegenerative leiomyoma (*arrowhead*) in a subserosal location of the posterior uterine wall

Degenerative leiomyomas demonstrate variable signal intensity and internal structure. On T2-weighted images, areas of degeneration are displayed with heterogeneous high signal intensity (Fig. 19.17). On T1-weighted images, they demonstrate inhomogeneous medium or high signal intensity. The type of degeneration, however, cannot be determined by MR imaging.

Necrotic areas ("red degeneration") may have variable signal intensity on either T1- or T2-weighted images, depending on the time of infarction (Togashi et al. 1989a). Calcification appears with low signal intensity on all kinds of sequences. A peripheral high signal intensity rim on T2-weighted images has been reported due to dilated vessels, lymphatics, or edema (Mittl et al. 1991).

Magnetic resonance imaging cannot reliably differentiate between leiomyomas and leiomyosarcomas. Both lesions may appear as heterogeneous masses with variable signal intensities.

Enhancement after administration of gadolinium chelates varies depending on the degree of cellularity and vascularization. Neither the detection rate nor the characterization of leiomyomas can be improved by contrast administration (HRICAK et al. 1992). However, contrast enhancement may assist the evaluation of patients who are candidates for treatment with gonadotropin-releasing hormone analogs.

Most leiomyomas are detected clinically and US is often used as a supplement to the gynecologic examination. However, US is normal in up to 22% of women with proven leiomyomas (GROSS et al. 1983). CT is not considered as a primary imaging modality for the diagnosis of leiomyoma due to very limited contrast between the lesion and uterine wall. MR imaging is the most accurate imaging modality in the assessment of leiomyoma (HRICAK et al. 1986a, 1992; ZAWIN et al. 1990; WEINREB et al. 1990; DUDIAK et al. 1988). It has a sensitivity of 92% in depicting leiomyomas as small as 5 mm and is particularly helpful in patients who are obese or in women with a retroverted uterus because US can be indeterminate. Its high specificity, especially in differentiating leiomyoma from adenomyosis, is another important advantage. Therefore, MR imaging is indicated when US is inconclusive or limited, in the search for submucosal lesions in infertile patients, for characterization of leiomyomas in the pretreatment situation, when myomectomy is planned, and in the evaluation and follow-up of patients treated with hormone analog treatment.

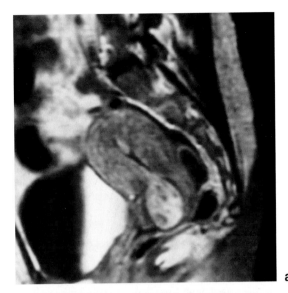

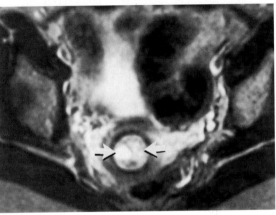

Fig. 19.18 a,b. Endometrial polyp. a Sagittal T1-weighted SE image after intravenous administration of gadolinium, showing a mass with heterogeneous enhancement prolapsing from the endometrial cavity into the cervical canal. b The axial T2-weighted SE image displays the widened endocervical canal with a heterogeneous high signal intensity mass (*arrows*), indicating degeneration in the endometrial polyp. (Courtesy of Hedvig Hricak, MD, San Francisco)

19.4.2.3
Endometrial Hyperplasia and Endometrial Polyps

Endometrial hyperplasia occurs secondary to the influence of unopposed estrogen. The endometrium thickens and becomes pseudopolypoid. In mild cases the pseudopolyps are microscopic but they may become as large as 5 cm in more severe cases. These hyperplastic endometrial projections may be sessile or pedunculated and most often arise from the uterine fundus or cornua. About 80% are found in women between 30 and 60 years of age and 10%–30% in patients with endometrial carcinoma. However, malignant changes are found only rarely in polyps (SCULLY 1982).

MR Imaging. Endometrial polyps display intermediate signal intensity on T1-weighted images and high signal intensity on T2-weighted images (Fig. 19.18). Therefore, they may be difficult to delineate from normal endometrium unless their signal on T2-weighted images is somewhat lower. In these cases, endometrial widening may be the only finding. As polyps enhance after gadolinium administration, their detection may be facilitated on postcontrast scans.

19.4.2.4
Gestational Trophoblastic Disease

Gestational trophoblastic disease encompasses a spectrum of tumors arising from placental villous tissue and ranging from the benign hydatidiform mole to the most malignant choriocarcinoma (BREWER et al. 1979; HAMMOND and PARKER 1970). The most sensitive laboratory marker is the elevation of human chorionic gonadotropin (HCG), which is not only useful for diagnosis but also for assessing response to treatment. Clinical symptoms mimic early pregnancy with hyperemesis, enlargement of the uterus, pain, and vaginal bleeding.

MR Imaging. A typical finding is the enlargement of the uterus by a heterogeneous mass that obliterates the uterine zonal anatomy usually seen on T2-weighted images and that may contain foci of hemorrhage and necrosis (Fig. 19.19). The mass is often hypervascular, displaying tortuous dilated vessels within the tumor and the adjacent myometrium. On T1-weighted images, the tumor may be either isointense to the adjacent myometrium or hyperintense when intralesional hemorrhage has occurred. Areas of necrosis demonstrate low to intermediate signal intensity on T1-weighted and high signal intensity on T2-weighted images (HRICAK et al. 1986a; BARTON et al. 1993). After intravenous application of gadolinium chelates the involved myometrium enhances and necrosis can be better differentiated from hypervascular tumor. After treatment with curettage and/or chemotherapy, there is usually a return of the uterus toward normal size and zonal anatomy. Recurrent tumor after therapy is characterized by similar features as the primary tumor, including heterogeneous high signal intensity and prominent vasculature.

19.4.2.5
Endometrial Carcinoma

Endometrial carcinoma is the most common gynecologic malignancy and accounts for approximately 7% of all cancers in women (American Cancer Society 1994). Most patients are postmenopausal and present in the sixth decade; however, up to 5% of tumors occur under the age of 40. Risk factors include nulliparity, positive family history, hypertension, and endocrine and metabolic disorders such as obesity, diabetes mellitus, and particularly the influence of unopposed estrogens. The latter may be administered as medication or produced endogenously either in the ovaries or by conversion of adrenal androstenedione.

About 85% of endometrial carcinomas are adenocarcinomas, and 15% contain squamous elements; less than 5% of endometrial malignancies are uterine sarcomas. Tumors may occur localized with a polypoid or exophytic character and only superficial attachment to the endometrium. Most endometrial carcinomas, however, grow diffusely and demostrate extensive invasion of the entire endometrium. Dif-

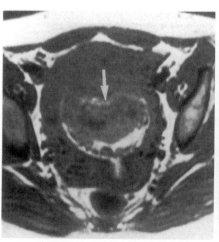 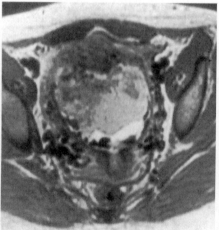 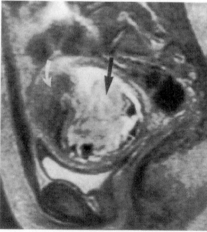

a   b, c

Fig. 19.19 a–c. Gestational trophoblastic disease (primary molar disease). **a** Axial T1-weighted MR image showing molar tissue (*arrow*) surrounded by blood in the endometrial canal. **b** T2-weighted MR image showing some increase in the signal intensity of molar tissue and increased adnexal and uterine vascularity. **c** The sagittal T2-weighted MR image demonstrates the tissue (*straight arrow*) and a contiguous hypointense area in the myometrium (*curved arrow*) (From Barton et al. 1993 with permission)

fuse tumor may then spread through the myometrium of the corpus and cervix and extend outside the uterus towards adjacent organs. Lymphatic spread is to the pelvic, para-aortic, and inguinal nodes. Distant metastases are found most often in the peritoneum, lung, liver, and supraclavicular lymph nodes.

The prognosis depends mainly on the depth of myometrial invasion, the presence and extension of lymph node metastases, and the histologic grading of the tumor. The incidence of lymphadenopathy is strongly related to the depth of myometrial invasion. Only 5% of patients with superficial myometrial invasion will have positive lymph nodes, as compared with up to 40% of patients with deep invasion (BORONOW et al. 1984).

Clinically, the most common symptom of endometrial carcinoma is abnormal uterine bleeding. Especially the onset of unexpected bleeding or spotting in postmentopausal women is suspicious and leads most patients to a prompt gynecologic examination. If the tumor secondarily obstructs the endocervical canal, hematometra or pyometra may occur.

Treatment of early (stage I) endometrial cancer consists of hysterectomy and lymphadenectomy, with or without radiotherapy. In more advanced stages radiation therapy may be preferred over surgery or may precede surgery.

19.4.2.5.1
CLINICAL STAGING

The clinical staging of endometrial cancer classically includes physical examination and fractional dilatation und curettage. A tissue sample from the endometrium is absolutely necessary to prove the diagnosis, and careful histopathologic examination of the curettage samples may give an indication for the presence of myometrial invasion. The depth of myometrial invasion, however, cannot be estimated by clinical investigation.

Extrauterine spread may be detected by the bimanual gynecologic examination, particularly when performed during anesthesia. Lymph node involvement, however, usually cannot be successfully assessed by clinical means. Hysteroscopy, used as an adjunct to physical examination, is being investigated as a staging technique. Clinical examinations may be supplemented by intravenous pyelography, barium enema, cystoscopy, and rectosigmoidoscopy, when the physical findings suggest possible involvement of the bladder or rectum or to rule out the presence of primary conditions of the

Table 19.3. Staging systems for endometrial neoplasms

TNM	Uterus	FIGO
T1	Tumor limited to corpus uteri	I
T1a	Tumor limited to endometrium	IA
T1b	Invasion less than or equal to half of the myometrium	IB
T1c	Invasion greater than half of the myometrium	IC
T2	Invasion of cervix but not beyond uterus	II
T2a	Endocervical glandular involvement	IIA
T2b	Cervical stromal invasion	IIB
T3 and/or N1	Local and/or regional spread	III
T3a	Tumor involves the serosa and/or adnexa and/or positive peritoneal cytology	IIIA
T3b	Vaginal involvement	IIIB
N1	Metastatic pelvic and/or para-aortic lymph nodes	IIIC
T4	Invades bladder and/or bowel mucosa	IV
M1	Distant metastases	IVB

urinary or gastrointestinal tract that may complicate therapy.

Clinical staging according to the system of the Federation Internationale de Gynécologie et d'Obstétrique (FIGO) is known to understage the disease in about 20% of cases, primarily due to the inability to evaluate the depth of myometrial invasion, intraperitoneal implants, and nodal and adnexal metastases. Therefore, a surgical FIGO staging system, which is equivalent to the TNM classification system, has been proposed (Table 19.3).

19.4.2.5.2
MR IMAGING

MR imaging is currently the most accurate pretherapeutic modality in staging histologically proven endometrial carcinoma as it not only allows for a reliable prediction of the depth of myometrial invasion, but also provides the highest accuracy in the detection of extrauterine extension and lymph node involvement. The MR appearance of endometrial carcinoma is nonspecific and may vary with individual tumor types and stages. The signal behavior of small tumors confined to the endometrium may be similar to the signal intensity of normal endometrium (HRICAK et al. 1987, 1991b; BELLONI et al. 1990). However, most often these tumors present on

T2-weighted images with decreased signal intensity compared with normal endometrium (Fig. 19.20c). It must be noted that these findings are not specific for endometrial carcinoma but may also occur in a similar fashion in other conditions such as endometrial polyps, adenomatous hyperplasia, and blood clots. HRICAK et al. (1991b) reported that in 81% of patients with endometrial carcinoma an abnormality within the uterine cavity was found. Endometrial carcinoma infiltrating the myometrium is usually characterized by regions of increased signal intensity within the low signal intensity of the junctional zone or within the outer myometrium.

Beside T2-weighted images in the sagittal and axial planes, optimal MR imaging requires gadolinium-enhanced dynamic studies (Figs. 19.20–19.22). Small tumors are better detected on early contrast-enhanced series due to increased contrast against normal endometrium. Compared with normal myometrium, endometrial carcinoma may be displayed with lesser or greater enhancement depending on the tumor vascularity and biology. Therefore, contrast-enhanced imaging is often very useful in determining the depth of myometrial invasion (YAMASHITA et al. 1993a,b; SIRONI et al. 1992b) (Figs. 19.20–19.22). In addition, contrast-enhanced imaging allows differentiation of viable tumor from necrosis or fluid.

The staging accuracies reported for stage I endometrial carcinoma range from 74% to 95%, with understaging primarily due to the presence of microinvasion (YAMASHITA et al. 1993a; SIRONI et al. 1992a; HRICAK et al. 1991b; CHEN et al. 1990; GORDON et al. 1989). The accuracy in differentiating tumors confined to the uterus from those extending outside the uterus was found to be 96%, with a sensitivity of 100% and a specificity of 71% (HRICAK et al. 1987).

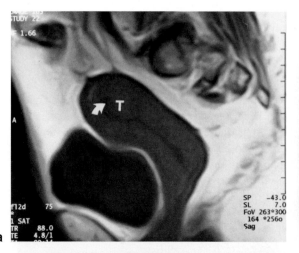

a

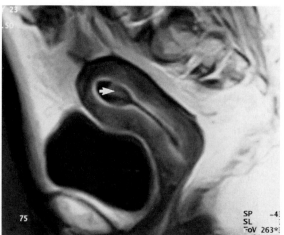

b

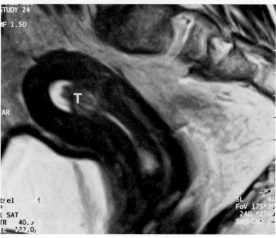

c

Fig. 19.20 a–c. Endometrial carcinoma stage FIGO IA (pT1a). Preoperative staging diagnosis was correctly established from dynamic contrast-enhanced MR imaging. a Sagittal T1-weighted GRE image: the tumor (*T*) cannot be distinguished by its intermediate signal intensity from the normal myometrium. Fluid and debris (*arrow*) within the uterine cavity are displayed with slightly lower signal intensity. b Sagittal T1-weighted GRE image from a dynamic contrast-enhanced sequence 75 s after intravenous administration of a gadolinium chelate: the carcinoma (*arrow*) is confined to the endometrial cavity and is clearly delineated from the strongly enhancing inner layer of the myometrium by its mild contrast uptake. In addition, there is clear delineation of the nonenhancing fluid and debris. c Sagittal T2-weighted FSE image: the tumor (*T*) displays intermediate signal intensity with good contrast in relation to the high signal intensity fluid and debris. The contrast between tumor and myometrium, however, is poor

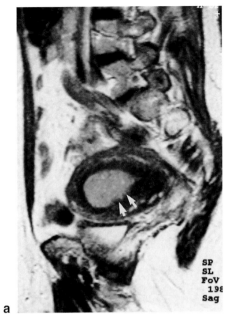
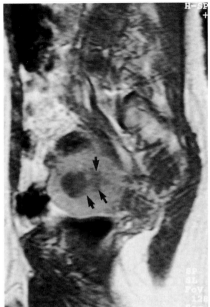

Fig. 19.21 a,b. Endometrial carcinoma stage FIGO IB (pT1b). **a** Sagittal T2-weighted FSE image showing increased thickness and intermediate signal intensity of the endometrial cavity and an irregular interface between endometrium and myometrium (*arrows*). **b** The corresponding sagittal T1- weighted GRE image 95 s after intravenous administration of gadolinium confirms the finding of an irregular endometrium/myometrium interface (*arrows*), indicating infiltration of the inner half of myometrium

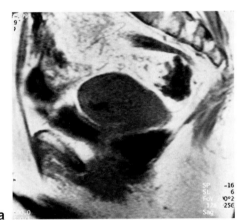
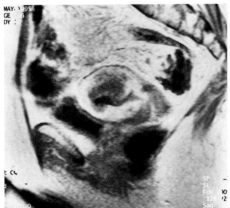

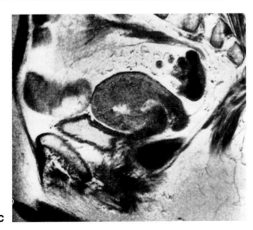

Fig. 19.22 a–c. Endometrial carcinoma stage FIGO IC (pT1c). **a** Sagittal T1-weighted GRE image shows an irregular internal structure of the uterus but the tumor extension within the corpus cannot be appreciated. Note the smooth outer contour of the uterus, indicating a tumor confined to the organ. **b** Sagittal T1-weighted GRE image 75 s post intravenous gadolinium administration: tumor infiltrating the inner and outer layer of the myometrium displays considerably less enhancement than normal myometrium. **c** Sagittal T2-weighted FSE image: compared with the contrast-enhanced T1-weighted image in **b** the delineation of tumor is considerably limited. Note the normal low signal intensity of the cervical stroma

19.4.2.5.3
STAGING WITH MR IMAGING

The MR staging of endometrial carcinoma follows the surgical FIGO staging system considering myometrial, extrauterine, and lymph node involvement.

Stage I. Endometrial carcinoma confined to the uterine corpus is classified as stage I. This group is further subdivided depending on the degree of invasiveness:

In *stage Ia.* the tumor is limited to the endometrium and may be delineated by its heterogeneous and lower signal intensity on T2-weighted images. In some cases only indirect signs such as increased thickness or lobulation of the endometrial cavity may be present. On T1-weighted dynamic contrast-enhanced series, the tumor displays in most cases a different enhancement pattern than normal endometrium and therefore may be better delineated than with T2-weighted images (Fig. 19.20). The most important criterion for stage Ia tumors is a completely intact junctional zone, or a sharp tumor – myometrium interface in patients with an indistinct junctional zone due to aging changes. An indistinct junctional zone in a postmenopausal woman alone must be considered with great caution to prevent overinterpretation.

Stage Ib endometrial carcinoma is defined by infiltration of the inner half of the myometrium. On MR imaging the most reliable indicator of myometrial invasion is disruption of the junctional zone. This sign, an irregular interface between endometrium and myometrium and/or abnormal signal intensity extending into the inner half of the myometrium, can be found in stage Ib disease (Fig. 19.21). Dynamic gadolinium-enhanced sequences in general have shown more reliable results than T2-weighted images in differentiating tumors of stage Ia and b from those with deep myometrial invasion (HRICAK et al. 1991b; ITO et al. 1994; YAMASHITA et al. 1993a; SIRONI et al. 1992a), with accuracy values ranging between 88% and 91%. However, in one study using nonenhanced images only, the accuracy was reported to be as high as 97% (HRICAK et al. 1987). The overall acuracy of MR imaging in staging endometrial carcinoma is 85% (HRICAK et al. 1991b). The gold standard for these data was pathologic sectioning, which may not always be completely reliable. In one study, cases were reported in which primary discrepancies between MR imaging and pathology after pathologic review subsequently showed agreement (SCOUTT et al. 1995).

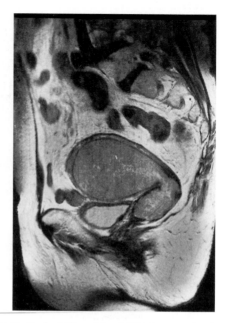

Fig. 19.23. Sagittal T2-weighted FSE image of endometrial carcinoma stage FIGO II (pT2). Expansively growing tumor mass of intermediate signal intensity in the uterine corpus, extending into the cervical stroma

Stage Ic endometrial carcinoma is characterized by invasion of the outer half of the myometrium. On T2-weighted images, the high signal intensity of tumor is seen in the deep layer of low signal intensity myometrium. On T1-weighted contrast-enhanced images the tumor is displayed in most cases with higher signal intensity than myometrium, but it may also present with lower signal intensity (Fig. 19.22).

Stage II. In this stage of endometrial cancer the tumor infiltrates the cervix but is limited to the uterus. Cervical involvement is most accurately diagnosed with T1-weighted dynamic gadolinium-enhanced sequences, which sensitively indicate tumor extension to the cervix and allow differentiation of viable tumor and debris. T2-weighted images are sensitive in tumor detection (Fig. 19.23) but less reliable in differentiating tumor from hemorrhage and debris.

Stage III. Stage III describes extrauterine tumor spread within the true pelvis but not invading the rectum and urinary bladder. In stage *IIIa* the tumor involves the serosa and/or adnexae and/or peritoneum (Fig. 19.24); in stage *IIIb* there is vaginal involvement. Usually, these findings can already be demonstrated on sagittal and axial T2-weighted images, and in most cases contrast-enhanced images do not improve staging accuracy.

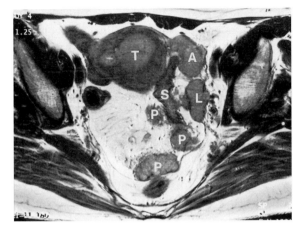

Fig. 19.24. Axial T2-weighted FSE image of endometrial carcinoma stage FIGO IIIC (pT3aN1). The tumor (*T*) displays intermediate signal intensity and involves the uterine corpus and left adnexa (*A*). In addition, there are lymph node (*L*) and peritoneal (*P*) metastases. *S*, Sigmoid

Stage IV. The disease involves the rectum and/or bladder or extends outside the true pelvis. The bladder and rectum are considered to be infiltrated when their wall demonstrates focal loss of low signal intensity on T2-weighted images.

Lymph node evaluation. Lymphatic spread primarily involves the pelvic nodes, later the para-aotic nodes, and rarely the inguinal nodes. As with cervical carcinoma, signal intensity is not reliable in differentiating benign (hyperplastic) and malignant nodes. Therefore, MR imaging relies on the size of lymph nodes, with most papers suggesting a transaxial diameter of 1.0 cm as a threshold for tumor involvement.

19.4.2.5.4
RECURRENT ENDOMETRIAL CARCINOMA

Recurrent endometrial carcinoma occurs in 70% of cases within the first 3 years after primary treatment. In patients who have not received radiation therapy, recurrence is most often seen in the pelvic side wall, in the vaginal apex, or in retained parametrium. After radiation therapy of the pelvis, recurrence is less likely to occur within the pelvis but rather in the abdomen, liver, lung, and skeleton.

On MR images, recurrent endometrial cancer appears with intermediate signal on T1-weighted images and high signal intensity on T2-weighted images. Recurrence can be differentiated from long-standing (≥1 year) radiation fibrosis, which is typically of low signal intensity on T2-weighted images.

However, differentiation of recurrent tumor from early radiation changes (granulation tissue) and inflammatory diseases may be impossible.

19.4.3
Diseases of the Uterine Cervix

19.4.3.1
Cervical Stenosis

Narrowing of the endocervical canal may occur in obstructing tumors, in senile atrophy, after infection, after radiation therapy, or as a result of interventions such as conization, cauterization, or cryosurgery.

MR Imaging. Benign cervical stenosis can be identified and located on sagittal or axial T2-weighted MR images. When the stenosis is secondary to obstructing tumor, the uterus is more frequently distended by retained uterine secretions, hematometra, or pyometra as in benign underlying disease. Depending on the quality of retention, the signal intensity of the uterine cavity varies. On T2-weighted scans, serous content images with very high signal intensity, whereas retentions with high protein or blood content display less signal intensity. In contrast, hemorrhagic or proteinaceous retentions may be identified by virtue of their increased signal intensity on T1-weighted images as compared with serous fluid.

19.4.3.2
Cervical Incompetence

Incompetence of the cervix may be congenital, associated with malformations of the uterus, or caused by low collagen content of the cervix, previous obstetric trauma, or multiple gestations (ANSARI and REYNOLDS 1987).

MR Imaging. As described by HRICAK et al. (1990), four MR imaging characteristics, which may occur alone or in combination, are suggestive of cervical incompetence: (a) the endocervical canal is shortened to less than 3 cm; (b) the width of the internal os is increased to more than 4 mm; (c) the endocervical canal is widened asymmetrically in association with normal or abnormally thin cervical stroma; and (d) the signal characteristics of the cervix have changed towards higher signal intensity.

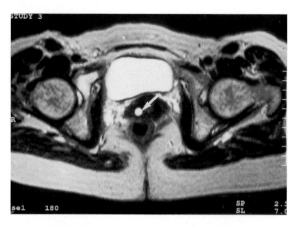

Fig. 19.25. Nabothian cyst. On the axial T2-weighted FSE image a well-defined 7-mm cystic lesion (*arrow*) is displayed with high signal intensity in the cervical stroma adjacent to the endocervical canal

19.4.3.3
Nabothian Cysts

Nabothian cysts are a common gynecologic finding caused by retention of mucus within the endocervical glands and clefts. The cysts are typically a few millimeters in size, rarely symptomatic, and usually require no treatment.

MR Imaging. Nabothian cysts are easily identified on sagittal or axial T2-weighted images as small foci of fluid-isointense high signal intensity within the cervix (Fig. 19.25). High signal intensity, small size, and well-defined margins allow differentiation of nabothian cysts from solid cervical neoplasms. They can also be distinguished from Gartner's duct cysts, which appear as tubular cystic structures in the upper vagina and less frequently within the uterine wall. Occasionally, nabothian cysts may become as large as 2–4 cm and mimic a cystic adnexal or perineal mass. Difficulties may occur in the differential diagnosis from small foci of cervical endometriosis or postbiopsy changes.

19.4.3.4
Cervical Carcinoma

Carcinoma of the cervix is the third most common malignant gynecologic tumor (after endometrial and ovarian cancer) (American Cancer Society 1994). It occurs more frequently in younger women of low socioeconomic standing. The average age at diagno-sis is about 50 years, with peaks at 38 and 62 years. Risk factors include early age at first intercourse, a high number of sexual partners, multiparity, cervical dysplasia, and a history of sexually transmitted diseases. Currently, strong evidence is suggesting human papillomavirus as a main cause of cervical carcinoma.

Carcinoma arises at the squamocolumnar junction which is located exocervically in young females. In these individuals cervical carcinoma grows predominantly exophytically and large parts of the tumor extend inferiorly into the vagina. In older women with atrophic cervices, however, the squamocolumnar junction is located in the endocervical canal. Tumors occurring inside the endocervical canal account for approximately 20% of cervical carcinomas, more commonly involve the supravaginal portion of the cervix, and frequently extend laterally through the cervical wall.

Two main histologic types of cervical carcinoma can be differentiated: squamous cell carcinoma, which accounts for 80%–90% of cases, and adenocarcinoma, which carries the worst prognosis. Other important prognostic factors are the volume and histologic grade of tumor, the location within the cervix (exo- versus endocervix), the depth of stromal invasion, adjacent tissue extension, and lymph node involvement at the time of treatment.

Clinically, the leading symptoms of cervical carcinoma are bleeding and vaginal discharge. Physical pelvic examination commonly reveals a more or less necrotic and bleeding tumor; in a number of patients, however, speculum examination may reveal a normal cervix when the carcioma is occult. In these cases, detection of cervical carcinoma is often based on exfoliative cytology (Papanicolaou smear). In cases with a grossly visible mass the definite diagnosis is made with biopsy. The main clinical information about local tumor spread is provided by the bimanual vaginal and rectal examination.

19.4.3.4.1
CLINICAL STAGING
The classical staging of cervical carcinoma is clinical and uses the FIGO classification (Table 19.4). The TNM staging classification is essentially based on the same criteria as the FIGO system (Table 19.4). In addition to the standard physical examination, FIGO staging may include examination under anesthesia, cystoscopy, rectosigmoidoscopy, barium enema, biopsy, intravenous pyelography, and chest radiogra-

Table 19.4. Staging systems for cervical neoplasms

TNM			Cervix	FIGO
T1			Limited to uterus	I
	T1a		Preclinical invasive carcinoma	IA
		T1a1	Depth ≤3 mm, horizontal spread ≤7 mm	IA1
		T1a2	Depth 3–5 mm, horizontal spread ≤7 mm	IA2
	T1b		Tumor greater than T1a2	IB
T2			Beyond uterus but not to pelvic side wall or lower third of vagina	II
	T2a		No parametrial invasion	IIA
	T2b		With parametrial invasion	IIB
T3			Extends to the pelvic wall and/or involves lower third of the vagina and/or hydronephrosis	III
	T3a		Lower third of vagina, not to pelvic side wall	IIIA
	T3b		Pelvic side wall and/or hydronephrosis	IIIB
T4			Tumor invades bladder mucosa or rectum; beyond true pelvis	IVA
M1			Distant metastasis	IVB

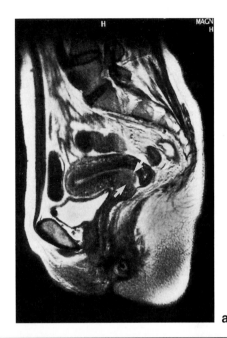

a

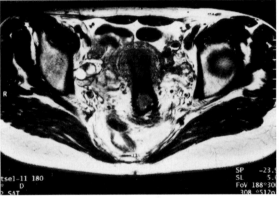

b

Fig. 19.26 a,b. Cervical carcinoma stage FIGO IB (pT1b). **a** On the sagittal T2-weighted FSE image tumor of intermediate to low signal intensity is demonstrated in the endocervical canal and anterior wall of the cervix (*arrows*). **b** The axial T2-weighted FSE image displays a 1.8-cm tumor in endocervical location. The intact low signal intensity stroma on both sides of the tumor indicates that the tumor is limited to the cervix. Note the high signal intensity of normal parametria

phy. However, when compared with intraoperative and pathologic findings, clinical staging shows errors in 20%–35% of cases, depending on the stage of disease (COBBY et al. 1990; KIM et al. 1990; CHUNG et al. 1981; HRICAK et al. 1996). In addition, up to 25% of patients have metastases to the locoregional pelvic or to the para-aortic lymph nodes that cannot be detected by clinical examination. Moreover, extension to the bladder or adjacent bowel is difficult to define by clinical means.

Accurate imaging evaluation of carcinoma of the cervix is, therefore, of paramount importance to determine which patients are potential candidates for radical hysterectomy and which have to be treated conservatively. The accuracy of CT in staging cervical carcinoma, however, is limited. In identifying parametrial involvement, CT has an accuracy of 55%–70% and the overall staging accuracy is as low as 45%–63% (ZAPF et al. 1988; KIM et al. 1990; SUBAK et al. 1995).

19.4.3.4.2
MR IMAGING

MR imaging performed at high field strengths is the most reliable pretherapeutic modality for the detection or exclusion of parametrial spread, overall tumor staging, and lymph node assessment (TOGASHI et al. 1989b; KIM et al. 1990; COBBY et al.

1990; SIRONI et al. 1991; LIEN et al. 1991a; GRECO et al. 1989; SCHEIDLER et al. 1998; HEUCK et al. 1997). Therefore, MR imaging plays a most important role in selecting patients for surgery or radiation therapy.

Cervical cancer appears as a relatively hyperintense mass on T2-weighted imaging, and is easily distinguishable from the normal low signal intensity cervical stroma (Figs. 19.26–19.28). As has been

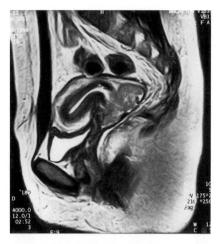

Fig. 19.27. Cervical carcinoma stage FIGO IIA (pT2a), sagittal T2-weighted FSE image. Large exophytic tumor of intermediate signal intensity infiltrating the cervical stroma, protruding into the vaginal lumen and infiltrating the upper third of the anterior vaginal wall

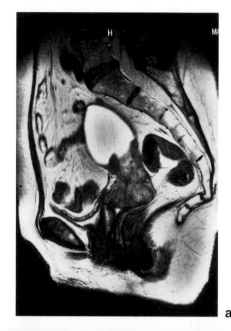

a

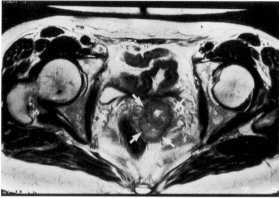

b

Fig. 19.28 a,b. Cervical carcinoma stage FIGO IIA (pT2a) with obstruction of the endocervical canal and fluid retention in the uterine body. **a** Sagittal T2-weighted FSE image showing tumor of intermediate signal intensity extending from the internal to the external os. Note the distended corpus uteri with high signal intensity of fluid in its cavity. **b** The axial T2-weighted FSE image displays the intermediate signal intensity of tumor infiltrating all cervical stroma but a small low signal intensity stromal rim (*arrows*): no parametrial involvement is noted

demonstrated by histopathologic correlation, the location and size of invasive tumor can be accurately determined even in clinically problematic lesions (HRICAK et al. 1988; TOGASHI 1989; LIEN et al. 1991; SIRONI et al. 1991; HEUCK et al. 1994; SCHEIDLER et al. 1998). The accuracy in determining the depth of stromal invasion is also high (about 80%) (KIM et al. 1990, 1993). Preinvasive disease, however, usually cannot be identified with MR imaging.

Parametrial invasion can be diagnosed when tumor extends through the entirety of the low signal intensity cervical stroma into the parametrium. If parametrial spread is subtle, it is more difficult to diagnose than in cases where a mass of similar signal intensity to the cervical tumor is found. Overall, in the assessment of parametrial invasion, MR imaging has an accuracy of 86%–92% (SCHEIDLER et al. 1998; KIM et al. 1990, 1993).

Intravenous administration of gadolinium chelates allows distinction between viable tumor and areas of necrosis; however, as contrast enhancement may render the tumor isointense to the surrounding cervical and parametrial tissue, it has not been shown to increase diagnostic performance in tumor depiction, in the definition of the depth of stromal invasion, or in the evaluation of early parametrial involvement. Nevertheless, contrast-enhanced imaging is helpful in the evaluation of tumor extension to the pelvic side wall or into adjacent organs such as the rectum or urinary bladder.

19.4.3.4.3

STAGING WITH MR IMAGING

The role of MR imaging in the diagnostic workup of cervical carcinoma is not to prove the presence of tumor, which is accomplished by biopsy or exfoliative cytology, but to exactly define the tumor extension in order to select the appropriate method of treatment.

Stage I. Stage I tumors are confined to the uterus. Preclinical invasive stage Ia tumors are characterized by either microsopic stromal invasion (stage Ia1) or macroscopic spread of ≤7 mm in the horizontal dimension or stromal invasion of ≤5 mm (stage Ia2). Many stage Ia tumors are not depicted on MR images due to their small size. Therefore, the cervical stroma appears widely normal on T2-weighted images, with a low signal intensity ring structure on axial scans.

In stage Ib carcinoma the tumor can be detected by the increased signal intensity remaining within the cervical ring (Fig. 19.26). In addition to the tumor size, the depth of invasion can be determined. In partial stromal invasion the uninvolved cervical tissue is demonstrated on T2-weighted images as a hypointense peripheral stripe. The presence of this stripe with a thickness of ≥3 mm is a very specific parameter (specificity 96%–99%) for the exclusion of parametrial invasion (HRICAK et al. 1988a; TOGASHI et al. 1989a; LIEN et al. 1991a; SIRONI et al. 1991; KIM et al. 1990, 1993; VANZULLI et al. 1994). Complete disruption of the low signal intensity cervical ring indicates full-thickness stromal involvement. In this situation, the exclusion of parametrial involvement is more difficult (VANZULLI et al. 1994). However, when the vaginal fornices are intact, the tumor is likely confined to the cervix.

Stage II. In stage II the tumor grows beyond the uterus but does not infiltrate the pelvic side wall or the lower third of the vagina.

Stage IIa tumors are characterized by infiltration of the upper vagina (less than two-thirds) in the absence of parametrial invasion (Figs. 19.27, 19.28). Vaginal infiltration is indicated by loss of normal low signal intensity or hyperintense thickening of the vagina. The sensitivity of MR imaging in the depiction of vaginal invasion is as high as 93% (HRICAK et al. 1988a).

Parametrial infiltration classifies the tumor as stage IIb cervical carcinoma. The infiltration occurs by direct spread from tumor of the endocervix or from tumor of the exocervix extending to the upper cervical canal or lower uterine body. In most cases with parametrial involvement, full-thickness stromal invasion is present. Confirmatory findings of parametrial invasion consist of small tumor extensions beyond the cervical contour or a tumor mass protruding into the parametrial space (Fig. 19.29). Microscopic parametrial invasion may be found in cases with broad full-thickness infiltration of the supravaginal cervix even when no paracervical tumor is found on MR images.

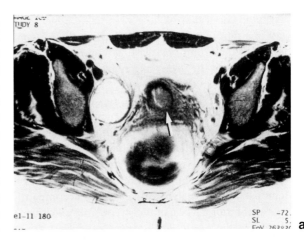

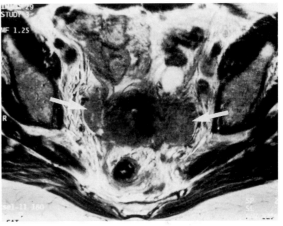

Fig. 19.29 a,b. Parametrial involvement in cervical carcinoma. **a** Axial T2-weighted FSE image of a stage FIGO IIB (pT2b) carcinoma. Note that there is posterior disruption of the low signal intensity cervical stroma (*arrow*) and infiltration of the parametria. **b** Axial T2-weighted FSE image of an advanced cervical carcinoma. There are bilateral tumor masses of intermediate signal intensity extending into the parametria (*arrows*)

Stage III. Stage III cervical carcinomas extend to the pelvic side wall, involve the lower third of the vagina, and/or cause hydronephrosis.

Involvement of the lower third of the vagina, consistent with stage IIIa, is indicated by the loss of normal hypointensity and thickening of the vaginal wall in its distal part. Commonly tumor spreads in continuity from the upper two-thirds to the lower third of the vagina.

Pelvic side wall extension (stage IIIb) is confirmed when solid tumor extends to either the pelvic musculature or the iliac vessels. However, fine strands of tissue between the tumor and pelvic muscles, even in the presence of fat tissue or the complete loss of parametrial high signal intensity associated with disrupted cervical stroma, may indicate pelvic side wall invasion (Togashi 1993). Hydronephrosis can be diagnosed if tumor is encasing the ureter, leading to dilatation of the ureter and renal pelvis.

Stage IV. If cervical carcinoma invades the bladder mucosa or rectum it is consistent with stage IV.

When the bladder is involved, the low signal intensity of normal muscular bladder wall on T2-weighted images is replaced by higher signal intensity tumor tissue (Fig. 19.30). Bullous edema may be demonstrated by a hyperintense band accompanying the interior surface of the (frequently disrupted) bladder wall.

Direct infiltration of the rectum is rarely found, probably because the rectum is separated from the posterior vaginal fornix by the pouch of Douglas. More frequently rectal involvement occurs by tumor spread along the uterosacral ligaments. Rectal invasion can be identified by segmental thickening and loss of low signal intensity of the anterior rectal wall, or by prominent strands between the main tumor bulk and the rectum.

Lymph Node Evaluation. Cervical carcinoma spreads to the parametrial lymph nodes first, followed by the obturator nodes and the internal and external iliac lymph node chains (Fig. 19.31). Signal intensity is not helpful in differentiating between benign and malignant nodes. Therefore, as in CT, the determination of metastatic infiltration of lymph nodes by MR imaging is based on their size. The size criteria for metastatic lymph nodes is currently under debate. Most authors have used a diameter of >1 cm as the threshold for metastatic lymph node involvement, achieving accuracy rates between 75% and 88% (Dooms et al. 1984; Kim et al. 1990; Togashi et al. 1989b; Zapf et al. 1988). With a minimal axial diameter of >1 cm as a sign of lymph node metastasis, Kim et al. (1994) reported a sensitivity of 62% and a specificity of 98%, with a resulting

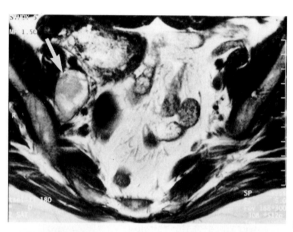

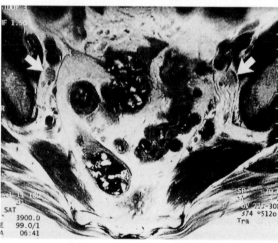

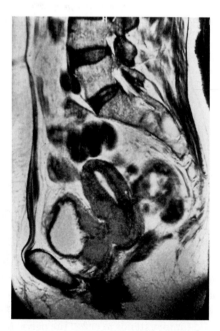

Fig. 19.30. Cervical carcinoma stage FIGO IV (T4). Intermediate signal intensity tumor has infiltrated the anterior walls of uterine body and vagina and has extended into the posterior bladder wall

Fig. 19.31 a,b. Pelvic lymph node metastases from cervical carcinoma. **a** Axial T2-weighted FSE image shows a metastatic lymph node of 3.3 × 3.5 cm in diameter posterior to the right external iliac vessels (*arrow*). **b** Axial T2-weighted FSE image of another patient displays one metastatic lymph node of less than 1 cm in diameter on each side (*arrows*) posterior to the external iliac vessels. (From Heuck et al. 1997)

accuracy of 93%. In a recent study utilizing high-resolution MR images obtained with a body phased-array coil and a threshold parameter of ≥8 mm for metastatic nodes, HEUCK et al. (1997) were able to achieve a sensitivity of 89% and a specificity of 91% in lymph node assessment.

19.4.3.4.4
RECURRENT CERVICAL CARCINOMA
VERSUS FIBROSIS

Recurrent cervical cancer may be found in up to 20% of cases. The presence of completely low signal intensity stroma around the endocervical canal and normal paracervical tissues excludes recurrence with a negative predictive value of 97% (HRICAK et al.

1993). A distinct mass of intermediate to high signal intensity on T2-weighted images is highly suspicious of recurrent tumor (positive predictive value 86%) (Fig. 19.32). One year or more after radiation or chemotherapy MR imaging greatly contributes to the distinction between residual or recurrent tumor and fibrosis (EBNER et al. 1988). In contrast to recurrent tumor, late fibrosis displays low signal intensity on T2-weighted images. However, early fibrosis, mainly containing granulation tissue with a high degree of vascularization, may be difficult or impossible to distinguish from residual or recurrent tumor, even if intravenous contrast medium is administered (EBNER et al. 1988, 1994).

19.4.4
Diseases of the Vagina

19.4.4.1
Anomalies of the Vagina

Congenital anomalies of the vagina include vaginal aplasia and atresia, vaginal duplication, and the presence of a vaginal septum. The normal vagina can be consistently visualized with MR imaging (HRICAK et al. 1988b). Vaginal agenesis may be partial or complete and is best displayed on T2-weighted images in sagittal and axial planes by the absence of normal vaginal musculature (Fig. 19.33). Vaginal duplication and septum are usually associated with other müllerian duct anomalies and can be clearly depicted on T2-weighted MR images (Fig. 19.9).

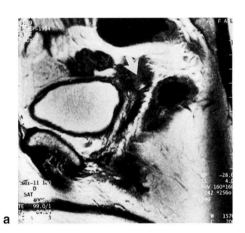
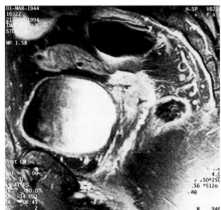

Fig. 19.32 a,b. Recurrent cervical carcinoma after radical hysterectomy. **a** Sagittal T2-weighted FSE image demonstrates a 3-cm mass at the upper end of the vagina, which, in part, displays intermediate signal intensity characteristic of cervical tumor (*arrow*). **b** Sagittal T1-weighted SE image with spectral fat suppression and after administration of a gadolinium contrast agent: the mass shows moderate contrast enhancement indicating viable tumor

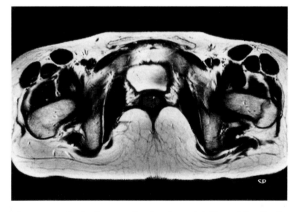

Fig. 19.33. Vaginal agenesis. On the axial T2-weighted FSE image the rectum (*R*) lies directly adjacent to the posterior wall of the urinary bladder (*B*). Note the absence of normal vaginal musculature between bladder and rectum

Fibrous bands at the introitus of the vagina and imperforate hymen are anomalies which commonly occur in isolation or may be associated with hydrocolpos or hydrometrocolpos. These accumulated secretions appear with low signal intensity on T1-weighted and high signal intensity on T2-weighted images; if they contain blood, they may be hyperintense on T1-weighted images.

Gartner duct cyst occurs along the wolffian duct remnant and is located anterolaterally within the vagina. Due to its proteinaceous content the cyst appears with high signal intensity on T1-weighted and medium to high signal intensity on T2-weighted images.

19.4.4.2
Bartholin's Cysts

Bartholin's cysts are located in the posterolateral parts of the lower vagina and the vulva, with diameters between a few millimeters and up to 5 cm. They are caused by retained secretions within the vulvovaginal glands and most commonly occur secondary to chronic inflammatory reactions or trauma. Usually the cysts are asymptomatic but they may cause considerable pain if they become infected ("bartholinitis").

MR imaging findings consist of low to intermediate signal intensity of retained fluid on T1-weighted and high signal intensity on T2-weighted images (Fig. 19.15). If the protein content is high, Bartholin's cysts may demonstrate high signal intensity on T1-weighted images. Infected cysts may display peripheral edema and/or contrast enhancement.

19.4.4.3
Vaginal Carcinoma

Vaginal carcinoma is a rare tumor accounting for less than 2% of gynecologic malignancies. The vast majority of vaginal cancers are adenocarcinomas. Clinical symptoms include pain, bleeding and discharge. The primary diagnosis of vaginal carcinoma is achieved clinically and histologically from biopsy.

MR Imaging and Staging. Due the high soft tissue contrast and multiplanar imaging capabilities MR imaging appears to be the most accurate imaging modality in the assessment of vaginal carcinoma. The MR imaging appearance of vaginal carcinoma is characterized by a high signal intensity mass on T2-

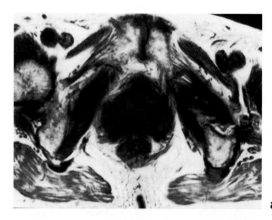

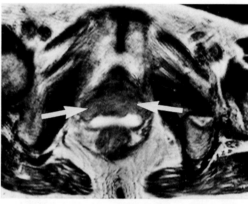

Fig. 19.34 a,b. Vaginal carcinoma. **a** The axial T1-weighted SE image shows a mass in the region of the lower third of the vagina. **b** On the corresponding T2-weighted FSE image there is a tumor of intermediate signal intensity (*arrows*) extending from the anterior wall of the vagina into the posterior wall of the urethra

weighted images that can be clearly differentiated from the normal low signal intensity of the vaginal wall (CHANG et al. 1988). Therefore the extent and location of vaginal carcinoma can be accurately assessed on T2-weighted scans while T1-weighted images are of limited value for tumor detection due to isointensity to normal vagina (Fig. 19.34). MR imaging findings, however, are not specific for vaginal carcinoma, and other tumors of the vagina may present similar findings.

Staging of vaginal carcinoma can be correlated to the clinical FIGO staging system or to the TNM classification system (Table 19.5):

Stage I tumor is confined to the vagina and displayed on T2-weighted images as a high signal intensity mass with a superficial location or with extensions of high signal intensity within the low signal intensity vaginal wall. The paravaginal fat

Table 19.5. Staging systems for vaginal cancer

TNM		FIGO
TX	Primary tumor cannot be assessed	
TO	No evidence of primary tumor	
Tis	Carcinoma in situ	0
T1	Tumor confined to vagina	I
T2	Tumor invades paravaginal tissues but does not extend to pelvic wall	II
T3	Tumor extends to pelvic wall	III
T4	Tumor invades mucosa of bladder or rectum and/or extends beyond true pelvis	IVA
M1	Distant metastasis	IVB

tissue appears to be distinct from the vagina and to have high signal intensity.

In stage II the tumor extends into surrounding tissue and the interface between fat and tumor is indistinct. The pelvic wall, bladder, and rectum are not involved.

Stage III vaginal carcinoma has reached the pelvic side wall and involves the obturator internus, piriformis, and/or levator ani muscles. In most cases the tumor extensions can be clearly indentified on MR images due to their contrast against fat and muscle tissues.

Stage IV tumors are characterized by infiltration of the bladder or rectum or by extension beyond the true pelvis. Infiltration of the bladder and rectum is indicated on T2-weighted images in sagittal and axial planes by disruption of the low signal intensity muscularis.

Sarcoma of the vagina is an extremely rare condition accounting for less than 0.4% of gynecologic tumors.

19.4.4.4
Secondary Tumors of the Vagina

Vaginal metastases are more common than primary vaginal carcinoma. Metastatic spread to the vagina most often results from carcinomas of the cervix, endometrium, or vulva. Rarely, metastases of other tumors, such as melanoma, breast cancer, or gastrointestinal tumors may be found.

MR Imaging. The appearance of vaginal metastases is very similar to that of vaginal carcinoma and cannot be reliably differentiated from the latter. There is even overlap with inflammatory processes involving the vagina. Metastasis of melanoma may display

high signal intensity on T1-weighted images due to paramagnetic contents of melanin.

The accuracy of MR imaging in the assessment of vaginal tumor spread has been reported to be as high as 92% (CHANG et al. 1988). In addition, MR imaging plays an important role in differentiating recurrent or metastatic tumor from radiation fibrosis in patients who have undergone radiation therapy. One year or longer after therapy, fibrosis displays low signal intensity on T2-weighted images, in contrast to viable tumor, which images with considerably higher signal intensity (EBNER et al. 1988).

References

American Cancer Society (1994) Cancer facts and figures. Atlanta: American Cancer Society

Ansari AH, Reynolds RA (1987) Cervical incompetence: a review. Reprod Med 32:161–171

Ascher SM, Arnold LL, Patt RH, Schruefer JJ, Bagley AS, Semelka R, Zeman RK, Simon JA (1994) Adenomyosis: prospective comparison of MR imaging and transvaginal sonography. Radiology 190:803–806

Barton J, McCarthy S, Kohorn E, Scoutt L, Lange R (1993) Pelvic MRI findings in gestational trophoblastic disease, incomplete abortion and ectopic pregnancy: Are they specific? Radiology 186:163–168

Baudouin CJ, Soutter WP, Gilderdale DJ, et al. (1992) Magnetic resonance imaging of the uterine cervix using an intra-vaginal coil. Magn Reson Med 24:196–203

Baumgartner BR, Bernardino ME (1989) MR imaging of the cervix: off-axial scan to improve visualization of zonal anatomy. AJR 153:1001–1002

Belloni C, Vigano R, del Maschio A, Sironi S, Taccagni GL, Vignali M (1990) Magnetic resonance imaging in endometrial carcinoma staging. Gynecol Oncol 37:172–177

Boronow RC, Morrow CP, Creasman WT, et al. (1984) Surgical staging in endometrial cancer: clinical-pathologic findings of a prospective study. Obstet Gynecol 63:825–832

Brewer JI, Halpern B, Torok EE (1979) Gestational trophoblastic disease: selected clinical aspects and chorionic gonadotropin test methods. Curr Probl Cancer 3:1–43

Brown JJ (1996) Gastrointestinal contrast agents for MR imaging. Magn Reson Imaging Clin North Am 4:25–35

Buttram VC, Gibbons WE (1979) Müllerian anomalies: a proposed classification (an analysis of 144 cases). Fertil Steril 32:40–46

Carrington BM, Hricak H, Nuruddin RN, et al. (1990) Mullerian duct anomalies: MR imaging evaluation. Radiology 176:715

Chang YCF, Hricak H, Thurnher S, et al. (1988) Evaluation of the vagina by magnetic resonance imaging. Part II. Neoplasm. Radiology 169:569–571

Chen SS, Rumancik WM, Spiegel G (1990) Magnetic resonance imaging in stage I endometrial carcinoma. Obstet Gynecol 75:274–277

Chung CK, Nahhas WA, Zaino R, et al. (1981) Histologic grade and lymph node metastasis in squamous cell carcinoma of the cervix. Gynecol Oncol 12:348–354

Cobby M, Browning J, Jones A, et al. (1990) Magnetic resonance imaging, computed tomography and endosonography in the local staging of carcinoma of the cervix. Br J Radiol 63:673–679

Cotran RS, Kumar V, Robbins SL (1989) Pathologic basis of disease, 4th edn. W.B. Saunders, Philadelphia

Demas B, Hricak H, Jaffe RB (1986) Uterine MR imaging: effects of hormonal stimulation Radiology 159:123–126

Dooms GC, Hricak H, Tscholakoff D (1986) Adnexal structures: MR imaging. Radiology 158:639–646

Dooms GC, Hricak H, Crooks LE, Higgins CB (1984) Magnetic resonance imaging of the lymph nodes: comparison with CT. Radiology 153:719–728

Dudiak CM, Turner DA, Patal SK, Archie JT, Silver B, Norusis M (1988) Uterine leiomyomas in the infertile patient: preoperative localization with MR imaging versus US and hysterosalpingography. Radiology 167:627–630

Ebner F, Kressel HY, Mintz MC, et al. (1988) Tumor recurrence venus fibrosis in the female pelvis: differentiation with MR imaging at 1.5 T. Radiology 166:333

Ebner F, Ranner G, Flückiger F (1994) Differenzierung von Narbengewebe und Tumorrezidiv nach Therapie von Tumoren des weiblichen Beckens. Radiologe 34:384–389

Ferenczy A, Winkler B (1987) Anatomy and histology of the cervix. In: Kurman R, ed. Blaustein's pathology of the female genital tract, 3rd edn. Springer, New York Berlin Heidelberg, pp 141–145

Forstner R, Hricak H (1994) Congenital malformations of uterus and vagina. Radiologe 34:397–404

Gauger J, Holzknecht NG, Lackerbauer CA, et al. (1996) Breathhold imaging of the upper abdomen using a CP-array coil: comparison with standard body coil imaging. Magma 4:93–104

Gordon AL, Fleisher AC, Dudley BS, et al. (1989) Preoperative assessment of myometrial invasion of endometrial adenocarcinoma by sonography (US) and magnetic resonance imaging (MRI). Gynecol Oncol 34:175–179

Greco A, Mason P, Leung AWL, et al. (1989) Staging of carcinoma of the uterine cervix: MRI-surgical correlation. Clin Radiol 40:401–405

Gross BH, Silver TM, Jaffe MH (1983) Sonographic features of uterine leiomyomas. J Ultrasound Med 2:401–406

Hammond CB, Parker RT (1970) Diagnosis and treatment of trophoblastic disease: a report from the Southeastern Regional Center. Obstet Gynecol 35:132–143

Hendrickson MR, Kempson RL (eds) (1980) Surgical pathology of the uterine corpus. W.B. Saunders, Philadelphia, p 452

Hermanek P, Scheibe O, Spiessl B, Wagner O (eds) (1992) UICC International Union Against Cancer. TNM Klassifikation maligner Tumoren. Springer, Berlin Heidelberg New York

Heuck A, Lukas P (1997) Gynäkologie. In: Reiser M, Semmler W (eds) Magnetresonanztomographie, 2nd edn. Springer, Berlin Heidelberg New York

Heuck A, Sittek H, Seelos K, Kreft B, Hermanns M, Reiser M (1994a) MRT des weiblichen Beckens: Turbo-Spin-Echo-(TSE)-Sequenzen im Vergleich mit konventionellen Spin-Echo-Sequenzen bei 0,5 Tesla. RöFo 160:538–545

Heuck A, Breinbauer A, Elsenhaus B, et al. (1994b) Orale Kontrastmittel in der MRT: Vergleich unterschiedlicher Wirkprinzipien. In: Lissner J, Margulis A (eds) MR '93. Schnetzler, Konstanz

Heuck A, Scheidler J, Sittek H, Müller-Lisse U, Kimmig R, Reiser M (1994c) MR imaging assessment of parametrial involvement in carcinoma of the cervix: value of T1-weighted fat-suppressed SE sequences. Radiology 193 (P):290

Heuck A, Scheidler J, Müller-Lisse U, Kimmig R, Brüning R, Reiser M (1995) Turbo-spin-echo, turbo-STIR and contrast-enhanced sequences in MR imaging of stage I endometrial carcinoma: a comparative study. Eur Radiol 5 (Suppl):143

Heuck A, Scheidler J, Kimmig R, Müller-Lisse U, Steinborn H, Reiser M (1997) Lymphknotenstaging beim Zervixkarzinom: Ergebnisse der hochauflösenden MRT mit einer Phased-Array-Körperspule. RöFo 166:210–214

Hricak H, Kim B (1993) Contrast-enhanced MR imaging of the female pelvis. J Magn Reson Imaging 3:297–306

Hricak H, Tscholakoff D, Heinrichs L, et al. (1986a) Uterine leiomyoma: correlation of MR, histopathologic findings, and symptoms. Radiology 158:385–391

Hricak H, Demas B, Braga C, et al. (1986b) Gestational trophoblastic neoplasm of the uterus: MR assessment. Radiology 161:11–16

Hricak H, Stern JL, Fisher MR, Shaperd LG, Winkler ML, Lacey CG (1987) Endometrial carcinoma staging by MR imaging. Radiology 162:297–305

Hricak H, Lacey CG, Sandles LG, et al. (1988a) Invasive cervical carcinoma: comparison of MR imaging and surgical findings. Radiology 166:623–631

Hricak H, Chang Y, Thurnher S (1988b) Vagina: evaluation with MR imaging. I. Normal anatomy and congenital anomalies. Radiology 169:169–174

Hricak H, Chang YCF, Cann CE et al. (1990) Cervical incompetence: preliminary evaluation with MR imaging. Radiology 174:821–826

Hricak H, Hamm B, Semelka RC, Cann CE, Nauert T, Secaf E, Stern JL, Wolf KJ (1991a) Carcinoma of the uterus: use of gadopentetate dimeglumine in MR imaging. Radiology 181:95–106

Hricak H, Rubinstein LV, Gherman GM, Karstaedt N (1991b) MR imaging evaluation of endometrial carcinoma: results of an NCI cooperative study. Radiology 179:829–832

Hricak H, Carrington B (1991c) MRI of the pelvis. Martin Dunitz, London, 1991

Hricak H, Finck S, Honda G, et al. (1992) MR imaging in the evaluation of benign uterine masses: value of gadopentetate dimeglumine-enhanced T1-weighted images. AJR 158:1043–1050

Hricak H, Swift PS, Campos Z, et al. (1993) Irradiation of the cervix uteri: value of unenhanced and contrast enhanced MR imaging. Radiology 189:381–388

Hricak H, Powell CB, Yu KK, Washington E, Subak LL, Stern JL, Cisternas MG, Arenson RL (1996) Invasive cervical carcinoma: role of MR imaging in pretreatment work-up-cost minimization and diagnostic efficacy analysis. Radiology 198:403–410

Huch Böni R, Haldemann Heusler R, Hebisch G, Krestin GP (1994) CT und MRT bei Entzündungen der weiblichen Genitalorgane. Radiologe 34:390–396

Ito K, Matsumot T, Nakada T, et al. (1994) Assessing myometrial invasion by endometrial carcinoma with dynamic MRI. J Comput Assist Tomogr 18:77–86

Kilkku P, Erkkola R, Gronroos M (1984) Nonspecificity of symptoms related to adenomyosis: a prospective comparative survey. Acta Obstet Gynecol Scand 63:229–231

Kim SH, Choi BI, Lee HP, et al. (1990) Uterine cervical carcinoma comparison of CT and MR findings. Radiology 175:45–51

Kim SH, Choi BI, Han JK, et al. (1993) Preoperative staging of uterine cervical carcinoma: comparison of CT and MRI in 99 patients. J Comput Assist Tomogr 17:633–639

Kim HK, Kim SC, Choi BI, Han MC (1994) Uterine cervical carcinoma: evaluation of pelvic lymph node metastasis with MR imaging. Radiology 190:807–811

Kotlus Rosenberg H, Sherman NH, Tarry WF, et al. (1986) Mayer-Rokitansky-Küster-Hauser syndrome: US aid to diagnosis. Radiology 161:815–819

Lee NC, Dicker RC, Rubin GL, Ory HW (1984) Confirmation of preoperative diagnoses for hysterectomy. Am J Obstet Gynecol 150:283

Lien HH, Blomlie V, Kjorstad K, et al. (1991a) Clinical stage I carcinoma of the cervix: value of MR imaging in determining degree of invasiveness. AJR 156:1191–1194

Lien HH, Blomile V, Trope C, Kaern J, Abeler VM (1991b) Cancer of the endometrium: value of MR imaging in determining depth of invasion into the myometrium. AJR 157:1221–1223

Malini S, Valdes C, Malniak LR (1984) Sonographic diagnosis and classification of anomalies of the female genital tract. J Ultrasound Med 3:397–404

Mark AS, Hricak H (1987) Intrauterine contraceptive devices: MR imaging. Radiology 162:311–314

McCarthy S, Tauber C, Gore J (1986) Female pelvic anatomy: MR assessment of variation during the menstrual cycle and with use of oral contraceptives. Radiology 160:119–123

McCarthy S, Scott G, Majumdar S, Shapiro B, Thompson S, Lange R, Gore J (1989) Uterine junctional zone: MR study of water content and relaxation properties. Radiology 171:241–243

Mittl RL, Yeh IT, Kressel HY (1991) High signal intensity rim surrounding uterine leiomyomas on MR images: pathologic correlation. Radiology 180:81–83

Netter FH (1977) Reproductive system. The Ciba Collection of Medical Illustrations 2:112

Nghiem HV, Herfhens RJ, Francis IR, et al. (1992) The pelvis: T2 weighted fast spin-echo MR imaging. Radiology 185:213–217

Pellerito JS, Mc Carthys SM, Doyle MB, et al. (1992) Diagnosis of uterine anomalies: relative accuracy of MR imaging, endovaginal sonography and hysterosalpingography. Radiology 183:795–800

Pels Rijcken TH, Davis MA, Ros PR (1994) Intraluminal contrast agents for MR imaging of the abdomen and pelvis. J Magn Reson Imaging 4:291–300

Randolph JR Jr, Ying YK, Maier DB, et al. (1986) Comparison of real-time ultrasonography, hysterosalpingography and laparoscopy/hysteroscopy in the evaluation of uterine abnormalities and tubal patency. Fertil Steril 46:28–32

Reinhold C, McCarthy S, Bret M, et al. (1993) Uterine adenomyosis: a prospective comparative analysis with endovaginal US and MR imaging. Radiology 189:300

Reinhold C, McCarthy S, Bret P, Mehio A, Atri M, Zakarian R (1996) Uterine adenomyosis: comparison of endovaginal US and MRI with histopathological correlation. Radiology 199:151–158

Scheidler J, Heuck A, Reiser M (1994) MR-Tomographie im Staging von Karzinomen des Uterus. Radiologe 34:377–383

Scheidler J, Heuck AF, Bruening R, et al. (1997a) Diagnostic impact of a circularly polarized phased-array coils for high resolution MR imaging of the female pelvis. Investig Radiol 32:1–6

Scheidler J, Heuck AF, Meier W, et al. (1997b) MR imaging of pelvic masses: efficacy of the rectal superparamagnetic contrast agent ferumoxsil. J Magn Reson Imaging (in press)

Scheidler J, Heuck AF, Steinborn M, et al. (1998) Parametrial invasion in cervical carcinoma: evaluation of detection at MR imaging with fat suppression. Radiology 206:125–129

Schwartz LB, Panageas E, Lange R, Rizzo J, Comite F, McCarthy S (1994) Female pelvis: impact of MR imaging on treatment decisions and net cost analysis. Radiology 192:55–60

Scoutt LM, McCauley TR, Flynn SD, et al. (1993) Zonal anatomy of the cervix: correlation of MR imaging and histological examination of hysterectomy specimens. Radiology 186:159–162

Scoutt LM, McCarthy SM, Flynn SD, et al. (1995) Clinical stage I endometrial carcinoma: pitfalls in preoperative assessment with MR imaging. Work in progress. Radiology 194:567–572

Scully RE (1982) Definition of endometrial carcinoma precursors. Clin Obstet Gynecol 25:39–48

Sironi S, Belloni C, Taccagni GL, et al. (1991) Carcinoma of the cervix: value of MR imaging in detecting parametrial involvement. AJR 156:753–756

Sironi S, Colombo E, Villa G, et al. (1992a) Myometrial invasion by endometrial carcinoma: assessment by MR imaging. AJR 158:565–569

Sironi S, Colombo E, Villa G, et al. (1992b) Myometrial invasion by endometrial carcinoma: assessment with plain and gadolinium-enhanced MR imaging. Radiology 185:207–212

Smith RC, Reinhold C, Lange RC, et al. (1992a) Fast spin-echo MR imaging of the female pelvis. Radiology 184:665–669

Smith RC, Reinhold C, Lange RC, et al. (1992b) Multicoil high-resolution fast spin-echo MR imaging of the female pelvis. Radiology 184:671–675

Sorenson SS (1987) Hysteroscopic evaluation and endocrinological aspects of women with müllerian duct anomalies and oligomenorrhea. Int J Fertil 32:445–452

Sorenson SS (1988) Estimated prevalence of müllerian anomalies. Acta Obstet Gynecol Scand 67:441–445

Subak LL, Hricak H, Powell CB, et al. (1995) Cervical carcinoma: computed tomography and magnetic resonance imaging for preoperative staging. Obstet Gynecol 86:43–50

Thurnher SA (1992) MR imaging of pelvic masses in women: contrast enhanced vs unenhanced images. AJR 159:1243–1250

Thurnher S, McPhillips M, von Schulthess K, Marincek B (1991) Staging des Zerixkarzinoms mit der magneti-schen Resonanztomographie. Anwendung von Gadolinium-DOTA bei 31 Patientinnen. RöFo 154:643–649

Togashi K, Nishimura K, Itoh K, et al. (1988) Adenomyosis: diagnosis with MR imaging. Radiology 166:111–114

Togashi K, Ozasa H, Konishi I, et al. (1989a) Enlarged uterus: differentiation between adenomyosis and leiomyoma with MRI. Radiology 171:531–534

Togashi K, Nishimura J, Sagoh T, et al. (1989b) Carcinoma of the cervix: staging with MR imaging. Radiology 171:245–251

Togashi K (1993) MRI of the female pelvis. Igaku-Shoin, New York

UICC, International Union Against Cancer (1997) TNM classification of malignant tumors, 5th edn (edited by Sobin LH and Wittekind C). Wiley-Liss, New York

Van Gils APG, Tham RT, Falke TH, Peters AA (1989) Abnormalities of the uterus and cervix after diethylstilbestrol exposure: correlation of findings on MR and hysterosalpingography. AJR 153:1235–1238

Vanzulli A, Sironi S, Pellegrino A, et al. (1994) MRI in stage I carcinoma of the uterine cervix: evaluation of residual uninvolved myometrium and pericervical tissnes. Eur Radiol 4:190–196

Weinreb JC, Barkoff ND, Megibow A, et al. (1990) The value of MR imaging in distinguishing leiomyomas from other solid pelvic masses when sonography is indeterminate. AJR 154:295–299

Yamashita Y, Harada M, Sawada T, Takahashi M, Miyazaki K, Okamura H (1993a) Normal uterus and FIGO stage I in endometrial carcinoma: dynamic gadolinium-enhanced MR imaging. Radiology 186:495–501

Yamashita Y, Mizutani H, Torashima M, et al. (1993b) Assessment of myometrial invasion by endometrial carcinoma: transvaginal sonography vs contrast-enhanced MR imaging. AJR 161:595–599

Zapf S, Halbsguth A, Schweden F, et al. (1988) Magnetresonanztomographie in der Diagnostik des Kollumkarzinoms. Computertomographie und histologische Korrelation. RöFo 148:34–37

Zawin M, McCarthy S, Scoutt LM, Comite F (1990) High-field MRI and US evaluation of the pelvis in women with leiomyomas. Magn Res Imaging 8:371–376

Subject Index

List of Contributors

ALBERT L. BAERT, MD
Professor, Department of Radiology
University Hospitals K.U. Leuven
Herestraat 49
B-3000 Leuven
Belgium

JELLE O. BARENTSZ, MD
Department of Diagnostic Radiology
University Hospital Nijmegen
P.O. Box 9101
6500 HB Nijmegen
The Netherlands

H.-J. BRAMBS, MD
Professor, Director, Department of Diagnostic Radiology
Radiologische Universitätsklinik und Poliklinik
Steinhövelstrasse 9
D-89075 Ulm
Germany

M. A. CUESTA, MD
Associate Professor of Endocrine Surgery
Director of Abdominal Surgery
Free University Hospital Amsterdam
de Boelenlaan
P.O. Box 7057
1007 MB Amsterdam
The Netherlands

TEDDO DOESBURG, MD
Research Fellow
Department of Radiology
Free University Hospital Amsterdam
de Boelenlaan
P.O. Box 7057
1007 MB Amsterdam
The Netherlands

THEODORUS H. M. FALKE, MD
Professor of Radiology
Department of Radiology
Free University Hospital Amsterdam
de Boelenlaan
P.O. Box 7057
1007 MB Amsterdam
The Netherlands

ROSEMARIE FORSTNER, MD
Zentralroentgeninstitut LKA Salzburg
Müllnerhauptstrasse 48
A-5020 Salzburg
Austria

STEPHAN GRYSPEERDT, MD
Department of Radiology
University Hospitals K.U. Leuven
Herestraat 49
B-3000 Leuven
Belgium

THOMAS HELMBERGER, MD
Department of Diagnostic Radiology
Klinikum Großhadern
Ludwig-Maximilians University
Marchioninistrasse 15
D-81377 München
Germany

ANDREAS HEUCK, MD
Assistant Professor
Department of Diagnostic Radiology
Klinikum Großhadern
Ludwig-Maximilians University
Marchioninistrasse 15
D-81377 München
Germany

NICOLAUS HOLZKNECHT, MD
Department of Diagnostic Radiology
Klinikum Großhadern
Ludwig-Maximilians University
Marchioninistrasse 15
D-81377 München
Germany

HEDVIG HRICAK, MD
Professor of Radiology and Urology
Department of Radiology
Abdominal Imaging Section
University of California, San Francisco
505 Parnassus Avenue
San Francisco, CA 94143-0628
USA

GABRIEL P. KRESTIN, MD
Professor of Radiology
Department of Diagnostic Radiology
University Hospital Zurich
Rämistrasse 100
CH-8091 Zürich
Switzerland

WOLFGANG LUBOLDT, MD, MSC
Department of Diagnostic Radiology
University Hospital Zurich
Rämistrasse 100
CH-8091 Zürich
Switzerland

GUY MARCHAL, MD
Professor, Department of Radiology
University Hospitals K.U. Leuven
Herestraat 49
B-3000 Leuven
Belgium

HANI B. MARCOS, MD
Clinical Research Fellow in MR Services
Department of Radiology
University of North Carolina
Chapel Hill, NC 27599-7510
USA

PATRICIA J. MERGO, MD
Assistant Professor
Division of Body Imaging and MRI
Department of Radiology
University of Florida College of Medicine
P.O. Box 100374
1600 SW Archer Road
Gainesville, FL 32610
USA

U. G. MÜLLER-LISSE, MD
Department of Diagnostic Radiology
Klinikum Großhadern
Ludwig-Maximilians University
Marchioninistrasse 15
D-81377 München
Germany

RAYMOND H. OYEN, MD, PhD
Department of Radiology
University Hospitals K.U. Leuven
Herestraat 49
B-3000 Leuven
Belgium

PABLO R. ROS, MD
Professor and Associate Chairman
Division of Body Imaging and MRI
Department of Radiology
University of Florida College of Medicine
P.O. Box 100374
1600 SW Archer Road
Gainesville, FL 32610
USA

ERNST J. RUMMENY, MD
Institut für Klinische Radiologie
Albert-Schweitzer-Strasse 33
D-48129 Muenster
Germany

MARTIN P. SANDLER, MD
Professor of Radiology and Radiological Sciences
Associate Professor of Medicine
Director of Nuclear Medicine
Vice-Chairman, Department of Radiology and Radiological
Sciences
Vanderbilt University School of Medicine
1161 21st Avenue South
Nashville, TN
USA

PETER SATTLEGGER, MD
Zentralroentgeninstitut LKA Salzburg
Müllnerhauptstrasse 48
A-5020 Salzburg
Austria

JÜRGEN SCHEIDLER, MD:
Department of Diagnostic Radiology
Klinikum Großhadern
Ludwig-Maximilians University
Marchioninistrasse 15
D-81377 München
Germany

RICHARD C. SEMELKA, MD
Director of MR Services
Associate Professor of Radiology
Department of Radiology
University of North Carolina
Chapel Hill, NC 27599-7510
USA

MARC STEINBORN, MD
Department of Diagnostic Radiology
Klinikum Großhadern
Ludwig-Maximilians University
Marchioninistrasse 15
D-81377 München
Germany

RUEDI F. THOENI, MD
Professor of Radiology
Department of Radiology
Box 0628
University of California
San Francisco, CA 94143-06208
USA

A. P. VAN GILS, MD
Assistant Professor
Department of Radiology
Central Military Hospital
Heidelberglaan 100
3584 CX Utrecht
The Netherlands

LIEVEN VAN HOE, MD
Departent of Radiology
University Hospitals K.U. Leuven
Herestraat 49
B-3000 Leuven
Belgium

MEDICAL RADIOLOGY
Diagnostic Imaging and Radiation Oncology

Titles in the series already published

MEDICAL RADIOLOGY
Diagnostic Imaging and Radiation Oncology

Titles in the series already published